Principles and Practice of Epidemiology

An Engaged Approach

Annette Rossignol, Sc.D.

Oregon State University

Boston   Burr Ridge, IL   Dubuque, IA   Madison, WI   New York
San Francisco   St. Louis   Bangkok   Bogotá   Caracas   Kuala Lumpur
Lisbon   London   Madrid   Mexico City   Milan   Montreal   New Delhi
Santiago   Seoul   Singapore   Sydney   Taipei   Toronto

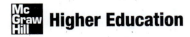

Higher Education

Published by McGraw-Hill, an imprint of The McGraw-Hill Companies, Inc., 1221 Avenue of the Americas, New York, NY 10020. Copyright © 2007. All rights reserved. No part of this publication may be reproduced or distributed in any form or by any means, or stored in a database or retrieval system, without the prior written consent of The McGraw-Hill Companies, Inc., including, but not limited to, in any network or other electronic storage or transmission, or broadcast for distance learning.

This book is printed on acid-free paper

1 2 3 4 5 6 7 8 9 0 FGR/FGR 0 9 8 7 6 5

ISBN-13: 978-0-07-286939-2
ISBN-10: 0-07-286939-9

Editor in Chief: *Emily Barrosse*
Publisher: *William R. Glass*
Sponsoring Editor: *Christopher Johnson*
Marketing Manager: *Pamela S. Cooper*
Developmental Editor: *Gary O'Brien*
Project Manager: *Carey Eisner*
Manuscript Editor: *Carole Crouse*
Design Manager and Cover Designer: *Cassandra Chu*
Text Designer: *Linda Robertson*
Art Editor: *Ayelet Arbel*
Illustrator: *Lotus Art*
Production Supervisor: *Richard DeVitto*
Composition: *10.5/12 Times by Carlisle Publishing Services*
Printing: *45# New Era Matte Plus, Quebecor World*

Library of Congress Cataloging-in-Publication Data

Rossignol, Annette.
    Principles and practice of epidemiology: an engaged approach/by Annette Rossignol.—
1st ed.
        p. cm.
    Includes bibliographical references and index.
    ISBN-10: 0-07-286939-9
    ISBN-13: 978-0-07-286939-2
    1. Epidemiology. I. Title

RA651.R67 2005
614.4—dc22

                                                                    2005055125

The Internet addresses listed in the text were accurate at the time of publication. The inclusion of a Web site does not indicate an endorsement by the authors or McGraw-Hill, and McGraw-Hill does not guarantee the accuracy of the information presented at these sites.

www.mhhe.com

For Philippe, Jacques-Philippe, and Alice-Louise

BRIEF CONTENTS

Preface   xv

1   Introduction   1

2   Historical Development   20

3   What Is an Epidemic?   35

4   Measuring Disease Frequency: Incidence Rate   63

5   Prevalence and Its Application to Screening Programs   102

6   Cumulative Incidence (Risk)   130

7   Design Strategies: Descriptive Studies   143

8   Causation   165

9   Design Strategies: Analytic Studies
Part 1— Intervention Studies   188

10   Design Strategies: Analytic Studies
Part 2—Observational Studies   206

11   Simple Analysis of Epidemiologic Data:
Effect Measures   228

12   Accuracy   250

Epilogue: Engaged Epidemiology   E–1
Appendix: Sample Answers to Review Exercises   A–1
References   R–1
Index   I–1

CONTENTS

Preface   xv

1 Introduction   1
   Definition of Epidemiology   3
   BOX 1.1: Causal Webs and Signed Digraphs   4
      Example of an Epidemiologic Study   8
   Comparisons   9
   Studying Human Populations   10
   Ethical Considerations   11
   BOX 1.2: Ethics Matters: The Nuremberg Code   12
   Population Perspective   14
   Objectives of Epidemiology   15
   BOX 1.3: The Epidemic Intelligence Service: Training the World's "Disease
      Detectives"   16
   BOX 1.4: The West Nile Virus—Epidemiology of a Rapidly Emerging
      Disease   17
   Summary   19
   Review Questions   19
   Review Exercises   19

2 Historical Development   20
   Acute Onset Versus Chronic Disease Epidemiology   23
   Development of Epidemiology as a Science   25
      Statistics   25
      Social Sciences   26
      Computer Technology   27
      Managerial Science   27
   BOX 2.1: Ethics Matters: Institutional Review Boards (IRBs)   28
   BOX 2.2: Practical Epidemiology in a Public Health Setting: Ethics
      and Partners   29
      The Case/Control Study   33
   Summary   33
   Review Questions   34
   Review Exercises   34

3 What Is an Epidemic?   35
   What Constitutes an Epidemic?   35
   BOX 3.1: Clinical Epidemiology   37
   Are Epidemics Always Obvious to the Populations Affected?   38
   How Can Epidemics Be Described Quantitatively?   41

BOX 3.2: Worldwide Disease Surveillance: Communicable Disease
Surveillance and Response (CSR)   44
    Other Aspects of Attack Rates   47
    Health Indicators   47
What Causes Epidemics?   48
BOX 3.3: Communication of Health Risks   50
Monitoring the Nation's Health: Goals and Surveillance   50
BOX 3.4: Ethics Matters: All the News That's Fit to Print—News Reporters
and Epidemiology   51
BOX 3.5: Practical Epidemiology in a Public Health Setting: Developing
a Public Health Surveillance System Using Data from the National
Health Interview Survey   52
    What Are the Leading Health Indicators?   54
Summary   54
Review Questions   56
Review Exercises   56
SPECIAL CASE STUDY: After-Action Report for the August 2003
Measles Investigation in Corvallis, Oregon   57

4   Measuring Disease Frequency: Incidence Rate   63
Definition of Incidence Rate   63
Restriction of Incidence Rates   64
Components of Incidence Rates   64
The Cohort Study   67
Calculation of Incidence Rates   67
    Example 1   67
    Example 2   68
    Example 3   68
    Example 4   69
BOX 4.1: National Situation of Dengue and Dengue Hemorrhagic Fever
in Thailand   69
Mortality Rates   72
    Age-Adjusted Incidence and Mortality Rates   73
        Example: The Process of Age-Adjustment   74
    Variation in Disease and Injury Frequency   75
    Morbidity and Mortality Worldwide   77
    Causes of Death According to Exposure Status 79
BOX 4.2: Obesity and the Super-Sized Industry   80
    Obesity in the United States   82
    Other Leading Causes of Death   83
BOX 4.3: Ethics Matters: Do Tropical Diseases Cause Poverty, or Does
Poverty Cause Tropical Diseases?   84
Epidemiology in Action: Disease Eradication   85
BOX 4.4: Global Program to Eradicate Malaria   86
BOX 4.5: Practical Epidemiology in a Public Health Setting: Ethical
Considerations and Tuberculosis Elimination   88

Summary   91
Review Questions   92
Review Exercises   93
SPECIAL CASE STUDY: Public Health in Afghanistan   96

5 Prevalence and Its Application to Screening Programs   102
   BOX 5.1: Ethics Matters: Baby Doe Regulations and the Care
     of Premature Infants   104
   Examples Illustrating How to Calculate Prevalence   107
     Example 1   107
     Example 2   107
   Screening Programs   108
   BOX 5.2: Practical Epidemiology in a Public Health Setting: Wisconsin's
     Oral-Health Screening Program   109
   Characteristics of a Good Disease or Risk Factor for
     which to Screen   112
   Characteristics of a Good Screening Test   114
   Characteristics of a Good Screening Program   116
   BOX 5.3: Numerical Example Demonstrating the Importance
     of Specificity in Determining the Predictive Value Positive
     of a Screening Program   117
   Lead Time   120
   Final Comment Regarding Screening Programs   121
   BOX 5.4: Weighing the Risks and the Benefits of Screening Programs   122
   Summary   123
   Review Questions   125
   Review Exercises   126

6 Cumulative Incidence (Risk)   130
   First Approach for Estimating Cumulative Incidence   130
     Examples Using the First Approach   131
   BOX 6.1: Ethics Matters: Business and Engaged Epidemiology   132
   Second Approach for Estimating Cumulative Incidence   133
   BOX 6.2: Theoretical Web of Causation for Ergonomic-Related
     Disability   134
     Examples Using the Second Approach   136
       Example 1   136
       Example 2   138
   BOX 6.3: Other Useful Proportions   139
   Overview of Measures of Disease/Injury Frequency   140
   Review Questions   140
   Review Exercises   141

7   Design Strategies: Descriptive Studies   143
    Objectives of Descriptive Studies   144
    Primary Uses of Descriptive Studies   144
        Quantifying Variation in Exposures and Health Statuses   144
        Examples of Descriptive Studies   144
    BOX 7.1: Practical Epidemiology in a Public Health Setting:
        Nutritional Anthropometrics Survey, Kono District, Sierra Leone   145
        Forming Hypotheses   148
    BOX 7.2: Practical Epidemiology in a Public Health Setting:
        Epidemiology on the Front Lines—Assessing the Mental
        Health Needs of Benton County, Oregon, Children   150
    Types of Descriptive Studies   153
        Case Reports and Case Series   153
    BOX 7.3: Ethics Matters: Us and Them—Public Health Ethics in
        an Age of "Otherness"   154
        Cross-Sectional Studies   157
        Correlational Studies   159
    Summary   163
    Review Questions   164
    Review Exercises   164

8   Causation   165
    Causation   165
    Criteria for Evaluating Causation   166
        1. How Strong Is the Association between Exposure and
           Outcome?   166
        2. Is the Association Biologically Credible?   166
        3. Are the Results of Epidemiologic Studies Generally
           Consistent with Respect to the Presence and Size of an
           Association between Exposure and Outcome?   166
        4. Is the Time-Response between the Exposure and the Health
           Outcome Appropriate?   167
        5. Is There a Dose-Response Relationship between the Exposure
           and the Health Outcome?   167
        6. Are the Henle-Koch Postulates Satisfied?   168
        7. Prelude to Intervention Studies   169
    A Model for Disease/Injury Causation   169
    Summary   172
    BOX 8.1: What Causes Cardiovascular Disease?   173
    BOX 8.2: Ethics Matters: Why Do Some Consumer Products Kill?   174
    BOX 8.3: Genetic Versus Environmental Causes of Disease   176
    BOX 8.4: The Epidemiologist as Forensic Scientist   178
    Review Questions   179
    Review Exercises   180
    SPECIAL CASE STUDY: Insights into Biocolonialism   181

9   Design Strategies: Analytic Studies
     Part 1—Intervention Studies   188
     Intervention Studies Versus Observational Studies   189
     Intervention Studies   191
     BOX 9.1: Practical Epidemiology In a Clinical Setting: Diabetes Mellitus—
       Overview of Clinical and Public Health Implications   192
     External Validity   195
     Adherence to the Intervention Protocol   196
     Lost-to-Follow-Up   197
     Examples of Preventive Trials   199
          1954 Poliomyelitis Vaccine Trial   199
          Newburgh-Kingston Dental Caries Trial   199
          Physicians' Health Study   200
     Example of a Clinical Trial   201
          Polyp Prevention Trial   201
     Vaccines and Social Change   202
     BOX 9.2: Ethics Matters: A Rift in the Rift Valley   202
     Summary   203
     Review Questions   204
     Review Exercises   205

10   Design Strategies: Analytic Studies
     Part 2—Observational Studies   206
     Cohort Studies   207
     Important Questions to Consider When Designing
       Cohort Studies   209
          Who Is Exposed?   209
          Sources of the Exposed Cohort   209
          Who Is Unexposed?   210
          Sources of the Unexposed Cohort   210
          How Are Data Collected?   211
          How Do Investigators Follow Up on Participants?   212
          How Are Data Analyzed?   212
     Examples of Cohort Studies   213
          The Nurses' Health Study   213
          *Coronary Heart Disease among Workers Exposed
            to Carbon Disulfide*   213
     Case/Control Studies   214
     Important Questions to Consider When Designing Case/
       Control Studies   215
          Who Is a Case?   215
          Sources of Cases   217
     BOX 10.1: Ethics Matters: Geographic Information Systems   218

Who Is a Good Control?   219
Sources of Controls   220
Examples of Case/Control Studies   222
Esophageal Cancer and Green Tea Consumption   222
Smoking and Carcinoma of the Lung   222
BOX 10.2: The Genetic Epidemiology of Lung Cancer and Smoking
(GELCS) Study   223
Cohort Versus Case/Control Studies   224
Summary   225
Review Questions   227

11   Simple Analysis of Epidemiologic Data: Effect Measures   228
BOX 11.1: Ethics Matters: Hypothesis Generation versus Hypothesis
Evaluation   229
Data Editing   231
Data Reduction   231
Data Analysis   232
Effect Measures   232
Cohort Studies   233
Cohort Studies with Count Denominators   233
Numerical Example of How to Estimate the CIR and the CID   234
Cohort Studies with Person-Time Denominators   234
Numerical Example of How to Estimate the IRR and the IRD   235
Ratio Measures Versus Difference Measures   236
Case/Control Studies   236
Numerical Example of How to Estimate an EOR   238
Summary   238
BOX 11.2: Program Evaluation   239
BOX 11.3: Ronald Ross's Model of Malaria Transmission   240
Review Questions   242
Review Exercises   243
SPECIAL CASE STUDY: Truly a Success? The Effects of the
1996 National Welfare Reform Act on Children's Health
in the United States   246

12   Accuracy   250
Precision   251
P-Value   251
Confidence Intervals   253
The Mathematical Relationship   255
Validity   255
External Validity   256

Internal Validity   257
  Comparison Biases   257
    Selection bias   257
      An Example of Selection Bias: Oral Contraceptives
        and Embolisms   259
    Confounding bias   260
    Prevention and control of confounding   261
      An Example of Confounding Bias: Hormone
        Replacement Therapy (HRT) and Coronary Heart
        Disease   265
  Information Biases   267
    Misclassification   267
    Observation bias   267
BOX 12.1: Practical Epidemiology in a Public Health Setting:
  An Alternative Method for Collecting Complex
  Occupational Histories   268
BOX 12.2: Ethics Matters: Domestic Violence in Lesbian
  Relationships   272
    Concluding Remark about Bias   273
Review Questions   274

Epilogue: Engaged Epidemiology   E–1
Appendix: Sample Answers to Review Exercises   A–1
References   R–1
Index   I–1

PREFACE

This book was written with four conceptual underpinnings in mind. First, a foundational book in epidemiology should teach the basic mathematical components of epidemiology, options in study design, primary types and sources of error in epidemiologic studies, and how to read and interpret the epidemiologic literature.

The second conceptual underpinning for the book centers on the importance of ethics in the work that epidemiologists perform. Each chapter has a stand-alone box titled "Ethics Matters." These boxes contain discussions of ethical issues associated either with epidemiology per se or with the application of epidemiology in understanding current challenges in public health. The objective of the "Ethics Matters" boxes is to encourage improved insights into the ethical responsibilities and questions involved in studying human populations, as epidemiologists do.

The third conceptual underpinning expresses the need for epidemiologists to embrace a global perspective and understanding when investigating public health concerns. A perceived separation between domestic and international health issues no longer is a realistic position to hold. Well-established diseases and emerging diseases once regarded as being "over there" now spread quickly with the massive, rapid movement of people from one region of the world to another. Examples of rapidly spreading diseases include West Nile fever, dengue hemorrhagic fever, and severe acute respiratory syndrome (SARS). Previously, HIV/AIDS was an example of a rapidly spreading disease, and despite its control in some countries, such as Uganda, it continues to spread rapidly in other countries, such as India. Pollution of local air or ocean regions also unites the global community in causing worldwide health and/or environmental challenges such as global warming or, as another example, radiation effects from the meltdown of a nuclear reactor in Chernobyl, formerly in the Union of Soviet Socialist Republics (USSR) now in Ukraine. Food grown in one country but sold in another may fail to meet local standards for pesticide residues or bacterial contamination. The dumping of hazardous wastes or of outdated pharmaceuticals by one country into another may create burdensome health and/or environmental problems far from the source of the hazardous materials or pharmaceuticals. The list of possible examples of local or regional health problems that have global repercussions is long and now includes the potential for severe health effects and injuries from bioterrorist activities.

The final conceptual underpinning for the book concerns the framework for discussing substantive epidemiology in contrast to epidemiologic methodology. Several chapters contain a report of a case study related either directly to an epidemiologic study or methodological challenge, or to a public health program or issue in which the application of epidemiologic expertise was required or at least advantageous. Experts in epidemiology and/or in other specialties within public health wrote a majority of these case studies, basing their contributions on their professional experiences in the "real-world" practice of epidemiology. Taken together, these studies provide the reader with valuable insights into how epidemiology is used in a variety of professional settings. In addition, they emphasize my belief that "knowing epidemiology" is not enough. Ideally, an epidemiologist or some other public health professional should understand the fundamental principles that underlie the application of epidemiologic methodology to help solve public health problems. I term this idea "engaged epidemiology" to emphasize the relationship between epidemiology and the betterment of society.

Annette Rossignol, Sc.D.

FEATURES—AT A GLANCE

Are you looking for an easy-to-follow approach to epidemiology? Working toward a stronger grasp at the mathematical components? Trying to understand an epidemiologist's role in the greater world? The features in *Principles and Practice of Epidemiology: An Engaged Approach* will help you do all that and more.

Mathematical Concepts

The basic mathematical concepts of epidemiology are presented clearly, using easy-to-follow, step-by-step instructions and numerous examples.

Feature Boxes and "Special Case Studies"

The feature boxes and "Special Case Studies" are contributed by practicing epidemiologists and other public health professionals. They highlight current hot topics, applications of epidemiology and real-life situations, and demonstrate the applications of epidemiology and perspectives in quantifying and controlling public health problems.

"Ethics Matters"

The "Ethics Matters" feature highlights ethical dilemmas faced by practicing epidemiologists and public health practitioners and stimulates critical thought.

Review Questions and Exercises

Closing each chapter with a review of key concepts and objectives, these features facilitate and support learning.

Online Learning Center

The Online Learning Center (www.mhhe.com/rossignol1e) that accompanies this text provides instructors with downloads of helpful ancillaries. For students, the Online Learning Center offers study aids, updated material, and other resources.

ACKNOWLEDGMENTS

The following instructors reviewed this book in various stages of development and through their suggestions and experience helped lay the groundwork for this text.

McKinley Thomas
Augusta State University

Lowell Sever
University of Texas–Houston

Dona Schneider
Rutgers University

Srijana Bajracharya
University of Maine at Presque Isle

Elias Duryea
University of New Mexico–Albuquerque

Wendy Stuhldreher
Slippery Rock University

Joanne Shields
East Tennessee State University

Beverly Tremain
Public Health Consultant, formerly of Truman State University

Jan Richter
University of Central Oklahoma

Richard Travis
James Madison University

Gerald Pyle
University of North Carolina–Charlotte

## CHAPTER 1

Introduction

The development and application of epidemiology was one of the most profound changes in public health to occur during the latter half of the twentieth century. At the core of this change was the widespread realization that factors such as lifestyle choices, nutrition, occupation, environment, and genetic/familial constitution alter the risk of disease and injury and that the amount of such alterations can be quantified.

Why was this change in the understanding of disease causation so revolutionary? Previous epidemiologic investigators, including John Graunt, William Farr, and John Snow, had demonstrated the value of using routinely collected data and new data to study disease in human populations. Nevertheless, until the mid–twentieth century, prevalent beliefs about disease causation continued to include the **miasma theory** (the idea that "bad odors" cause disease) and the idea that moral and/or religious turpitude causes disease. Although those ideas about disease causation were rather vague, each lent itself to certain effective disease-control strategies. For example, water-drainage and solid-waste-disposal projects associated with the sanitary movements in the latter part of the nineteenth century and the early twentieth century resulted in marked reductions in the rates of infectious and vector-borne diseases. Similarly, prohibitions against tobacco and alcohol use, habits deemed by some people as morally offensive, prevented chronic diseases such as lung cancer and liver disorders.

Neither of those two theories about disease causation, however, offered an adequate explanation for why certain diseases occur more often in some populations than in others or suggested satisfactory measures for preventing disease. Similarly, neither theory could erode the widely held belief that disease, and especially **chronic disease** (disease caused by the accumulation of exposure over a long period of time and/or disease of long duration), occurs randomly, that is, unpredictably. It followed that any efforts to predict a disease whose occurrence was random would prove futile.

Other theories of disease causation were more promising. The **contagion theory** of disease causation, probably introduced centuries ago by physicians in ancient Rome, posited that some human diseases are caused by pathogens, biologic agents that reproduce inside a human host. In 1546, the term "contagion" was first used and the theory popularized. It was then that Fracastorius, a physician living in the Italian city-state of Verona, published his book, *Des Res Conatagiosa,* in which he described how seminaria contagium (germs) could be transferred from one person to another. He described three types of contagion: direct person-to-person contagion, contagion through "fomes" (clothing or other objects on which a germ could survive, now called **fomites**), and contagion "at a distance."

Perhaps best known among the pioneers of the contagion theory are Louis Pasteur, Robert Koch, and Koch's teacher, Friedrich Gustav Jacob Henle, writing during the latter part of the nineteenth century and the early twentieth century. Among his many accomplishments, Pasteur is remembered for inventing the bacteria-killing process called pasteurization and for identifying the infectious agent of and developing a vaccine for rabies.

Henle and Koch, both well known in the field of microbiology, developed the **Henle-Koch postulates.** The Henle-Koch postulates became the standard for establishing causation for infectious diseases that have short **incubation times** (a short time between a person's exposure to an infectious agent and the onset of disease). Infectious diseases that have short incubation times are one category of **acute diseases,** diseases whose symptoms occur shortly after exposure. The postulates state that to be a cause of disease, the infectious agent must be able to be isolated from all cases of a disease, grown in culture in a laboratory, and, when injected into a susceptible host, cause the disease. In addition, the infectious agent must be able to be isolated from these new cases and grown in culture. Associated with the idea that some biologic agents cause disease was the observation that people living in crowded conditions were more apt to develop disease than were people living in less crowded areas.

The **epidemiologic triad** (the dynamic interaction of agent, host, and environment to produce disease or injury) offered a theoretical as well as practical underpinning for understanding human illness (Figure 1.1). The triad first was used to explain how infectious agents interact with a susceptible person (host) to produce disease given **permissive environmental conditions** (environments that allow the biologic agent to survive and come into contact with a person). The epidemiologic triad, although not yet known by that phrase, was articulated clearly by an American pathologist, Theobald Smith, in his 1934 book, *Parasitism and Disease.* The triad later was extended as a framework for understanding noninfectious diseases. Closely associated with the concept of the epidemiologic triad is the idea of **person, place, and time:** The agent, host, and permissive environment must interact at the "right" place and time to result in disease or injury.

Epidemiology, by quantifying the predictability of acute and chronic infectious and noninfectious diseases in populations, demonstrated that control of those maladies is possible, at least in theory. In addition, because many diseases result in part from

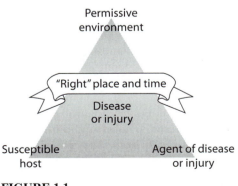

FIGURE 1.1
Epidemiologic triad.

lifestyle choices, epidemiology offered hope that individuals could manage part of their individual risks of disease.

DEFINITION OF EPIDEMIOLOGY

What is **epidemiology?** Epidemiology is the foundational science of public health. Much as a yardstick measures length, epidemiologic investigations measure and compare the frequencies of disease, injury, and other health-related events in human populations. Epidemiology is concerned with understanding the distribution, causes, and occurrence of ill health in human populations, often studying populations in which ill health is occurring at a high ("epidemic") proportion. Epidemiologic investigations embrace a characteristic methodology or sequence of questions not unlike that of certain board or card games in which the identity of some person or object must be determined through asking a series of questions. This analogy is depicted in Figure 1.2.

No longer restricted to identifying relationships between health-related events and their immediate predecessors, epidemiologists endeavor to understand the complex interactions of factors that result in disease or injury as those factors occur, disappear, and then reoccur, often over a span of decades. In their landmark publication, *Principles of Epidemiology,* MacMahon and Pugh (1970) refer to this complex interaction of factors as a **web of causation.** A web of causation depicts associations between causes and their health consequences while at the same time explicitly placing those associations within their economic, social, cultural, and/or political contexts. Understanding these contexts often provides insights into how certain factors (causes/preventives of adverse health outcomes) exert their effects. In addition, understanding these contexts can enhance the development and implementation of effective disease- and injury-control programs.

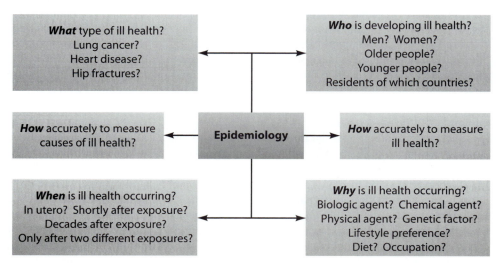

FIGURE 1.2
Questions asked during epidemiologic investigations.

The populous state of Kerala in southwest India provides an illustrative example. An effective strategy for reducing family size in Kerala was increasing the education of girls and women. That education created opportunities for women, thereby placing them in a better position to make choices with respect to their reproductive health. Providing education about reproductive choices in the absence of female education and literacy more generally was not as effective a strategy in reducing family size. Increased female literacy had a greater impact on family size, even though the association between knowledge of family-planning options and family size is more obvious and seemingly direct.

Epidemiologists study different parts of causal webs in an attempt to learn which factors in the web directly or indirectly exert positive or negative effects on health outcomes within the web. Only recently have they begun to appreciate the importance of evaluating causal webs in their entirety (Agar 1996; Pearce 1996; Susser and Susser 1996a; Susser and Susser 1996b). Box 1.1 and Figures 1.3 through 1.5 present examples of causal webs to elucidate some of the many factors that interacted to produce diabetes, the *Titanic* disaster, and severe acute respiratory syndrome (SARS). Intervening on only

---

BOX 1.1

CAUSAL WEBS AND SIGNED DIGRAPHS

Figures 1.3 through 1.5 depict examples of causal webs. Understanding the causal web in which an exposure-outcome relation occurs is of paramount importance if the results of epidemiologic studies are to be used intelligently in the planning of programs to prevent or control disease or injury. The difficulty in relying on an exposure-outcome relation for program planning, in the absence of knowledge concerning the causal web in which the relation is a part, is the possibility of developing a program that focuses on a part of a causal web that will not lead to an improvement in health status. As an example, in the state of Kerala, in southern India, a highly successful program to reduce family size focused on the (school) education of women, rather than on greater access to birth control options or education about birth control. Increased education provided these women with increased options, such as establishing micro-enterprises and greater power over sexual and reproductive activities. Understanding the causal web concerning family size provided the program planners with the insight to identify the education of women as the pivotal variable whose increase would lead to a reduced family size. In general, understanding how the different components of causal webs interact with one another within a system can provide invaluable insights into how differences in the strengths of the interactions among variables affect the frequency of disease or injury.

Eventually, epidemiologists will be able to improve their reliance on causal webs by relying more on **signed digraphs.** A signed digraph is a system model that shows the components of the system and the positive or negative interactions among the components (see Figure 1.6 on page 8). Often these interactions form loops, or chains of interactions that feed back on themselves. Thus the interactions affect each other either directly or indirectly through other components of the system. For a more complete description of signed digraphs, see http://oregonstate.edu/~rossignp/.

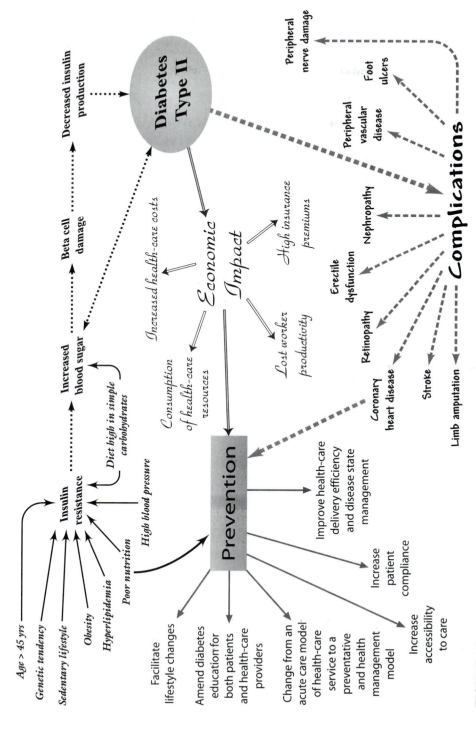

FIGURE 1.3

Web of causation: Diabetes Type II.

Source: Mark Clayton.

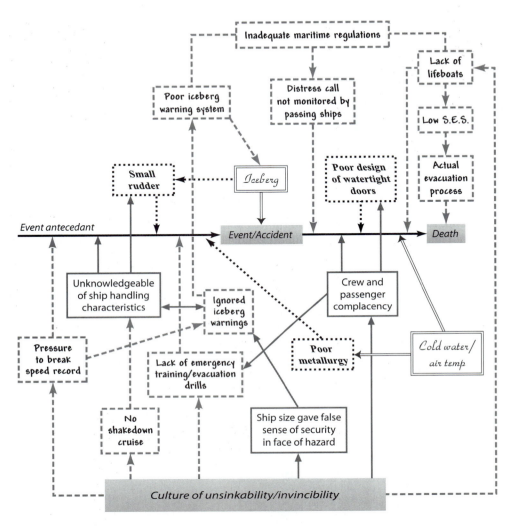

FIGURE 1.4

Web of causation: Profile of the *Titanic* disaster.

Source: Deb Fell Carlson, Julie Norton, Sandee Holmes, and Tony Brace.

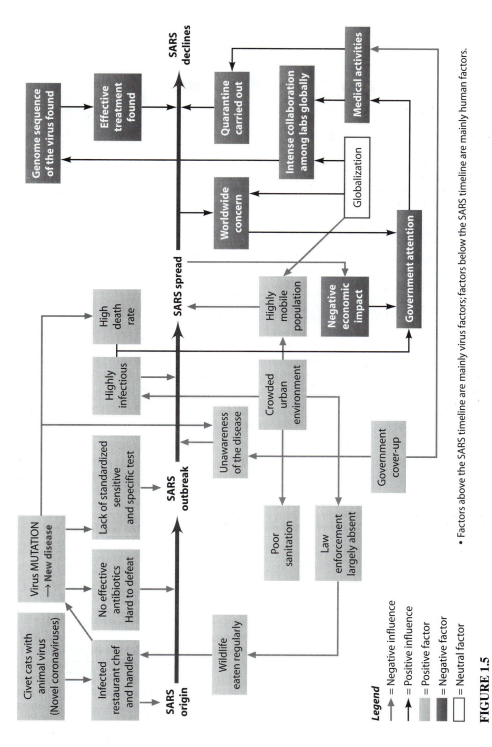

FIGURE 1.5

Web of causation: Severe acute respiratory syndrome (SARS).

Source: Jingmin Liu.

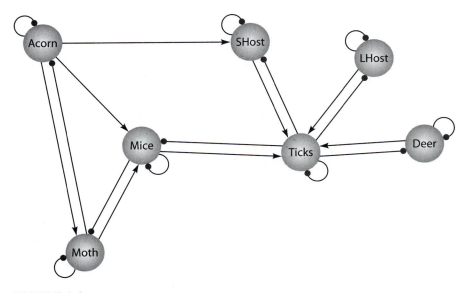

FIGURE 1.6
Signed digraph of a Lyme disease vector-host community.

In the signed digraph, circles represent variables; lines (or links) represent interactions (with arrows indicating positive effects, and small, dark circles indicating negative effects). Curved lines with small, dark circles are self-regulating effects. The variable "Lhost" are large hosts (mostly deer); the variable "Shost" are small hosts (mostly raccoons, foxes, and skunks). Lyme disease is an infection caused by *Borrelia burgdorferi,* a type of bacterium called a spirochete, which is carried by deer ticks. Gypsy moths are part of the vector-host community because they eat oak trees. Moths, in turn, are food for white-footed deer mice that harbor Lyme disease ticks. *Source:* From Orme-Zavalete and Rossignol 2004.

one or two components of a causal web often is sufficient to decrease disease or injury. Those components may be thought of as leverage points, factors whose modification substantially weakens the disease- or injury-producing capability of the causal web.

EXAMPLE OF AN EPIDEMIOLOGIC STUDY

The Pennsylvania Department of Health and Centers for Disease Control and Prevention (CDC) investigated an outbreak of hepatitis A among patrons of a restaurant ("Restaurant A") in Monaca, Pennsylvania. As of November 20, 2003, approximately 555 persons with hepatitis A had been identified, including at least 13 Restaurant A food service workers and 75 residents of six other states who dined at Restaurant A. Three people died. Analysis of the hepatitis A virus obtained from three of the patrons indicated that all three viruses were identical.

Among 207 persons with hepatitis A who were interviewed and who ate at Restaurant A only once during the 2–6 weeks (the typical incubation period for hepatitis A) before illness, dates of illness onset were between October 14 and November 12. These 207 patrons reported eating food prepared in Restaurant A during September 14–October 17; a total of 181 (87%) persons reported eating at Restaurant A during October 3–6. All infected Restaurant A food service workers became ill after October 26, suggesting that a food service worker could not have been the source of the outbreak. However, during late October–early November, these ill food service workers were working in Restaurant A when they could have been infectious. For this reason, immune globulin (to protect against hepatitis A) was provided to approximately 9,000 persons who ate food from Restaurant A during this time or had exposures to ill persons involved in the outbreak. The restaurant has been closed.

A study was conducted to identify menu item(s) or ingredient(s) associated with illness. A case-patient was defined as a person who had illness onset during October 14–November 12, had laboratory confirmation of acute hepatitis A virus (HAV) infection (positive Immunoglobulin M anti-HAV), reported eating food prepared at Restaurant A during October 3–6, and had eaten only once at Restaurant A during the 2–6 weeks before illness onset. A comparison group ("controls") was studied also and included persons without hepatitis A who either had dined with case-patients at Restaurant A or were identified through credit card receipts as having dined at Restaurant A during October 3–6. Controls with a previous history of hepatitis A, hepatitis A vaccination, or receipt of immune globulin within two weeks after eating Restaurant A food were excluded from the study. Enrolled case-patients and controls were asked about Restaurant A food that they had eaten.

The median age of the 181 case-patients in the study was 34 years (range: 4–73 years), and that of the 83 controls was 28 years (range: 2–81). Of 133 menu items, only chili con queso and mild salsa were associated significantly with illness. Mild salsa was eaten by 94% of case-patients, compared with only 39% of controls. Chili con queso was eaten by 15% of case-patients, compared with only 3% of controls. Both menu items associated with illness contained uncooked or minimally heated fresh green onions. Among 11 case-patients who reported not eating mild salsa, seven ate at least one of the other 52 menu items that contained green onions. Of 103 ingredients used at the restaurant, 12 were associated with illness. Of these, 10 had been consumed by less than 50% of case-patients. Eating a menu item containing green onions was reported by 98% of case-patients, compared with only 69% of controls. Eating a menu item containing white onions also was associated with illness. However, among the 176 case-patients who reported eating white onions, 174 (99%) also ate green onions. Among the four case-patients and 28 controls who reported not eating green onions, white onions were not associated with illness.

The Food and Drug Administration (FDA), CDC, and the state health departments investigated the source of the green onions associated with this outbreak and how they became contaminated with HAV. Preliminary trace-back information indicates that green onions supplied to Restaurant A were grown in Mexico.

Source: Quoted with minor modifications and abbreviated from V. Dato, A. Weltman, K. Waller, M. A. Ruta, A. Highbaugh-Battle, C. Hembree, S. Evenson, C. Wheeler, T. Vogt, "Hepatitis A Outbreak Associated with Green Onions at a Restaurant—Monaca, Pennsylvania, 2003," *Morbidity and Mortality Weekly Report,* November 21, 2003, Dispatch.

COMPARISONS

At the core of epidemiology is the idea of comparisons. Epidemiologists strive to quantify relative differences in disease frequency among human populations according to certain quantifiable and variable characteristics of those populations. For example, an epidemiologist might be interested in quantifying health outcomes in sedentary populations and comparing these outcomes with those in more physically active populations. Only in comparing populations having different levels of physical activity can the effect of physical activity on health be quantified.

In the identification of a characteristic as a cause or a preventive of a health out-come, the range of values for which that characteristic is causal or preventive also is important. For instance, smoking a half-pack of cigarettes each day is detrimental to health compared with nonsmoking but beneficial to health compared with smoking two packs of cigarettes each day.

Similarly, consumption of alcoholic beverages is associated with an increased risk of coronary heart disease and stroke at high levels of consumption, perhaps because of an association between the lack of good nutrition and high alcohol intake. In contrast, alcohol consumption appears to be a preventive for coronary heart disease, stroke, and mortality (death) from all causes at more moderate levels of consumption (Goldberg 2003; Liao et al. 2000; Mukamal et al. 2003; Thun et al. 1997).

STUDYING HUMAN POPULATIONS

Most epidemiologists study human populations. This aspect of epidemiology is funda-mental, for at least two reasons. First, findings from epidemiologic studies reflect actual disease experiences in humans. In some other fields of inquiry, in which animals or in vitro (laboratory or "test-tube") systems are studied, extrapolation of study results to humans can be problematic. This difficulty arises because humans and animals may differ with respect to their physiologic responses to certain exposures. For example, it would be unproductive to study the causes of human heart disease using a guinea pig model, because guinea pigs do not develop heart disease.

The second reason the epidemiologic focus on studying disease in humans is fun-damental pertains to the routes and the dosages of the **exposures** under study. "Expo-sures" refers to any of the actual or supposed causes and preventives of disease and/or injury in human populations. Investigators who use animal models to study human dis-eases must be concerned about whether the doses of exposures or the routes of expo-sure they use are appropriate and applicable to human populations. For example, an investigator might expose study animals to a considerably higher dose of an assumed cause of human disease than the dose to which people normally (that is, in usual situ-ations) are exposed. The purpose of using a high dose of exposure for animal models often is to shorten the time interval between exposure and disease, thereby reducing the time and the costs needed to complete a study. The question that arises in these studies is whether people, because of their lower doses of exposure, would respond physio-logically in the same ways in which the highly dosed study animals responded.

A similar question arises when investigators, using animal models, alter the typical route of exposure (inhalation, ingestion, or dermal absorption). For instance, an investi-gator might inject an animal with a substance that causes disease in humans through inhalation. The question of whether the same study results would have occurred if the investigator had caused the study animals to inhale the harmful substance instead of being injected complicates the interpretation of the study results. Because epidemiolo-gists study people, the results from epidemiologic studies reflect human health effects of doses and routes of exposure that actually occur in human populations.

Like data generated by other fields of science, data collected during epidemiologic investigations need to be reviewed critically, with the goal of evaluating the accuracy of the data and its relevance to understanding and/or solving a public health problem. This dispassionate viewpoint facilitates identification of the strengths and the limitations in a set of data and reins in unwarranted enthusiasm regarding research findings.

ETHICAL CONSIDERATIONS

Integral to epidemiology are the ethical constraints on what types of studies can be conducted, what populations can be studied, and what methods can be employed. For instance, epidemiologists cannot ethically assign study subjects to receive a cause of disease in order to measure the associated health effects, nor can they refrain from offering the best available treatment to study subjects, when that treatment is known. In addition, epidemiologic studies can be conducted only on volunteers, people who have given their informed and voluntary consent to participate in the study.

There are examples of unethical studies involving human subjects in both the medical and the epidemiologic literatures. Examples of unethical studies include the Tuskegee Syphilis Study and the radiation experiments conducted by the United States from the 1940s through the 1970s. In the Tuskegee study, initiated in 1932, 399 African American men with syphilis were followed for forty years. The objective of the study was to learn about the **natural history** of syphilis. The natural history of a disease is the usual pattern of symptoms and pathology associated with the disease from its inception until cure, remission, or death. In the Tuskegee study, the subjects were denied treatment for syphilis even after an effective treatment (penicillin) was found. The legacy of this study is apparent even now, as some African Americans still cite the Tuskegee study as a primary reason for their distrust of medicine and public health in the United States (Gamble 1997).

In the radiation experiments of the 1940s through the 1970s, over four thousand medical experiments, all involving the exposure of people to radiation, were conducted on thousands of human subjects, often without the subjects' knowledge or consent. At least seventy-nine of the experiments recruited children and infants (sometimes orphans) or fetuses, and other experiments targeted subjects who had low economic statuses and/or were perceived as being mentally challenged (Pasternak and Cary 1995). Some experiments were continued even after subjects, suffering from the adverse physiologic effects of their radiation exposures, requested that the investigators end the study. A significant percentage of the radiation experiments was funded by the U.S. Pentagon or by other governmental agencies, even though the **Nuremberg Code** had been adopted worldwide in 1949 (see Box 1.2) (International Military Tribunal 1950; Shuster 1997). The Nuremberg Code was developed in response to unethical medical experimentation on people held captive by the German military during World War II. The code lists ten ethical principles that should be followed whenever people are used in scientific experiments.

BOX 1.2

ETHICS MATTERS: THE NUREMBERG CODE

Background: Quotations from the United States Holocaust Memorial Museum

The "Doctors Trial"

On December 9, 1946, an American military tribunal opened criminal proceedings against 23 leading German physicians and administrators for their willing participation in war crimes and crimes against humanity. In Nazi Germany, German physicians planned and enacted the "Euthanasia" Program, the systematic killing of those they deemed "unworthy of life." The victims included the mentally retarded, the institutionalized mentally ill, and the physically impaired. Further, during World War II, German physicians conducted pseudoscientific medical experiments utilizing thousands of concentration camp prisoners without their consent. Most died or were permanently crippled as a result. Most of the victims were Jews, Poles, Russians, and also Roma (Gypsies). After almost 140 days of proceedings, including the testimony of 85 witnesses and the submission of almost 1,500 documents, the American judges pronounced their verdict on August 20, 1947. Sixteen of the doctors were found guilty. Seven were sentenced to death. They were executed on June 2, 1948. (www.ushmm.org/research/doctors/index.html)

History of the Nuremberg Code

On August 19, 1947, the judges of the American military tribunal in the case of the USA vs. Karl Brandt et al. delivered their verdict. Before announcing the guilt or innocence of each defendant, they confronted the difficult question of medical experimentation on human beings. Several German doctors had argued in their own defense that their experiments differed little from previous American or German ones. Furthermore they showed that no international law or informal statement differentiated between legal and illegal human experimentation. This argument worried Drs. Andrew Ivy and Leo Alexander, American doctors who had worked with the prosecution during the trial. On April 17, 1947, Dr. Alexander submitted a memorandum to the United States Counsel for War Crimes which outlined six points defining legitimate research. The verdict of August 19 reiterated almost all of these points in a section entitled *Permissible Medical Experiments* and revised the original six points into ten. Subsequently, the ten points became known as the "Nuremberg Code." Although the code addressed the defense arguments in general, remarkably none of the specific findings against Brandt and his codefendants mentioned the code. Thus the legal force of the document was not well established. The uncertain use of the code continued in the half century following the trial when it informed numerous international ethics statements but failed to find a place in either the American or German national law codes. Nevertheless, it remains a landmark document on medical ethics and one of the most lasting products of the "Doctors Trial." (www.ushmm.org/research/doctors/code_expl.htm)

Box 1.2 continued

The Nuremberg Code

Permissible Medical Experiments

The great weight of the evidence before us is to the effect that certain types of medical experiments on human beings, when kept within reasonably well-defined bounds, conform to the ethics of the medical profession generally. The protagonists of the practice of human experimentation justify their views on the basis that such experiments yield results for the good of society that are unprocurable by other methods or means of study. All agree, however, that certain basic principles must be observed in order to satisfy moral, ethical and legal concepts:

1. The voluntary consent of the human subject is absolutely essential. This means that the person involved should have legal capacity to give consent; should be so situated as to be able to exercise free power of choice, without the intervention of any element of force, fraud, deceit, duress, overreaching, or other form of constraint or coercion; and should have sufficient knowledge and comprehension of the elements of the subject matter involved as to enable him to make an understanding and enlightened decision. This latter element requires that before the acceptance of an affirmative decision by the experimental subject there should be made known to him the nature, duration, and purpose of the experiment; the method and means by which it is to be conducted; all inconveniences and hazards reasonably to be expected; and the effects upon his health or person which may reasonably come from his participation in the experiment.
2. The experiment should be such as to yield fruitful results for the good of society, unprocurable by other methods or means of study, and not random and unnecessary in nature.
3. The experiment should be so designed and based on the results of animal experimentation and knowledge of the natural history of the disease or other problem under study that the anticipated results will justify the performance of the experiment.
4. The experiment should be so conducted as to avoid all unnecessary physical and mental suffering and injury.
5. No experiment should be conducted where there is an a priori reason to believe that death or disabling injury will occur; except, perhaps, in those experiments where the experimental physicians also serve as subjects.
6. The degree of risk to be taken should never exceed that determined by the humanitarian importance of the problem to be solved by the experiment.
7. Proper preparations should be made and adequate facilities provided to protect the experimental subject against even remote possibilities of injury, disability, or death.
8. The experiment should be conducted only by scientifically qualified persons. The highest degree of skill and care should be required through all stages of the experiment of those who conduct or engage in the experiment.

Box 1.2 continued

9. During the course of the experiment the human subject should be at liberty to bring the experiment to an end if he has reached the physical or mental state where continuation of the experiment seems to him to be impossible.
10. During the course of the experiment the scientist in charge must be prepared to terminate the experiment at any stage, if he has probable cause to believe, in the exercise of good faith, superior skill, and careful judgment required of him, that a continuation of the experiment is likely to result in injury, disability, or death to the experimental subject.

Source: International Military Tribunal 1950.

More recent studies focusing on the ethics of conducting **drug trials** of HIV/AIDS treatment and transmission in sub-Saharan Africa emphasize the difficult ethical issues that arise when conducting research on human subjects. In a drug trial, the research investigator gives some subjects a newly developed therapeutic agent and other subjects a comparison treatment agent (typically "standard or usual care"). The investigator then compares the health outcomes of the subjects in each group. The goal of the trial is to determine whether the newly developed therapeutic agent results in greater improvements in health outcomes than does the comparison treatment.

As examples of the kinds of difficult ethical questions that arise in drug trials of this type are the following: Should drug trials be conducted among subjects living in countries that will not be able to benefit from the results of the trial because of economic constraints? In those same countries, do investigators incur an ethical responsibility to offer ongoing health services to (often economically poor) people and/or their families after their participation in an epidemiologic study? If they do, for how long should such services be offered? Who should pay for those services? Would the offering of such services undermine the voluntary nature of participation in the study by constituting a benefit that could not be refused? Those questions are particularly material in situations in which a tacit promise of such services has been made because of the cultural norms and expectations of the country or region in which a study is being conducted (Angell 2000; Annas and Grodin 1998; Bayer 1998; De Zoysa, Elias, and Bentley 1998; Lurie and Wolfe 1997).

POPULATION PERSPECTIVE

Another dominant feature of epidemiology is its **population perspective.** Unlike the medical/clinical sciences that focus on individual people's welfare, epidemiology strives to understand the causes of disease and injury in populations of people. Whereas the clinician strives to treat ill health in a single individual, epidemiology attempts to understand and improve health in a population. This difference in perspective has several profound implications.

First, the results of epidemiologic studies are intended to benefit entire populations, with the goal of improving their average levels of health. Epidemiology does not seek specifically to improve the health of any one individual as would a clinician treating a patient.

Second, the risks to good health identified in epidemiologic studies apply to populations and not to particular individuals. As an example, the overall **risk** (probability) of dying from heart disease in the United States in 2001 was 29 percent. That risk summarizes a feature of the U.S. population and not a feature of any one person: Each person's individual risk of dying from heart disease is either 100 percent (dies from heart disease) or 0 percent (does not die from heart disease).

And, third, the effective strategies for preventing disease and injury suggested by epidemiologic studies typically are population-based rather than based on the needs of a particular individual. For instance, banning tobacco advertisements from television in the United States is one strategy for attempting to reduce tobacco use among the population of television viewers. That strategy does not target individual viewers in the same sense as a clinician's prescribing medication to decrease a person's cravings for nicotine.

The population perspective of epidemiology embodies what is known as the **public health perspective,** the view that places the good of populations above the good of individuals, *given that all ethical constraints are met.* This latter clause differentiates the public health perspective from a straight utilitarian model of ethics. The utilitarian theory, often summarized as "the greatest happiness for the greatest number of people," allows for people to be treated badly as long as the happiness created for others is larger. Neither epidemiology nor public health embraces that concept.

OBJECTIVES OF EPIDEMIOLOGY

The primary objective of epidemiology is to identify causes of disease and injury that have practical applicability in preventing ill health in human populations. For example, knowing that active or passive exposure to tobacco smoke (relative to no exposure to tobacco smoke) causes lung cancer readily identifies a preventive for lung cancer (reduce exposure to tobacco smoke).

On the other hand, knowing that women with germ-line mutations in BRCA1 and BRCA2 genes have an estimated 56 percent risk of breast cancer by age 70 years may not suggest a practical primary preventive strategy, other than prophylactic breast removal, at least not within the current state of knowledge (Struewing et al. 1997). Such information may still be valuable for breast cancer prevention because new knowledge about gene-therapy opportunities may offer practical avenues for prevention in the future.

Other uses for epidemiology include measuring the extent of **morbidity** (state of ill health) and mortality in human populations, elucidating the **natural history** of human diseases (typical progression of disease from its initiation until cure, remission, or death), and measuring the efficacy of new treatments or preventives of disease and injury.

Each of the objectives of epidemiology complements the overall epidemiologic goal of controlling disease and injury in human populations. Control may occur through early detection and treatment of ill health, identification of the causes/preventives of ill health, the design of effective programs or strategies, and/or improvement of clinical care and access to health care. Cornerstones of these activities include the Epidemic Intelligence Service, which is headquartered at the Centers for Disease Control and Prevention (see Box 1.3); state and local departments of public health; academic programs

---

BOX 1.3

THE EPIDEMIC INTELLIGENCE SERVICE: TRAINING THE WORLD'S "DISEASE DETECTIVES"

RACHEL WOODS, M.P.H.

The Epidemic Intelligence Service (EIS) is headquartered at the Centers for Disease Control and Prevention (CDC) in Atlanta, Georgia. EIS is a unique two-year postgraduate program of service and on-the-job training for health professionals interested in the practice of epidemiology. Individuals in the program are officially called EIS Officers, but because of their outstanding work on epidemic diseases all over the world they have been fondly known as "disease detectives."

The EIS program was established in 1951 as a response to potential biological warfare, as during the Korean War. EIS has been a cornerstone of public health ever since. Today, graduates of the EIS program are working all over the world. They are in local, state, national, and international health agencies, medical organizations, and schools of public health. They have been on the front lines of major epidemics such as smallpox and AIDS, have assisted in the surveillance and understanding of chronic diseases and injuries, and more recently have responded to bioterrorism in the United States.

The program educates medical doctors, veterinarians, researchers, and scientists through intensive two-year assignments. Once in the program, officers receive on-the-job training by participating in epidemiologic investigations, research, and public health surveillance. They serve the epidemiologic needs of state health departments and disseminate vital public health information to the media and the public. EIS officers present epidemiologic papers at scientific and medical conferences and publish their work in the scientific literature. After completing the program, approximately 70 percent of EIS officers pursue careers in public health, 20 percent enter academia, and fewer than 10 percent enter private practice.

EIS officers serve in a variety of locations, including field assignments to state and local health departments and to the centers, institutes, and offices of the CDC. Although international work may be part of any EIS assignment, no two-year assignment is based outside the United States. Since the program's beginning, officers have worked on over 10,000 epidemiologic studies and investigations and each year assist with approximately 100 investigations by request of states and other countries.

Over the past fifty years, EIS officers have played a pivotal role in combating the root causes of major epidemics all over the world. For more information about the program or how to apply to be an EIS officer, view the EIS Web site at www.cdc.gov/eis.

in epidemiology; and national agencies such as the National Institutes of Health and the Environmental Protection Agency.

Epidemiologic methods and the epidemiologic perspective now are being used to identify and solve a broader range of public health problems than in the past. For example, epidemiology is being used in health services research to better understand the epidemiologic bases for cost containment in managed care organizations. Epidemiology also is being used in clinical settings to evaluate standards and outcomes of care and to help define "quality care." More and more, the ability to "think epidemiologically" is being rewarded with improved patient management in health services settings, development of more effective programs in health promotion settings, improved targeting of inspection and regulatory protocols by public and governmental agencies, and reduced workers' compensation premiums in industrial arenas. In addition, epidemiology is being used to aid understanding of the newly emerging and reemerging diseases such as the West Nile virus (described in Box 1.4), dengue hemorrhagic fever, and tuberculosis.

Epidemiology became a "household word" following the terrorist attacks on the World Trade Center in New York City and the Pentagon in Washington, D.C., on September 11, 2001, as the need for increased surveillance of public food and water supplies and of unusual clusters of disease (for example, pulmonary anthrax) surfaced. Epidemiology, with its new responsibilities associated with anticipating, identifying, and responding to terrorist and bioterrorist events, is featured prominently in the United States Office of Homeland Security, created on November 25, 2002.

BOX 1.4

THE WEST NILE VIRUS—EPIDEMIOLOGY OF A RAPIDLY EMERGING DISEASE

Disease associated with the West Nile virus first was identified among birds in Uganda in 1937. The virus was spread by mosquitoes and, initially, had the potential to cause only mild disease. In addition, transmission of the virus was inefficient, making an epidemic of the disease among birds unlikely. In the early 1990s, part of the DNA of the virus mutated, resulting in a virus that spread more efficiently. The new virus, now referred to as the "Old World" West Nile virus, began to appear in birds in other regions of Africa and in Europe. Still, the virus caused only mild disease and did not kill its avian hosts. In 1998, however, a new strain of the virus, the "New World" West Nile virus, appeared in Israel. Infected birds began to die.

In 1999, the New World West Nile virus was found in Queens in New York City and, from there, started to spread rapidly. It infected not only birds (primarily crows, house sparrows, and blue jays) but also horses and people. People in five states in the northeastern region of the United States became infected. By 2002, the virus, perhaps again genetically altered, had been identified in forty-three states, killing thousands of birds (mostly crows) and about one-third of the approximately 13,000 infected horses. The virus also killed 216 people and caused disease in an additional 3,775. Most of the deaths occurred among older individuals.

Box 1.4 continued

Additional Considerations

The rapid development and spread of the West Nile virus probably was unparalleled in the history of human disease until the recent emergence of severe acute respiratory syndrome (SARS). (Figure 1.5 shows a web of causation for SARS.) The Chinese Ministry of Health first reported SARS to the World Health Organization on February 11, 2003. Over the course of several months, SARS, caused by several strains of novel coronaviruses, spread from its initiation point in Guangdong Province, China, to Hong Kong and at least twenty-five other countries. The working hypothesis is that SARS, originally an animal virus, first infected humans working at the Dongyuan meat market, where workers and recently killed animals commingle in extremely crowded conditions. The rapid spread and high percentage of cases who die (about 1 percent in people aged 24 years or younger to more than 50 percent in people aged 65 years or older) from SARS raises the worrisome question of what other new infectious and/or zoonotic diseases may arise from the interactions and sometimes-relentless intrusions of people into new environments.

The preponderance of academic thought in the medical and public health communities in the United States during the 1970s was that infectious and vector-borne diseases, at least in economically developed countries, no longer were major public health problems. Since that time, morbidity and mortality from nosocomial infections have reached epidemic proportions in the United States; tuberculosis associated with HIV/AIDS has reemerged as a substantial public health problem; HIV/AIDS has become a leading cause of mortality, especially in sub-Saharan African countries but also among certain populations in the United States; and the fear that bioterrorist activities may involve the use of anthrax, possibly smallpox, or other infectious agents has led public health agencies to develop emergency response plans for a widespread bioterrorist event. In addition, it now is better understood that some viruses can cause cancers, such as hepatitis C causing liver cancer, the human papillomavirus causing cervical cancer, and perhaps the Epstein-Barr virus causing Hodgkin's lymphoma. Inflammatory processes may be involved in some cases of heart disease; and the helicobacter pylori bacterium can cause stomach ulcers in humans. Further, *giardia* and *cryptosporidium,* both protozoan parasites, are increasingly contaminating drinking-water supplies. For example, in 1993, *Cryptosporidium* contamination of the municipal water system in Milwaukee, Wisconsin, caused over 400,000 people to become ill, of whom 70 died. These relatively recent findings regarding the effects of infectious agents in the etiology of both acute and chronic diseases, coupled with the rapid increase in pathogenic bacteria that show multiple antimicrobial-resistance, raise sobering questions about the public's ability to prevent and/or control the health impacts of infectious agents.

Source: "West Nile Virus," www.cdc.gov/ncidod/dvbid/westnile/qa/overview.htm (accessed December 6, 2002).

SUMMARY

Epidemiology, as the fundamental science of public health, is empowering. It provides a framework in which to view public health problems and identify solutions in a way that no other scientific field provides.

As you read through and study the chapters in this book, it might be helpful to ask yourself the following: How does the material in each chapter pertain to my professional goals? What content areas of the epidemiologic literature provide essential information for my field of interest? How can the creative application of epidemiology be used to elucidate the underpinnings and challenges in public health, health services, and public policy? How can I use epidemiology to help me become a more competent, successful professional?

REVIEW QUESTIONS

1. List several different ideas about what factors cause disease. How is each of those ideas related to the prevention of disease and injury?
2. Define "epidemiology." What are the primary differences and similarities between acute- and chronic-disease epidemiology?
3. List several advantages and disadvantages in using epidemiology instead of animal-based science to study the causes of human disease and injury.
4. List several of the ethical questions that arise in epidemiologic research. How can those ethical questions be resolved? Should epidemiologists be required to adhere to a professional code of ethics?
5. Define "population perspective."
6. List the major objectives of epidemiology, and provide examples of each objective. What kinds of questions can epidemiology help to answer in the diverse specialty areas of public health such as health services administration, health promotion and education, environmental health and science, international health, minority health, and maternal and child health?
7. What is the "Nuremberg Code"? Summarize the content of the code. Of what significance, if any, is the code historically and today? To what human research situations does the code apply?

REVIEW EXERCISES

1. Draw a web of causation that depicts the social, political, and other influences on an important public health problem.
2. List potential applications of epidemiology to your selected professional field, and compare those applications with applications in other fields.
3. Identify five World Wide Web sites that provide quality information for your professional field.

CHAPTER 2

Historical Development

The history of epidemiology often is traced to Hippocrates, whose scrolls, written approximately 2,400 years ago, were translated and published as a treatise titled *On Airs, Waters, and Places.* The treatise included novel, epidemiologic ideas. For example, Part I of the Treatise, as translated by Francis Adams, states:

> Whoever wishes to investigate medicine properly, should proceed thus: in the first place to consider the seasons of the year, and what effects each of them produces for they are not at all alike, but differ much from themselves in regard to their changes. Then the winds, the hot and the cold, especially such as are common to all countries, and then such as are peculiar to each locality. We must also consider the qualities of the waters, for as they differ from one another in taste and weight, so also do they differ much in their qualities. In the same manner, when one comes into a city to which he is a stranger, he ought to consider its situation, how it lies as to the winds and the rising of the sun; for its influence is not the same whether it lies to the north or the south, to the rising or to the setting sun. These things one ought to *consider* [emphasis added] most attentively, and concerning the waters which the inhabitants use, whether they be marshy and soft, or hard, and running from elevated and rocky situations, and then if saltish and unfit for cooking; and the ground, whether it be naked and deficient in water, or wooded and well watered, and whether it lies in a hollow, confined situation, or is elevated and cold; and the mode in which the inhabitants live, and what are their pursuits, whether they are fond of drinking and eating to excess, and given to indolence, or are fond of exercise and labor, and not given to excess in eating and drinking. (classics.mit.edu/Hippocrates/airwatpl.1.1.html)

It seems remarkable that few advances in epidemiologic insights were published until 1662 when John Graunt, an Englishman, published *Natural and Political Observations Made Upon the Bills of Mortality* (Graunt 1662). (An original copy of the *Observations* is located in the Salisbury Cathedral in Salisbury, United Kingdom.) The British epidemiologist Major Greenwood interpreted this delay in the evolution of epidemiologic theory to the treatise's omission of the need to *quantify* the magnitude of a link between a cause of disease and the disease. The treatise included only the idea that a person's environment or lifestyle needed to be "considered." No amount of "considering" would usher in epidemiology. Only a quantitative approach to studying human diseases would bring about this evolution (Greenwood 1935).

In his *Observations,* Graunt published analyses of the weekly reports of births and deaths in London. Among his findings were that the number of male births exceeded the number of female births, the **infant mortality rate** (number of children who die during the first year of life per 1,000 live births in a year) was high, and there was **seasonal variation** (differences in the frequency of disease or injury by month) in the number of deaths.

Graunt's work was remarkable for two reasons. He was the first person to recognize fully the public health value of analyzing routinely collected data about human health status. Second, he used those routinely collected data to quantify and compare the distribution of health events (in this case, births and deaths) in a population. Those two advances contributed materially to the development of epidemiologic methods.

Accolades for developing the quantitative bases for epidemiology also belong to William Farr and John Snow who were contemporaries in the nineteenth century. In 1839, and for forty years thereafter, Farr was responsible for medical statistics in the Office of the Registrar General for England and Wales. In that capacity, he developed a system for routinely assembling vital statistics on the health of the population. Using those data, he undertook studies comparing mortality among subsets of the population according to marital status, occupation, and area of residence. Farr documented the fact that most prisoners who died in jail did so from disease and not from execution (Halliday 2000).

One of Farr's most significant contributions was his understanding of the value of quantifying the size of a **population at risk.** A population at risk is the number of susceptible people in which health-related events occur. With that new idea, Farr was able to compare the *relative frequency* of health outcomes in different populations and not only the *relative numbers* of health events, as illustrated in Table 2.1. Farr also provided insights into the potential **biases** (systematic errors) likely to be present in epidemiologic studies, especially biases related to how study participants should be selected and what factors, such as age or prior health status, could cause study findings to be in error.

TABLE 2.1

Comparison of the Relative Frequency and Relative Number of a Health-Related Event

Gender	Number of a Health-Related Event	Size of the Population at Risk
Male	50	500
Female	70	1,000
Gender	Relative Number of the Event	Relative Frequency of the Event
Male	50	50/500 = 0.10 or 10%
Female	70	70/1,000 = 0.07 or 7%

Note: Notice that comparing the *relative number* of the health-related event may suggest that the event occurs more often in females than in males, because the number 70 is larger than the number 50. Comparing the *relative frequency,* however, shows that the event occurs more often in males than in females as a proportion of the total numbers of males and females in the population.

Twenty years after Farr began his work, John Snow, perhaps the most renowned of the early epidemiologists, initiated his landmark studies of cholera (Snow 1855). His studies culminated in the demonstration that cholera was being transmitted through London's public water supplies (Vinten-Johansen et al. 2003). (Snow, whose picture is available at www.jsi.com, is the physician remembered for administering chloroform to Queen Victoria during childbirth.)

Snow began his work with the realization that different sections of London experienced vastly different numbers of death from cholera. Sections of London with the highest number of cholera deaths were connected to water supplied by either the Lambeth Company or the Southwark and Vauxhall Company. Both companies obtained their water from a severely polluted point in the Thames River, after the river had flowed through London. By 1854, the Lambeth Company had changed its water source to a point in the Thames upstream from London. This water source was relatively free of sewage and other pollution. After that change, cholera deaths in the areas supplied by the Lambeth Company or the Southwark and Vauxhall Company began to decline. Snow realized that the reduction in cholera deaths could have occurred for reasons other than the change in water source; that is, there could have been differences other than the water supply that may have affected cholera deaths in the sections of London served by those two companies.

During a terrible cholera epidemic of 1854, Snow observed that the relative number of cholera deaths was considerably higher in sections of London served only by the Southwark and Vauxhall Company than in sections served only by the Lambeth Company. In particular, in an area around Broad Street and Golden Square, over five hundred fatal cases of cholera occurred within ten days.

Snow also observed that the relative number of cholera deaths in a district of London served by both companies was midway between the numbers of deaths for districts having a sole water provider. Houses in this district were connected to one of the two water companies almost by chance, because the connections had been established during a period of fierce competition between the two companies.

Snow's genius lay in his next set of observations. He realized that he had an opportunity to conduct a definitive test of the hypothesis that the source of water was responsible for cholera deaths. All he needed to do was determine which water company served each house in which a cholera death occurred within the region served by both companies. The numbers of cholera deaths, divided by the total numbers of houses served by each company, would demonstrate whether there was a difference in the relative frequency of cholera deaths according to water source.

Snow's house-to-house survey of cholera deaths yielded the following data:

Water Company	Number of Houses	Relative Number of Cholera Deaths	Relative Frequency of Cholera Deaths (number of deaths per 10,000 houses)
Only Southwark and Vauxhall	40,046	1,263	315
Only Lambeth	26,107	98	37
Remaining sections of London	256,423	1,422	59*

*1,422/256,423 = 55 deaths/10,000 houses. The reason for this discrepancy is not clear.

Within the London district served by both water companies, the relative frequencies of cholera deaths were 315 deaths/10,000 houses and 37 deaths/10,000 houses for houses connected to the Southwark and Vauxhall Company and the Lambeth Company, respectively. Other explanations for the difference in cholera deaths were unlikely because few other differences existed between the residents and their houses served by each company. After his investigation, Snow removed the handle on the Broad Street water pump. The pump was used by the general public as a source of water and supplied by the Southwark and Vauxhall Company. Snow's sterling contribution to epidemiologic methods was his insight that ideas concerning suspected causes of disease can be tested by observing and quantifying naturally occurring situations.

Snow's idea that dirty water may be a cause of cholera did not carry over into a similar concern that "dirty air" may be a cause of disease. Snow served as an expert witness for the big industries of his time in support of the belief that polluted air was not causing ill health.

A poignant historical illustration of a strong relationship between a person's occupational environment and the diseases and injuries from which he or she is apt to suffer is provided in Upton Sinclair's novel *The Jungle,* published in 1906 (Sinclair 1981). In Chapter 9, Sinclair describes the difficult working conditions within the U.S. meatpacking industry at the beginning of the twentieth century:

> There was another interesting set of statistics that a person might have gathered in Packingtown—those of the various afflictions of the workers. When Jurgis (a recent immigrant to the United States) had first inspected the packing plants with Szedvilas, he had marveled while he listened to the tale of all the things that were made out of the carcasses of animals, and of all the lesser industries that were maintained there; now he found that each of these lesser industries was a separate little inferno, in its way as horrible as the killing beds, the source and fountain of them all. The workers in each of them had their own peculiar diseases. And the wandering visitor might be skeptical about all the swindles, but he could not be skeptical about these, for the worker bore the evidence of them about on his own person—generally he had only to hold out his hand.

Sinclair continues by describing the ailments of the workers' hands, including amputations among men who worked at the stamping machines, thumbs that were stubs because of repeated cuts among the butchers and beef-boners, and fingers eaten away by acid among the wool-pluckers. The workers also suffered from occupationally induced or transmitted diseases such as rheumatism and tuberculosis.

The links between occupation and disease and injury, described in Sinclair's novel, were easily identified because a large proportion of the workers engaged in a work activity were affected by the ailment at about the same time. The links were unmistakable even without the use of specialized, epidemiologic methods. Understanding the less obvious relationships between suspected causes of disease and health outcomes would have to wait until those methods were developed.

ACUTE ONSET VERSUS CHRONIC DISEASE EPIDEMIOLOGY

Early epidemiologic studies typically entailed investigations of acute onset diseases. **Acute onset disease epidemiology** emphasizes the study of diseases that have short incubation or **latent periods** (a short time period between exposure to the causal agent and the onset of disease). Acute onset infectious diseases include the childhood immunizable diseases such as measles, mumps, and rubella; typhoid fever; cholera; foodborne outbreaks; and influenza. Epidemics of these diseases often are easily recognizable because the **incident cases** of disease (newly occurring cases) cluster in time and space close to the source of the causal agent. An example of a large foodborne outbreak of hepatitis A associated with eating green onions was described in Chapter 1.

Other acute onset diseases cluster in time but not necessarily in a defined geographic location because the infectious agent spreads rapidly from one person to another. As an example, the **pandemic** (global epidemic) of influenza in 1918–1919 killed between 20 million and 40 million people worldwide and was one of the most disastrous disease outbreaks in recorded human history. Fully one-fifth of the world's population was infected. The pandemic was deadliest for people between the ages of 20 and 40 years, unlike most influenza epidemics that kill primarily young children and the elderly. (See, for example, www.stanford.edu/group/virus/uda/.)

Starting in the early 1950s, epidemiologists, typically clinicians or statisticians by education and training, began investigating chronic diseases. The characteristic clustering in time and space associated with acute onset diseases differs substantially from the temporal and spatial patterns observed for the **chronic diseases,** such as the cancers and diseases of the heart. For chronic diseases, there typically is a long interval between first exposure to a causal agent(s) and the occurrence of disease.

The long latent period associated with chronic diseases is a primary impediment to identifying their etiologies (causes). For example, the long latent period means that people die from other ailments before the disease under study has had time to occur and be diagnosed. In addition, recall of past exposure fades, and medical and exposure records become unavailable. To exacerbate the difficulties in identifying the causes of chronic diseases is the fact that some chronic diseases, such as brain cancer or cardiac amyloidosis, have low incidence rates which makes case-finding burdensome, insidious onsets of signs and symptoms, and multiple and interacting etiologies. (Cardiac amyloidosis, a disease that occurs four times more often in the Black population in the United States than in the White population, is a disorder in which protein builds up in tissues and organs, causing the heart to beat erratically or fail completely.) For those reasons, it usually is more difficult to identify the causes of chronic diseases than it is to identify the causes of acute onset diseases.

Notwithstanding those differences between acute and chronic diseases, the methodologic advances and insights gained by studying the acute onset diseases have been instrumental in the development of methods designed specifically for studying chronic diseases and **late sequelae** (health outcomes occurring long after the time of first exposure) of infectious diseases such as polio and polio syndrome diseases or chicken pox and shingles. Among those methods is the measurement and comparison of **attack rates.**

An attack rate, discussed further in Chapter 3, is the percentage of a **population** (any identifiable group of people) that develops disease shortly after exposure to a causal agent. Such an exposure is called a **point exposure** because people are affected at about the same time and location by the same causal agent. Attack rates were the first **measures of disease frequency** (quantifications of the magnitude of disease or injury occurrence in a population). Measures of disease frequency are as essential to chronic disease epidemiology as they are to acute onset epidemiology in the evaluation of relationships between exposures and health outcomes.

DEVELOPMENT OF EPIDEMIOLOGY AS A SCIENCE

Before about 1950, essentially all epidemiology was acute onset epidemiology. Then, in the 1950s, Sir Richard Doll and A. Bradford Hill, in a series of stunning studies of English physicians, published their landmark findings pertaining to tobacco use and lung cancer (Doll and Hill, 1950). Those studies formed the nucleus of nascent **modern epidemiology.** Epidemiologic thought developed quickly in the 1960s and 1970s, with codification of methodologies specific to the study of the chronic, emerging, and remerging diseases. The 1980s brought further refinements of epidemiologic methodology and the emergence of the epidemiologic "specialties," such as nutritional epidemiology, occupational epidemiology, and environmental epidemiology.

More recently, epidemiology has focused not only on the study of chronic diseases but also on the emerging and reemerging diseases such as HIV/AIDS, Ebola, tuberculosis, dengue hemorrhagic fever, West Nile virus, mad cow disease, and severe acute respiratory syndrome (SARS). In addition, the new epidemiology has relied more heavily on developing novel methods to measure exposures accurately and to identify physiologically harmful doses of exposure; it also has strengthened the methodological tools available for quantifying the magnitude of interactions among exposures that result in disease. In the United States and elsewhere, epidemiologists have been called upon to participate in a wide variety of activities related to homeland security. Those activities include enhanced disease surveillance, protection of food and water supplies, and development of plans to respond to bioterrorist events.

The new epidemiology has foundations in a number of other fields in addition to acute onset epidemiology and knowledge of biology, medicine, and pathology. Those fields included statistics, the social sciences, computer technology, and the managerial sciences (Figure 2.1). In addition to those areas, development of epidemiology relied upon the case/control study, the hallmark **analytic study design** (a hypothesis-evaluating study) of modern epidemiology.

What did each of the following fields contribute to the development of modern epidemiology?

Statistics

Essentially all of epidemiology is **population-based.** Epidemiologists study groups of people, looking for causal associations between exposures and health outcomes in those groups. For example, an epidemiologist might ask whether populations having higher levels of high-density lipoproteins (HDLs; the "good" cholesterol) have lower rates of cardiac problems than do comparable populations having lower levels of HDLs. Epidemiologists might also inquire whether the magnitude of association between HDLs and cardiac outcomes is the same for populations having differing levels of homocystein and C-reactive protein (both suspected causes of poor cardiac

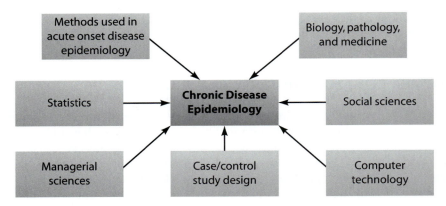

FIGURE 2.1
Academic and practical roots of chronic disease epidemiology.

outcomes). Because epidemiologists study groups of people rather than individuals, the data epidemiologists collect require a **statistical analysis** (a mathematical analysis based on groups of objects).

Social Sciences

Social sciences such as sociology, psychology, and anthropology are foundational fields for epidemiology because the vast majority of epidemiologic studies are **observational** (studies in which an epidemiologist collects information about people's existing exposures and health outcomes but does not change people's exposure statuses as occurs in experiments). Epidemiologists must understand the social processes and forces that result in some individuals' having certain exposures while other people lack those exposures. Sometimes the exposures that people have are partly or largely determined by conditions outside their immediate control. For example, few people choose to live in poverty. Nevertheless, as far as the epidemiologic perspective is concerned, those exposures are preexisting rather than newly assigned or **randomly allocated** by an investigator.

Random allocation means that an investigator decides which subjects receive certain exposures based on a process in which every subject in the study has the same probability as has any other subject of receiving a particular exposure. Assignment of particular subjects to specific exposures is determined by "chance." Random allocation of exposure occurs in an **experiment** and is the defining characteristic of an experiment. As mentioned previously, most epidemiologic studies are observational and thus do not involve the random allocation of exposure(s) to the groups whose health outcomes are to be compared. Random allocation of exposure is ethical only when an exposure is a suspected preventive or cure for an adverse health outcome. In epidemiology, most studies seek to determine the etiology of adverse health outcomes. Suspected etiologic factors ethically cannot be randomly allocated to study participants.

Computer Technology

The development of computer technology was central to the development of epidemiology. Epidemiologists often study large groups of people (several hundred thousand people) and collect numerous data over time for each person. Because the data management and analysis requirements for these large studies are extensive, the implementation of large studies needed to await the development of computer hardware and associated software capable of storing, managing, and analyzing large amounts of data.

There are numerous software programs available to facilitate the analyses of epidemiologic data. (See, for example, www.ehdp.com/vitalnet/episw.htm.) In addition, novel analytic methods are being developed as both the theory and the substantive knowledge of epidemiology are understood better. Advances in computer technology offer exciting opportunities for epidemiologists to improve their measurements and understanding of the ways in which variables interact as a system in facilitating or preventing disease and injury in human populations.

Managerial Science

The managerial sciences have been important in the development of modern epidemiology for several reasons. First, epidemiologists study volunteers and therefore must manage the "volunteer process" that encourages potential study subjects to participate in studies. Participating clinical, university, and/or community sites' **Institutional Review Boards (IRBs),** also known as **Human Subjects Committees,** must approve the plan for enrolling study subjects into an epidemiologic study, as well as the other aspects of a study design, before the initiation of the study. IRBs first were set up on a wide-scale basis during the 1970s partly in response to increasing numbers of epidemiologic studies and several alleged abuses of subjects in epidemiologic and other investigations involving human subjects.

The responsibilities of IRBs are to protect the rights of human subjects in research studies; assure that subject participation is voluntary and informed; and evaluate the adequacy of safeguards for protecting the confidentiality of data collected as part of a study, including an assurance of the anonymity of study subjects, to the extent that the law allows (see Boxes 2.1 and 2.2). The procedures for obtaining IRB approvals can be a time-, money-, and energy-consuming managerial undertaking, particularly when many clinical sites or universities are involved in a study.

The second reason the managerial sciences have been important in the development of epidemiology pertains to the actual conduct of the study. Once an epidemiologic study is initiated, an investigator must keep the investigative team working together and the study subjects interested in voluntarily continuing their participation for the duration of the study. An epidemiologist's managerial skills are particularly tested if the study involves collecting information from thousands of study subjects who were treated in a multitude of different clinical settings over an extended period of time.

BOX 2.1

ETHICS MATTERS: INSTITUTIONAL REVIEW BOARDS (IRBs)

The roles of Institutional Review Boards (IRBs) are to protect the rights of human subjects in research studies; assure that subject participation is voluntary and informed; and evaluate the adequacy of safeguards for protecting the confidentiality of data collected as part of a study, including an assurance of the anonymity of study subjects. Almost every university and health services facility has an in-house IRB.

The Nuremberg Code (Box 1.2) delineates the expected ethical standards for experiments involving human subjects. Although the code provides the overall structure for deciding ethical issues in human studies, issues arise for which the code may not provide a definitive answer.

For example, in studies involving children as study subjects, what constitutes "voluntary, informed consent"? At what age or level of maturity is a child able to give his or her own voluntary informed consent? Is the consent of one parent sufficient, or must both parents consent? What if the parents live apart from each other because of a separation? Suppose the study subject is an adult whose mental or emotional functioning capabilities are compromised. Who consents in that situation? Or, perhaps the potential study subject is a person with Alzheimer's disease who is suffering from severe cognitive deficits. Who, if anyone, is entitled morally to provide informed, voluntary consent for that person? Can prisoners give informed, voluntary consent? What factors undermine the voluntary and/or informed nature of consent?

In some cultures, a woman is not permitted to make decisions about participating in a scientific study (nor is she permitted to make decisions about other personal issues, such as the use of family resources or the timing and frequency of sexual encounters). Either the woman's husband or her father makes those decisions. When conducting research in that kind of cultural setting, is it ethically acceptable for an epidemiologist from the United States (a country in which women are permitted to make decisions about participating in a research study) to take a father's or a husband's informed, voluntary consent to mean that the woman has given her own informed, voluntary consent?

Issues arise also with respect to the confidentiality of data and the anonymity of study subjects. For example, at times, courts subpoena data collected as part of an epidemiologic study. Thus, study subjects, who believe that both their names and their personal data will be kept confidential, find that the courts have access to those data for use in legal proceedings. In fact, voluntary, informed consent forms now regularly include the disclaimer that the subjects' data will be kept confidential *to the extent that the law allows.*

As another example of questions related to confidentiality, should the confidentiality of data be honored when a public harm, such as the transmission of HIV to sexual partners, is likely? Should the sexual contacts of study subjects with sexually transmitted diseases be notified of their increased risk of disease? (That question is explored in detail in Box 2.2.) Should information regarding planned illegal activities,

Box 2.1 continued

such as personal assault or other violent crimes, that is discovered during the course of data collection be included among the data that are "confidential"?

Difficult ethical issues regarding human studies remain. For example, how does an epidemiologist prioritize among ethical obligations and responsibilities when those obligations and responsibilities conflict? Who, if not an individual epidemiologist or an IRB, decides which ethical constraints or imperatives have priority over others? Which obligations or responsibilities are unwavering and which subject to modification based on "special" circumstances?

On April 14, 2003, new federal rules to protect the privacy of patients and their medical records went into effect. These new rules, initially issued in a 1996 law entitled the Health Insurance Portability and Accountability Act (HIPAA), require healthcare providers to limit the disclosure of personal health information to the "minimum necessary" to meet a certain objective. Violations of the new law are punishable by both civil and criminal penalties of up to a $250,000 fine and ten years in prison.

The effects of the new law on the availability of health information to researchers, including epidemiologists, may be profound. Some clinical care settings are refusing to share health information with researchers, even if the information pertains to patients treated ten or fifteen years previously. Other clinical care centers no longer are willing to provide researchers with medical data that formerly were provided freely. In addition, for research in progress, some investigators are quickly trying to obtain permission from study subjects who had not been told that their health information was being used for research purposes.

The new law raises once again a basic ethical question: Do people have a responsibility to share their personal health information for the betterment of society because they themselves have benefited from the services and opportunities afforded by living in that society?

BOX 2.2

PRACTICAL EPIDEMIOLOGY IN A PUBLIC HEALTH SETTING: ETHICS AND PARTNERS

PAUL ETKIND, DR.P.H., M.P.H.

LOCAL SERVICES COORDINATOR, BUREAU OF COMMUNICABLE DISEASE CONTROL, MASSACHUSETTS DEPARTMENT OF PUBLIC HEALTH

Identifying exposed and susceptible people, and then informing them of their risk of infection and offering appropriate services with which to act on this information, is at the heart of public health disease control strategies. It seems to be a straightforward concept until it is applied to sexually transmitted infections (STIs).

Box 2.2 continued

This strategy, currently called Partner Services (PS), was first suggested as a tool for venereal disease (as it was known then) prevention in 1910 and was adopted as a standard tool of public health venereal disease programs in the early 1940s. It was initially called Contact Tracing, but has had other names in different times, such as CARE (Contact Awareness and Referral for Exposure), CTPRN (Counseling, Testing, Partner Referral and Notification), PCRS (Partner Counseling and Referral Service), and PN (Partner Notification), as the focus and scope of the service changed. Regardless of its name, the process begins when a person who has been diagnosed as having an STI is interviewed by a public health professional (often called a Disease Intervention Specialist, or DIS), and information about the partner(s) is requested. The DIS will then try to locate the partner using information provided by the infected individual. When located, the partner is informed of their exposure to infection and is offered medical evaluation and treatment as well as personalized risk reduction education to help prevent future infections. However, the social, political and medical implications of the HIV/AIDS epidemic have produced a view that that this disease is different from other STIs and that PS can pose additional, unwarranted risks to people.

Arguments supporting the special nature of HIV/AIDS that make PS inappropriate to use as a prevention tool include the following:

- **HIV/AIDS is not curable.** This contrasts with the "traditional" bacterial STIs (upon which the medical model of STI prevention was based), against which antibiotics are effective.
- **Prophylactic treatment to prevent HIV infection is generally not available.** Prophylactic antibiotic treatment of bacterial STIs is routine for partners.
- **HIV/AIDS is fatal.** Other STIs, bacterial or otherwise, are generally not fatal.
- **HIV/AIDS generates a greater degree of stigma.** Although people with HIV/AIDS and people with "other" STIs share many characteristics and come from similar if not the same populations, the "other" STIs do not invoke the same degree of stigma and discrimination.
- **People with HIV/AIDS frequently have minimal access to the health care system for ongoing care of a life-long infection.** This contrasts with the care required for bacterial STIs, which usually require only episodic, short-term care. Such care is available from a number of sources including but not limited to emergency rooms, walk-in centers, family planning clinics, and publicly funded STI clinics.
- **There is a fear that the process of eliciting information about partners will be mandatory or coercive.** Curiously, this concern is most often stated in relation to HIV/AIDS but not for other STIs.
- **There is a fear that PS data collection may create a registry of infected and at-risk people that would be maintained by a government agency.** There is mistrust regarding government use of data it collects, particularly among people and communities that already face discrimination in their lives. The history of the Tuskegee Project reinforces this mistrust. Once again, though, this concern is most often specific to HIV/AIDS.

Box 2.2 continued

- **There is a fear that personal relationships will be adversely affected.** This, too, is more often HIV/AIDS-specific.
- **There are fears of violence in acts of retribution subsequent to partners being notified.** This is true for both HIV/AIDS and "other" STIs.

Thus, an argument can be made that PS will be a disservice to people named as partners if there is no guarantee of medical and social services to deal with such news. This may add to other personal and social issues that partners are trying to cope with, such as sexism, racism, homophobia, poverty, educational deprivation, addiction, etc. Critics ask if notifying someone of their potential HIV-infection status, and providing focused education about risks and disease, outweigh the possible negative consequences to that person's life.

The question of whether or not PS is an ethical practice depends on whether it can adhere to ethical principles in order to maximize acceptance and impact as well as whether it can actually achieve its stated goals. The attributes of ethical public health practice include the following:

- **Respect for autonomy**—it must be voluntary and there is buy-in for participation
- **Beneficence**—it enhances the welfare of all
- **Justice**—there is an equitable distribution of risks and benefits
- **Veracity**—there is full disclosure of relevant information
- **Privacy**—the right of a person to determine the extent to which his/her thoughts will be communicated to others
- **Confidentiality**—no disclosure occurs without consent
- **Fidelity**—the public health professional and Program keeps its word regarding what it will do with the information
- **Protects vulnerable people and populations without being paternal**—the individual and the community participate in designing the service and setting parameters
- **No conflict of interest**—the information is used only for what it is intended and not used for other, unrelated purposes

Does the practice of PS meet these standards of ethical conduct? Properly conducted partner services are done in the following manner:

- **PS is always voluntary.** No one is forced to use or participate in the service.
- **The STI interviewer must verify that the source of information about partners is actually infected.** This protects against ruses, scams and malicious intentions by people who would try to perpetrate a false notification as part of a personal dispute.
- **Notification is done face-to-face.** It is essential that the person being informed is the person who was named as the partner. This cannot be assured if notification is done via the mail or a telephone call.
- **Notification is done in private.** Notification is done wherever that person feels comfortable and it respects the need for and importance of his/her privacy.
- **Partners are notified of their possible exposure.** They are not told they have an infection. They will not know that until evaluated by a clinician.

Box 2.2 continued

- **Options for medical care are offered.** The partner is told how to obtain a clinical evaluation. Thus, this is a gateway service that links people with the healthcare system.
- **Partners are informed of risks that they may not have previously recognized.** We know that many people continue to misunderstand risks for HIV/AIDS and other STIs. Exposure notification is a "teaching moment." In addition, partners have an opportunity to recognize risks to or from their other partners.
- **The source of information is never revealed or acknowledged.** The DIS is trained to never reveal names or to even use pronouns. When asked "Who named me?" or "Where did you get this information?" the answer is always "From someone who cares for your health and wellbeing."
- **Records are not kept on partners.** Demographic and risk behavior information may be kept for program evaluation purposes, but personal identifiers about partners are not retained in any registry.
- **Safety is paramount.** PS is not an "all or none" process. A person with an STI is free to name only those partners he/she feels comfortable or safe to name. If they fear that a partner may pose a threat of physical abuse or retaliation as a result of being named and informed of exposure to an STI, that name does not need to be divulged. The interviewer will not and cannot force anyone to name all partners.

Does properly conducted PS achieve its goals? The answer is "yes" to some and it is still a work in progress to others. Despite the fact that PS has been discussed for almost a century and practiced for more than 60 years, its evaluation is still not comprehensive. There are some things that we do know.

- It can be conducted in an ethical fashion that strikes a balance between the rights of individuals and the disease prevention needs of the population.
- It has a history of success in disease prevention and control.
- Recent studies have shown that PS does not pose dangers to relationships as feared or postulated.
- The value of early intervention cannot be overemphasized.
- Risk reduction education is a worthy service.

How many people currently infected with HIV, or sick with AIDS, would have objected to being told years ago that they were at risk of infection and had an opportunity to reduce future risks? How many infections might have been prevented? PS is not a "cure-all" to the HIV/AIDS, or to the "other STI" epidemic. Widespread adoption of the practice will not, in itself, halt these diseases. However, we cannot overlook its use because it does not address every need and situation of those who are infected. Should we routinely wait to apply appropriate, proven control measures until profound social and political inequities are resolved so as to be absolutely certain that there will be no negative effects on the individual? Do we do this in any aspect of public health? If that is to be the choice, then we will all be guilty of letting the band play on.

Source: Originally published in part by Paul Etkind, "Should Partners of HIV-Infected People Be Notified?" *Epidemiology Monitor* 13, no. 10 (1992): 4, 7.

The Case/Control Study

A **case/control study,** discussed in detail in Chapter 10, is one of the two main types of observational studies in epidemiology. In a case/control study, the exposure histories of a group of people having a particular disease or injury are compared with the exposure histories of a group of people who do not have that particular disease. (These people may have some other disease or injury but not the disease or injury under investigation.) The objective of a case/control study is to identify past exposures that differ between the case and control groups and that therefore may be a cause/preventive of the cases' disease or injury.

The centrality of the case/control study in modern analytic epidemiology resides in its facility for studying diseases that have long latent periods, such as the chronic diseases, without having to follow large numbers of people over long periods of time. For example, without the availability of the case/control study, an investigator who wanted to study the causes of bladder cancer might have to study people **prospectively** (forward in time) for thirty or forty years (the latency period for bladder cancer) unless data for people exposed to known or suspected causes of bladder cancer thirty or forty years earlier were available for analysis. A case/control study design has a clear advantage in terms of time and costs over a prospective study design for studying diseases, such as bladder cancer, that have long latent periods.

SUMMARY

Taken together, the foundations of modern epidemiology facilitated the development of the most powerful and effective science for determining the distribution and determinants of ill health in human populations. No other field of inquiry has been able to equal epidemiology's record of successes in understanding human disease and injury etiology (MacMahon 1979).

The evolution of epidemiology is a triumph for public health: Epidemiology has become the basic science of population-based studies involving human subjects and health. What additional advances in epidemiology might be expected in the future? Surely such advances will include the following:

- Improved methods for accurately quantifying the dose and duration of exposures including toxicants, nutrients, patterns of physical activity, and lifestyle variables that increase the risk of disease or injury
- Better understanding of the interactions between genetic factors and other exposures in causing ill health
- Enhanced protocols for disease surveillance resulting in earlier recognition of the beginning of epidemics or of emerging or reemerging diseases and hence earlier initiation of disease-control procedures
- Increased knowledge of preclinical physiologic indicators that predict later disease
- Development of more-inclusive analytic methods for quantifying the effects of exposures on health status, taking into account the broader social systems within which those exposure and health outcomes occur

- Improved incorporation of qualitative (in contrast to quantitative) data into epidemiologic research
- Assemblage and sharing of large databases both domestically and internationally
- More rigorous methods for solving health outcomes related to violence and injuries, such as improved methods for quantifying actual "periods of risk"
- Increased use of epidemiology by health-care organizations to prevent ill health, improve the efficiency and outcomes of caregiving, and reduce costs
- Expanded integration of epidemiologic data forming clinical, preventive, and public health policies

It will be exciting to reflect upon the evolution of epidemiology in the years ahead. Will the epidemics of today come under control? What new epidemics will occur? What specific contributions will epidemiologists make toward improving people's health both domestically and globally? What contributions to epidemiology will you make?

REVIEW QUESTIONS

1. Who were the early founders of epidemiologic methods? What were their contributions to epidemiology?
2. What is the "latent period" of a disease? How do the latent periods differ between the acute and the chronic diseases? Why are those differences important with respect to identifying the causes of the acute and the chronic diseases?
3. Define "modern epidemiology." List the major fields of study that allowed modern epidemiology to develop. What did each of those fields contribute to epidemiology?
4. Define "case/control study." Why are case/control studies of particular importance in chronic disease epidemiology?

REVIEW EXERCISES

1. Reread Box 2.1 ("Ethics Matters: Institutional Review Boards"). Then, list five situations involving epidemiologic research in which an ethical conflict might arise.
2. Go to http://cme.nci.nih.gov/. Complete the National Institutes of Health Institutional Review Board (IRB) Tutorial, and print your certificate of course completion.

## CHAPTER 3

What Is an Epidemic?

What constitutes an epidemic of disease or injury? Are epidemics always obvious to the populations affected? How can epidemics be described quantitatively? What causes epidemics? How can surveillance systems monitor a population's health status? Those are several of the questions that lie at the core of epidemiologic inquiry. Each question will be discussed in turn with the goal of understanding some of the fundamental perspectives of epidemiologists.

WHAT CONSTITUTES AN EPIDEMIC?

In general, an **epidemic** is a state of excess frequency of a disease, an injury, or some other health-related event (see, for example, Box 3.1). The meaning of "excess" is variable and depends upon which standard is used to determine "usual" frequency. For example, relative to the statistics for White infants in the United States, the perinatal mortality rate in the Kiev area of the Ukraine, a newly independent country that was formerly part of the Soviet Union, occurred at epidemic levels in the early 1990s. The **perinatal mortality rate** (number of infants of at least twenty weeks' gestation who die within seven days of birth among all live births of at least twenty weeks' gestation plus stillbirths) in Kiev was between 32 and 36 deaths per 1,000 infants, compared with 9.7 deaths per 1,000 White infants in the United States, more than a threefold increase (Little et al. 1999). Using the worldwide perinatal mortality in 1900 as the standard, however, the perinatal mortality rate in Kiev in the 1990s probably was not excessive.

As another example, the **infant mortality rate** (the number of infants who die during the first year of life per 1,000 live births during the same year) in the 1990s exceeded 30 per 1,000 in a number of South and Central American countries. Those countries included Bolivia, Brazil, Colombia, Dominican Republic, Ecuador, El Salvador, Guatemala, Guyana, Haiti, Honduras, Nicaragua, Paraguay, and Peru (Pan American

Health Organization 2000). In contrast, overall infant mortality in the United States was 7.2 per 1,000 live births in 1997. Within the United States, infant mortality in 1997 was more than twice as high among African American infants as among White infants. Thus, infant mortality is occurring at epidemic proportions among many South and Central American countries compared with the overall infant mortality in the United States. Within the United States, however, African American infants have an infant mortality rate that is excessive compared with the rate for White infants (National Center for Health Statistics 2002).

Another example of an epidemic is the rate of tuberculosis among people living in the United States–Mexico border region. In this 2,000-mile region, the rate of tuberculosis is six times the overall rate of tuberculosis in the United States (U.S. Department of Health and Human Services 2000).

Often, the concept of what is excessive depends upon the frequency of disease or injury within the same geographic area at different times. For example, in Romania, 32,915 measles cases and 21 deaths occurred between November 1996 and June 1998 compared with only 131 measles cases in the four months preceding November 1996, and 223 cases from July through December 1998 (Hennessey et al. 1999). Most of the epidemic cases occurred among unvaccinated children less than two years old and among vaccinated school-aged children.

In this example, the time periods for which the measles frequencies were compared were different. Not only were the periods of different durations, but also the particular months that were included in each period differed. If the **expected numbers** of measles cases were proportional to the duration of the period of observation, adjustments in the comparisons of measles frequency easily could be made. An expected number is the number of cases that would have been observed if there were no epidemic, that is, if the number of cases were constant throughout the time period studied. If measles occurrence displays a seasonal or cyclic pattern, the inclusion of different months within the time periods compared could lead to a **biased comparison,** that is, a comparison that is erroneous because it contains a systematic error. (In this example, the error would be comparing the numbers of measles cases among different months that, even in the absence of an epidemic, would be expected to have higher or lower numbers of cases because of the biology of measles and its transmission.)

Many acute onset diseases and injuries display marked seasonal variation in frequency. For example, fireworks-related burn injuries occur more frequently in July than in other months within the United States. The explanation for this pattern of occurrence is the sale and use of fireworks associated with the July 4 U.S. Independence Day festivities. On the other hand, fireworks-related burn injuries occur more frequently (approximately 78 percent of all fireworks-related burns) in the spring in Greece, coinciding with the Greek Orthodox celebration of Easter (Vassilia et al. 2004).

Similarly, some acute onset infectious diseases, such as influenza, follow marked seasonal variation in occurrence, with months of high incidence followed by months of essentially zero incidence. In some contexts, such as in planning for the health needs to care for influenza victims, it may be useful to regard the winter occurrence of influenza in the United States as an epidemic of influenza. In other contexts, it may be preferable to compare the winter rates of influenza from one year to another to establish whether influenza in any given year is occurring at a frequency that is excessive.

BOX 3.1

CLINICAL EPIDEMIOLOGY

Clinical epidemiology is the application of epidemiologic methods to study disease progression and treatment outcomes. Thus, clinical epidemiology is concerned with questions pertaining to diagnostic, prognostic, therapeutic, and preventive challenges encountered in the clinical delivery of care to populations. Clinical epidemiologic studies usually are conducted within a health-care setting. The following example, taken from burn treatment facilities in Iran, illustrates the use of clinical epidemiology to evaluate the treatment and prognosis for patients with large burn wounds.

Example from Burn Treatment Units in Iran

REZA ALAGHEHBANDAN, M.D., BAHRAM GROOHI, M.D., AND ABDOLAZIZ RASTEGAR LARI, PH.D.

Burn injury is one of the most common forms of trauma in Iran as an economically developing country. Infection, which contributes significantly to morbidity as well as to excess cost for hospitalized patients, is the most common cause of death following burn injury.

Among all infections, *Pseudomonas,* especially *P. aeruginosa,* is the most important, common, resistant, and dangerous organism in burn patient infections. Despite advances in medical and surgical care, the prognosis remains poor with a mortality rate of about 80% in patients infected with *P. aeruginosa. P. aeruginosa* has been the most prevalent bacteria and "classic pathogen" in Iranian burn centers for over 20 years. Various studies have shown that the prevalence of *P. aeruginosa* infections/contaminations consistently was over 70% among burn patients in Iran, which is considerably higher than the prevalence of infection in other burn treatment units as reported in the professional literature. Thus, *P. aeruginosa* infections/contaminations may be viewed as an epidemic in Iranian burn units.

Multi-drug resistance of *P. aeruginosa* has compounded the seriousness of this pathogen in burn treatment units. In 1996, 45% of *Pseudomonas* infections were resistant to ciprofloxacin, 48% to amikacin, and 88% to gentamicin. By year 2000, however, the resistance to ciprofloxacin, amikacin, and gentamicin significantly increased to 85%, 90%, and 98%, respectively. In addition, the prevalence of *P. aeruginosa* resistance to other common antibiotics such as ceftizoxime, carbenicillin, ceftazidim, co-trimoxazole, and tetracycline increased dramatically to over 90%.

The magnitude of antibiotic resistance profile of *P. aeruginosa* in Iranian burn units is among the most troubling profiles reported in the literature. For this reason, it is necessary for physicians to limit their use of antimicrobial agents in hospital settings and especially in burn units. In addition, microbiological surveillance of burn patients must be performed periodically to identify the types of organisms infecting these patients and to facilitate the appropriate choice of antibiotic prophylaxis.

Source: Original title of work is "*Pseudomonas Aeruginosa* in Burn Wound Infections and Its Resistance to Antibiotics in Iran: Epidemiology of an Emerging and Increasing Problem." Article includes findings from the published study: Rastegar Lari, A., Bahrami Honar, H., and Alaghehbandan, R. 1998. Pseudomonas in Tohid Burn Center, Iran. *Burns* 24 (7):637–41.

As mentioned previously, what constitutes an epidemic depends upon which reference point or baseline is used for determining whether disease or injury frequency is excessive. Disease or injury frequency can be excessive based on comparisons over time, between different geographic regions, or among different subgroups of a population. Regardless of which comparison frequency is used, establishing the existence of an epidemic always involves quantifying the **relative frequency** of disease or injury among the population of interest with at least one other comparative frequency. Relative frequency is the magnitude of disease or injury occurrence in one population compared with the magnitude of disease or injury occurrence in another population.

ARE EPIDEMICS ALWAYS OBVIOUS TO THE POPULATIONS AFFECTED?

The time frame for epidemics varies. Some epidemics begin and end within the time span of a few weeks or months. Others evolve over decades. The United States was in the midst of a large epidemic of ischemic heart disease in the 1950s and early 1960s with few people even aware of the problem.

Similarly, the frequency of lung cancer among men in the United States increased fifteenfold between 1930 and 1990 before beginning to decline. Yet few people recognized the enormity of the epidemic until it was well under way. As women acquired the tobacco habit, they too had increasing rates of lung cancer. The epidemic among women began in the 1970s, and in 1987, lung cancer surpassed breast cancer as the leading cause of cancer mortality among women in the United States (Figure 3.1).

An epidemic of lung cancer began to appear in low-income countries following the increased export of cigarettes to those countries that began in the mid-1960s and 1970s. The increase in tobacco exports followed the U.S. Surgeon General's reports on the adverse health effects of smoking, which caused tobacco companies to seek new markets for their products. Thus, lung cancer, which once was epidemic primarily in high-income countries, now is **pandemic** (a worldwide epidemic; that is, an epidemic of disease or injury that is occurring simultaneously in many regions of the world). An estimated 18 percent of all cancer deaths worldwide are attributable to cancer of the lung, making lung cancer the leading cause of cancer mortality worldwide (International Agency for Research on Cancer 2000). Given today's pandemic of lung cancer, it is interesting to note that lung cancer was regarded as a medical rarity at the beginning of the twentieth century.

Other epidemics are easily recognizable. The epidemics of acute onset infectious and vector-borne diseases in the United States in the 1600s, 1700s, and 1800s were obvious to the populations affected. For example, a ship from Barbados brought yellow fever to Philadelphia in 1699. Among the city's population of 4,000, approximately one-third developed the disease, and 220 people died from it. Beginning in the summer of 1793, Philadelphia was devastated repeatedly by yellow fever. In the epidemic of 1793, approximately 13,000 of Philadelphia's population of 36,871 fled the city. Most

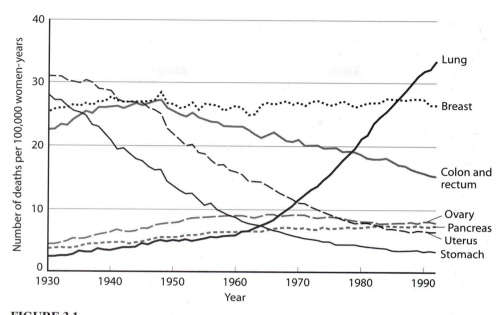

FIGURE 3.1

Cancer mortality rates in women in the United States.

In epidemiology, rates are expressed as the number of health-related events per unit of time. The unit of time used is **person-time.** Examples of person-times are "person-years" (the most commonly used measure of person-time) "person-months," "man-years," and "women-years." Person-time is discussed in more detail in Chapter 4.

Sources: Adapted from Dresler 1998; Parker et al. 1997.

who remained who had not contracted the disease previously, and thus were not immune to it, contracted the disease. Four-thousand-forty-four people (11 percent of the population) died within a few months.

As another example, smallpox struck repeatedly in the eastern cities. In Boston in 1721, among the population of 15,686 people, 5,998 previously had had smallpox, and 1,843 people fled the city to escape the disease. Among the remaining population, 5,545 contracted smallpox (71 percent of the remaining susceptible population). In one of the first vaccination efforts following Cotton Mather's inoculation of his son during the smallpox epidemic of 1721, the **case fatality** (percentage of cases who die from a disease or an injury) was 10 percent among unvaccinated persons and 1.5 percent among vaccinated persons (Boylston 1726).

In the early 1800s, mortality from "autumnal fevers" (mostly malaria) in Savannah averaged approximately 70 deaths per 1,000 persons each year. In response, and consistent with the **miasma theory of disease causation** (that "bad-smelling" air and water cause disease), the city eliminated all wet cultures of rice near Savannah in 1818, resulting in an immediate decline in malaria mortality to 26 deaths per 1,000 people each year (Gamble 1900).

Shyrock, citing data from the *Report on an Inquiry into the Sanitary Condition of the Labouring Population of Great Britain* (London, 1842) provides a particularly poignant description of the epidemics in U.S. cities in the mid-1900s, writing that

> The American of 1840 read with horror of Scottish tenements, where whole families crowded into single rooms, were provided with no running water, and paid their rent by selling their own dung heaps accumulated in the courts below. Yet, at home, in New York City, more than half the population lived in similarly overcrowded tenements, and some 25,000 people occupied the damp and dismal cellars of these same buildings. In Cherry Street, to be specific, a five-story tenement occupying only two ordinary building lots, housed 120 families, which included more than 500 individuals. I say merely "individuals" for under such circumstances one can hardly speak of them as "human beings." Similar conditions obtained in the slums of other American cities, and if it were desirable these could be described ad nauseam.
>
> As might be expected, such circumstances made disease problems more acute as well as more obvious. The tragic history of the major endemic diseases, typhus, typhoid, and tuberculosis, is familiar enough. So far as can be judged from the imperfect bills of mortality, urban death rates rose ominously during the first half of the nineteenth century. New York City, which was most inundated by poor immigrants and which grew most rapidly, again affords a striking example. In 1810, the crude death rate had been reported as about 21 per 1,000; by 1857, it had risen to around 37—an increase of almost 80 percent within 50 years (Boldan, 1916). Rates were lower in Philadelphia, but higher in New Orleans. What an increasing mortality implied in morbidity rates, to say nothing of "subclinical illness," is obvious enough. (Shyrock 1937)

Thus, epidemics can be silent or manifest, precipitous or slowly evolving. What makes a disease or an injury "epidemic" is its excessive frequency relative to a comparative frequency, regardless of how fast or obviously the epidemic unfolds.

An interesting parallel to the epidemics of infection and vector-borne diseases in the United States during the 1600s, 1700s, and 1800s is provided by the recent September 2005 flooding of New Orleans, Louisiana. A news release from Oregon State University, entitled "Aftermath Could Give Rise to Disease Epidemics," offers an insight into this parallel:

> Public health, sanitation facilities, and civil infrastructure that suffered massive damage in New Orleans and other parts of the Gulf Coast are more than just modern conveniences. Historically, they were what helped that region conquer the recurring epidemics of insect-borne tropical diseases that were once common and could return.
>
> There is one other period in New Orleans history when civil structure broke down, people were displaced from their homes, and basic support systems collapses, says Phil Rossignol, a professor of public health entomology at Oregon State University. It was after the Civil War, and it led directly to a series of epidemics, especially yellow fever, that killed tens of thousands of people.
>
> "From a historical perspective, New Orleans and some other southern ports like it were not always a very healthy place to live," Rossignol said. "It was the arrival of a comprehensive public health infrastructure, good sewers, water supply, and housing that made it possible to get rid of diseases like cholera, yellow fever, malaria, and dengue fever."

"But these diseases are still around, they are very deadly and very opportunistic. People should remember that as we work to rebuild this area."

The process of disruption itself can be a health concern, Rossignol said.

"In times of intense stress such as this, it's not unusual for people to hoard and collect things, sometimes in ways that can be conducive to disease transmission, " he said. "There can be a lot of financial problems, people relocate to new areas and often aren't able to manage the details of home maintenance and hygiene the way they used to."

The last major breakout of yellow fever in the United States actually occurred in New Orleans in 1905, following on the heels of a string of epidemics in the years after the Civil War. During two yellow fever outbreaks in 1867 and 1878, thousands died in New Orleans and many more fled the city.

The ways to combat these health concerns and epidemics, Rossignol said, was first pioneered about that same time in the construction of the Panama Canal.

"The French had been the first to try and build the canal across Panama, and failed largely because of health problems and disease epidemics," Rossignol said. "When the Americans took over in the early 1900s, the first thing they did was spend several years working on mosquito control and public health infrastructure. Only then were they able to inhabit the area safely and construct the canal."

HOW CAN EPIDEMICS BE DESCRIBED QUANTITATIVELY?

Epidemiology is a quantitative science. Thus, the basis for describing an epidemic is quantitative. The easiest epidemic to summarize quantitatively is an epidemic associated with an acute onset disease in which the exposure occurs as a point exposure. A point exposure is a cause of disease that affects a group of people at approximately the same point in time. Examples of point exposures are exposure to a foodborne pathogen (a bacterium, a virus, or some other infectious agent capable of causing disease) during a dinner banquet and exposure to an infective person at a social gathering. An infective person is capable of transmitting a pathogen to another person. Not all *infected* people are *infective,* or they may be infective for only part of time they are infected.

The shapes of graphs plotting the numbers of new cases versus time after exposure are quite similar for many acute onset infectious diseases from point exposures (Figure 3.2). In these graphs, although the majority of cases occur relatively early in the epidemic, the curve is **skewed to the right;** that is, there is a small proportion of cases that occurs later after the time of exposure. The kind of graph in which the number of new cases is plotted by time after exposure is called an **epidemic curve.**

Figure 3.3 shows the epidemic curve for an epidemic outbreak of *Escherichia coli* 0157 in Lanarkshire, United Kingdom, in 1996. Note the rapid increase in cases early in the outbreak and then the "tail" of cases that occurred later in the epidemic, similar to the hypothetical outbreak depicted in Figure 3.2.

The epidemic curves for other diseases are **skewed to the left** (the majority of cases occur relatively late in the epidemic and only a small proportion of cases occur soon after the time of exposure), and still other epidemic curves are **bimodal** (have

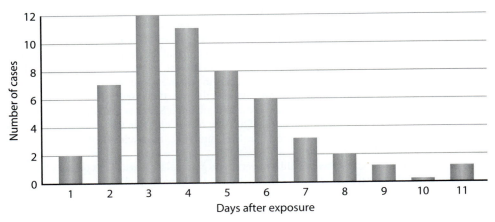

FIGURE 3.2
Graph depicting a hypothetical epidemic curve for an acute onset disease from a point
exposure such as a foodborne bacterium.

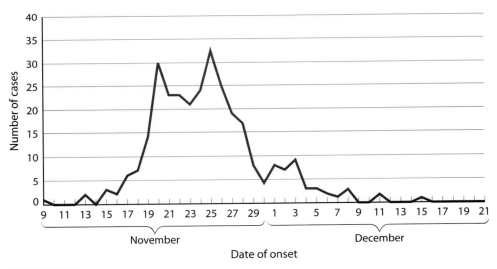

FIGURE 3.3
Epidemic curve for the foodborne outbreak of *Escherichia coli* 0157 in Lanarkshire in 1996,
all cases.
Source: Venters 2001. Reproduced with permission from the BMJ Publishing Group.

two time periods associated with a large proportion of the cases) or even **multimodal**
(several time periods having a large proportion of cases). The shape of an epidemic
curve and the distribution of cases by date of disease onset can help identify the source
of an infectious disease outbreak, especially if the typical **incubation periods** (times
from exposure to a pathogen to the onset of illness) for suspected pathogens are

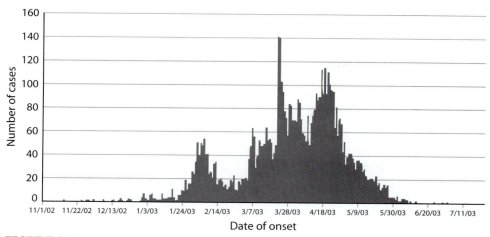

FIGURE 3.4

Probable cases of SARS by week of onset worldwide* (*n* = 5,910), 1 November 2002–10 July 2003.

*This graph does not include 2,527 probable cases of SARS (2,521 from Beijing, China), for whom no dates of onset are currently available.

Source: www.who.int/csr/sars/epicurve/epiindex/en/index1.html.

known. The shape of the curve and the distribution of cases are helpful because the dates of disease onset reflect the typical length and distribution of a pathogen's incubation period.

As mentioned previously, epidemics of disease associated with eating contaminated food typically mirror the epidemic curves depicted in Figures 3.2 and 3.3. An example of a bimodal (or even a trimodal) epidemic curve is the outbreak of severe acute respiratory syndrome (SARS) that began in November 2003 (Figure 3.4). In the epidemic curve, the first mode, occurring in late January to mid-February 2003, are cases from the People's Republic of China (PRC), where the SARS epidemic began. (Note that the graph does not include 2,521 cases from Beijing, PRC, for whom no dates of onset were available.) The later mode contains primarily cases occurring in countries other than the PRC as the disease spread from infective people, traveling by air, to people in other countries. The rapid spread of SARS by airline passengers underscores the need for a **worldwide surveillance system** to alert the global community to the presence of **emerging** (new) and **reemerging** (resurging) diseases (see Box 3.2).

Figure 3.5 shows the epidemic curve for an outbreak of bloody diarrhea in a remote region of Cameroon during 1997–1998. The epidemic curve has multiple modes of cases. The presence of many disease modes suggests that person-to-person transmission of the disease occurred as infective people moved from one village to another, initiating new epidemics as they traveled.

Often an **attack rate,** one measure of disease frequency, is used to summarize the magnitude of an acute onset disease that occurs from a point exposure. An attack rate

BOX 3.2

WORLDWIDE DISEASE SURVEILLANCE: COMMUNICABLE DISEASE SURVEILLANCE AND RESPONSE (CSR)

About CSR: The Challenge

Epidemics and newly-emerging infections are on the move as never before, threatening the health of people around the world and affecting travel and trade in the global village. Globalization, climate change, the growth of megacities and the explosive increase in international travel are increasing the potential for rapid spread of infections. Deforestation and urban sprawl bring humans and animals in closer contact and allow animal pathogens to "jump species" more easily and new epidemics to emerge.

Many of these epidemics, such as cholera and meningitis, recurrently challenge health systems in countries with limited resources. Others, such as influenza and dengue, have an increasing potential to create new pandemics. The return of yellow fever threatens large cities in the developing world, while the emergence and rapid spread of drug-resistant tuberculosis and malaria increase treatment costs dramatically. Travel, trade and tourism are all affected by emerging and epidemic disease threats, which could be used to cause intentional epidemics (bioterrorism).

WHO's Mandate

In 2001, the World Health Assembly, recognizing the threats to public health posed by epidemic-prone and emerging infections, adopted the resolution "global health security—epidemic alert and response" which made specific recommendations to WHO and its Member States:

- Resolution to the World Health Assembly 2001
- Background Report

The Vision of CSR

Every country should be able to detect, verify rapidly and respond appropriately to epidemic-prone and emerging disease threats when they arise to minimize their impact on the health and economy of the world's population.

CSR's Strategy

Working with its partners, the Department of Communicable Disease Surveillance and Response (CSR) aims to reach global health security following three strategic directions. **The International Health Regulations (IHR)** are the overall framework for CSR's strategy, the only global regulatory framework agreed by the international community to support.

Box 3.2 continued

Contain Known Risks: Focusing on the leading epidemic and emerging diseases, CSR develops and strengthens specific global surveillance and response networks for poverty-associated diseases such as cholera, dysentery, influenza, meningococcal meningitis, plague, viral hemorrhagic fevers (Ebola, Lassa), "mad cow" disease, anthrax and others.

Respond to the Unexpected: Rapid, effective response to outbreaks relies on timely alert and response mechanisms. CSR's epidemic intelligence system gathers and verifies outbreak information daily from around the world and coordinates international responses to outbreaks of global importance.

Improve Preparedness: Focusing particularly on resource-poor countries, CSR supports the strengthening of national capacity for alert and response through a multidisease or integrated approach. It provides tools, expert assistance and carefully-tailored training to enhance skills in laboratory diagnosis, field epidemiology and public health mapping. A WHO office in Lyon, France, is dedicated to further improving laboratory infrastructure and epidemiology capacity in developing countries.

Source: Quotation from the CSR home page at www.who.int/csr/about/en, where additional information is available.

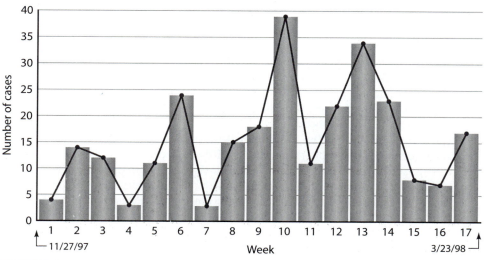

FIGURE 3.5
Epidemic curve for an outbreak of bloody diarrhea, Cameroon, 1997–1998.
Source: Cunin et al. 1999.

is defined as the number of people who develop the disease of interest divided by the size of the **population at risk** for developing the disease. The population at risk for developing the disease is the number of exposed people who could develop the disease being studied. As an example, suppose 50 people attend a birthday party. Forty-six people eat some cake, and 23 of the people who ate cake became sick. The attack rate is (23 ill people) divided by (46 people who ate the cake), or $23/46 = 0.50$, or 50 percent. The implied comparison attack rate in this example is 0 percent; that is, in a nonepidemic situation, 46 people might reasonably expect to eat cake without any person becoming ill. The population at risk of developing the disease must truly be **at risk** (capable of developing the disease under study). For an infectious disease, all individuals in the population at risk must be potential candidates for being a new case of disease. In other words, they must be susceptible to infection by the infectious agent in question and not immune because of prior infection or vaccination.

The phrase "attack rate" can be confusing because an attack rate is not a true rate in the mathematical sense. An attack rate is a proportion. Proportions are mathematical expressions of the form $(a/(a + b))$. An attack rate equals $(a/(a + b))$:

a = the number of people at risk of developing a disease who develop the disease

b = the number of people at risk of disease who do not develop the disease

In contrast, all true **rates** have as a denominator some unit of time (Elandt-Johnson 1975). For example, the rate of a car might be "55 miles per hour." It is not relevant how long the car travels at 55 miles per hour; the rate is the same. As mentioned previously, in epidemiology, rates are expressed as the number of health-related events per unit of time. The unit of time used is **person-time.** Examples of person-times are "person-years" (the most commonly used measure of person-time) "person-months," "man-years," and "women-years." Person-time is discussed in more detail in Chapter 4.

In an attack rate, the reference to time means the time between exposure to a disease- or injury-causing agent and the time marking the end of the **period at risk.** The period at risk is the interval of time during which the disease could occur as a result of the exposure under study. Notice that the time period at risk is different from person-time. The denominator of an attack rate is the *number* of people at risk of developing the health event of interest and not the amount of *person-time* in which a certain number of health-related events occurred.

The above notwithstanding, it is important to appreciate that the terminology used to refer to certain epidemiologic measures of disease or injury occurrence, such as attack rates, sometimes varies. This variation stems partly from the relative newness of epidemiology as a science. With respect to attack rates, some epidemiologists refer to attack rates as true rates, whereas others prefer to call attack rates proportions. This lack of consensus among epidemiologists can be confusing to the student trying for the first time to grasp the salient features of epidemiology. To help alleviate this confusion, students of epidemiology should focus on the *concepts* and *mathematics* that underlie the fundamentals of epidemiology regardless of any variation in the phrases used to express these fundamentals.

Other Aspects of Attack Rates

Usually attack rates, and all other measures of disease frequency, are **category-specific;** that is, each measure pertains to people who have certain characteristics, such as age and/or gender, in common. For example, the attack rate of salmonella infection following exposure to contaminated food might be 10 percent for people between the ages of 30 and 59 years and 25 percent for people between the ages of 60 and 79 years. The attack rates, 10 percent and 25 percent, are age-specific attack rates. In this example, the "category" is age.

Another question to consider when calculating an attack rate is what constitutes a "new case" of disease or injury. Attack rates measure the proportion of a population that develops a certain health outcome (are "new cases") among the population at risk of developing the health outcome over a specified period of time after exposure. New cases, often referred to as **incident cases,** are newly diagnosed cases of the health outcome of interest. For a person to be regarded as a "new case of disease," a clinician or some other knowledgeable person must make and record the diagnosis. People with disease whose symptoms are mild or people who lack access to health care may not be diagnosed and therefore not counted as new cases. The effect of not identifying all new cases of disease is a decrease in the magnitude of the calculated attack rate.

A concept related to identifying all new cases is the necessity of defining a homogeneous health outcome. In calculating an attack rate, all people who are counted as new cases must have the same disease or injury; that is, there must be a homogeneous disease entity for which the attack rate is being calculated. Including as "new cases" people who have different diseases not only inflates the magnitude of the attack rate but also hinders investigations into the cause of the disease outbreak because different diseases have different etiologies.

Health Indicators

Most diseases are age-related, and many are gender-related. In some countries, such as the United States, racial or ethnic heritage, or a person's self-identification with a particular racial or ethic heritage, may be an **indicator** of variation in disease frequency. Disease or injury indicators are variables that are associated with an increase or a decrease in disease or injury frequency but may not in themselves be a cause of the disease or the injury; that is, indicators are variables that are associated with a cause of a health outcome and mark or "indicate" the presence of the cause. As an example, knowing which people in an epidemiologic study identify themselves as "first-generation Chinese Americans" might indicate certain health-related dietary preferences that differ from the dietary preferences of people who self-identify with other populations. Similarly, knowledge of peoples' religious affiliations may indicate preferences in diet or other health-related behaviors. For example, members of The Church of Jesus Christ of Latter-day Saints (Mormons) generally are expected to avoid the use of tobacco and alcoholic beverages.

Other health indicators, such as levels of physical activity, substance abuse, and unprotected sexual activity, are more closely related to the physiologic causes of future disease or injury, and so are often regarded as **risk factors** for disease or injury. For example, unprotected sexual activity in women is associated not only with pregnancy but also with acquiring sexually transmitted diseases, including HIV/AIDS.

Globally, one of the most commonly used health indicators is a country's or a population's infant mortality rate (IMR). IMRs are particularly sensitive to changes in a population's risk factors for disease and injury, including access to health care; availability of food and potable water; basic sanitary conditions; increases in infectious and vectorborne diseases; and the presence of war or civil unrest. For that reason, changes in IMFs often predict subsequent changes in the entire population's health status. Worldwide, the estimated IMFs for 2003 ranged from 199.00 infant deaths per 1,000 live births in Mozambique to 3.30 infant deaths per 1,000 in Japan. The estimated IMR for the United States in 2003 was 6.75 (the *CIA World Factbook 2003,* at www.odci. gov/cia/publications/factbook/).

As is always true for epidemiologic studies, the quality of data, the study results, and interpretations of study results must be reviewed critically. A critical evaluation of a study, discussed in more detail in Chapter 12 and elsewhere, involves anticipating and preventing aspects of a study's design, data collection processes, and data analyses that result in errors. With respect to worldwide infant mortality rates, a critical evaluation might include an assessment of how complete the numbers of infant deaths and births are for each country. For example, were the numbers of deaths and births underestimated? Were those numbers accurate for urban populations but scant for rural populations? Were infant deaths caused by factors associated with a stigma, such as HIV/AIDS or cholera in some countries, underreported? Were deaths to female infants reported in populations that favor the birth of males? Those and other questions regarding the quality of reported epidemiologic data on IMRs must be addressed to gauge the accuracy of the data and hence its comparability and interpretation for each country.

WHAT CAUSES EPIDEMICS?

The causes of epidemics, and indeed the causes of disease and injury in general, are the subject of continued investigation. The simple explanation for what causes epidemics and pandemics pertains to the dynamics and timing of population exposures to factors that cause disease or injury, and to the population's biologic susceptibility to those health outcomes. (See the Special Case Study "After-Action Report for the August 2003 Measles Investigation in Corvallis, Oregon," which follows Chapter 3, for a description of how epidemiology was applied to contain an outbreak of measles on a college campus.) Etiologic factors for human diseases include biologic agents, chemical agents, physical agents, nutritional factors, lifestyle choices, characteristics of the host, and environmental factors. (See Table 3.1 for examples of etiologic factors). For a disease or an injury to be considered epidemic or pandemic, the proportion of the population that becomes ill must exceed the "expected" or baseline level of the illness in the population. Communication to the public of which agents *are* or *may be* harmful to

TABLE 3.1

Examples of Etiologic Factors for Human Diseases and Injuries

Etiologic Category	Examples*
Biologic agents	Certain bacteria; viruses; prions; rickettsia; "slow" viruses: age of exposure including in utero exposure
Chemical agents	Lead; mercury; certain pesticides; hydrogen cyanide; "nerve gas"; certain prescription medications; fluorine gas; arsenic
Physical agents	Asbestos; trauma including burns, gunshots, motor vehicle crashes; ionizing and nonionizing radiation; high-voltage electricity
Nutritional factors	Overly high/low caloric intake; low protein; vitamin deficiencies; calcium intake; sodium intake; saturated fat intake
Lifestyle choices	Exercise level; tobacco use; alcoholic beverage intake; dietary preferences; seat belt use; bicycle helmet use
Host characteristics	Genetic factors; immune status; gender; concurrent disease; level and types of natural and supplemented estrogens; social support; response to stress
Environmental factors	Heat; cold; certain allergens; air pollution or inversions; occupational exposures; contaminants in drinking water

*Some of the examples could have been placed into more than one etiologic category; for example, the common house mite could be listed under biologic agents or under environmental factors.

human health (risk communication) is a special field of study that has its own successes and failures (see, for example, Box 3.3 and www.psandman.com). Box 3.4 provides an example in which the communication of risk probably had untoward consequences.

As an example of a pandemic, the 1918–1919 outbreak of influenza resulted when small changes to a protein in a bird influenza virus permitted transmission of the virus to humans, and then allowed human-to-human transmission of the virus (Gamblin et al. 2004). Because humans previously had not been exposed to the avian influenza virus, and so did not have any immunity to it, essentially all people were susceptible to the disease. As a result, an estimated 20 million people worldwide died from the influenza.

Similarly, viruses that caused the "Asian influenza" pandemic in 1857 and the "Hong Kong influenza" pandemic in 1968 came from birds. (The names for those strains of influenza reflect the geographic region in which the influenza first was identified.) It remains to be seen whether the outbreak of chicken influenza in east Asia in 2004, which has infected humans, will be capable of being transmitted from one person to another and hence have the potential to cause epidemics or a pandemic.

The more complete explanation for what causes many epidemics or pandemics focuses on the complex, interacting, and often poorly understood social, economic, and political systems and subsystems in which the dynamics of exposures and diseases or injuries occur. For example, overcrowded living conditions cause epidemics of both infectious diseases, such as tuberculosis, and injuries, such as traffic-related trauma. Factors associated with living in poverty—including lack of access to clean drinking water and to basic sanitation such as human-waste removal, nutritional challenges, and inaccessibility to basic health services such as immunizations, pharmacologic products,

---

BOX 3.3

COMMUNICATION OF HEALTH RISKS

. . . some reasons why scientists typically use poor communication techniques when talking with nonscientists.

1. Many scientists don't approve of communicating with nonscientists.
2. Many scientists don't expect themselves to be able to communicate.
3. Many scientists over-value rationality, and mistrust—and even disdain—emotion.
4. Many scientists disavow their own emotions. This may lead them to project their emotions onto the public and the media.
5. Many scientists fail to allow for the public's mistrust.
6. Many scientists collude with the public's desire to be over-reassured.
7. Many scientists do not trust the public.
8. Many scientists see themselves as outside the communication process.
9. Many scientists don't notice when they have gone beyond their expertise.
10. Many scientists forget to start where their audience is.

Source: Jody Lanard and Peter M. Sandman, "Scientists and the Public: Barriers to Cross-Species Risk Communication," The Peter Sandman Risk Communication Web site: Risk = Hazard + Outrage, posted January 4, 2004, at www.psandman.com, where a copy of the full document is available.

---

and treatment options—cause epidemics. Lack of education and little empowerment over personal choices, such as the timing and number of sexual encounters, also cause epidemics. As an example of the latter, in general, males are the "gatekeepers" of the current pandemic of HIV/AIDS in sub-Saharan Africa, which has resulted in as many as one-third of adults in some countries being infected with HIV. Many infected women became infected by their husbands while unable to negotiate the use of condoms or a proscription against extramarital sexual encounters.

Apropos of the importance of adopting a systems perspective in epidemiology, MacMahon and Pugh (1970) wrote that "in descriptive epidemiology there is nowhere a more obvious need for the development of quantitative measures than in the consideration of social arrangements and relationships." Attending to that need remains as a paramount goal in understanding the societal bases for disease and injury occurrence.

MONITORING THE NATION'S HEALTH: GOALS AND SURVEILLANCE

The U.S. National Center for Health Statistics, using data from the **National Health Interview Survey,** has developed a new surveillance system to provide an expedient data release system for health-status, health-care, and health-related behavior indicators (see Box 3.5). The National Health Interview Survey is designed as a weekly

BOX 3.4

ETHICS MATTERS: ALL THE NEWS THAT'S FIT TO PRINT*– NEWS REPORTERS AND EPIDEMIOLOGY

Few news reporters or other professionals working in mass media news coverage have the education necessary to know how critically to evaluate the strengths and weaknesses of epidemiologic studies. They often lack even a rudimentary understanding of epidemiologic terminology and research methods. Partly for that reason, these professionals may convey information regarding the findings from epidemiologic studies that is misguided. Some reporters may even "sensationalize" findings from an epidemiologic study, whether inadvertently or otherwise.

What ethical responsibilities do reporters and other mass media professionals have to "get the story right"? The Preamble to the Code of Ethics for the Society of Professional Journalists provides some insight into this question.

> Members of the Society of Professional Journalists believe that public enlightenment is the forerunner of justice and the foundation of democracy. The duty of the journalist is to further those ends by seeking truth and providing a fair and comprehensive account of events and issues. Conscientious journalists from all media and specialties strive to serve the public with thoroughness and honesty. Professional integrity is the cornerstone of a journalist's credibility. Members of the Society share a dedication to ethical behavior and adopt this code to declare the Society's principles and standards of practice.

Further, as the first-listed ethical principle, the code requires news reporters to "test the accuracy of information from all sources and exercise care to avoid inadvertent error. Deliberate distortion is never permissible" (www.spj.org/ethics_code.asp).

Questions about accurate reporting of findings from epidemiologic studies are not merely academic. The case of Bendectin serves to illustrate the point. Bendectin was a prescription drug given to pregnant women during the 1970s to alleviate pregnancy-related nausea. One epidemiologic study was published that showed an association between Bendectin and congenital heart disease.[†] In their article, the authors stated that additional studies were needed to determine whether or not the association was causal. In interviews with reporters, the primary author reiterated his view that the study results were preliminary and in need of verification. Some reporters, however, reported the study's findings as demonstrating a definitive association between Bendectin and congenital heart disease. As a result, some women (many women? it is not known how many) chose to undergo elective abortions out of concern that their taking Bendectin had caused heart disease in their fetuses. It is not known how many healthy fetuses were aborted. More accurate reporting might have reduced unnecessary abortions. To date, it remains unclear whether or not Bendectin can cause congenital heart disease although the preponderance of the evidence suggests that it does not.

---

*The masthead logo of the *New York Times:* "All The News That's Fit to Print," 1896.

[†]K. J. Rothman, D. C. Fyler, A. Goldblatt, and M. B. Kreidberg. "Exogenous Hormones and Other Drug Exposures of Children with Congenital Heart Disease," *American Journal of Epidemiology* 109, no. 4 (1979): 433–39.

BOX 3.5

PRACTICAL EPIDEMIOLOGY IN A PUBLIC HEALTH SETTING: DEVELOPING A PUBLIC HEALTH SURVEILLANCE SYSTEM USING DATA FROM THE NATIONAL HEALTH INTERVIEW SURVEY

HANYU NI, PH.D.

The National Health Interview Survey (NHIS) has been conducted annually since 1955 by the National Center for Health Statistics (NCHS) of the Centers for Disease Control and Prevention (CDC). It has been a primary source of information on the health status, health behaviors, and health care access and utilization of the United States household population. Although the survey was designed to measure the trends in health and health care for the United States population, a shortcoming of the NHIS in the past had been the lack of an expedient data release system to meet data needs for public health surveillance.

The monitoring and ultimate prevention of adverse health outcomes in the United States is predicated on the availability of timely information. In 1997, the NHIS was redesigned and included many key measures of health currently needed by public health workers and health policy makers. The mode of data collection was also modified to utilize a computer assisted personal interviewing (CAPI) system. The CAPI system has reduced the need for certain types of data editing and thus expedited the process of data collection and editing. Because of the complexity of the NHIS, however, the final release of annual weighted microdata files and documentation from the NHIS still occurs about 12–18 months after data collection. Additionally, although the results from the NHIS have been released to the public in a variety of forms including CDC publications and journal manuscripts, these release mechanisms have not been timely because health policy makers had to wait about two years following data collection to receive the analytical results. This time frame is obviously not suitable for effective public surveillance.

To improve the access to the most recent data from the NHIS, a plan was developed in 2000 to evaluate the feasibility of the early release of a subset of key health measures using several months of data. The first step was to conduct an extensive literature review to identify the health indicators that policy makers, health-care providers, the general public, and health researchers are most interested in. The design structure and core questionnaire items from the current NHIS were also reviewed to compile a list of **sentinel health indicators** available from NHIS data. Sentinel health indicators are health-related variables that are sensitive to early changes in a population's health status and thus serve as harbingers of future changes. Initial results from an evaluation study indicate that earlier release of certain health measures on a quarterly or semi-annual basis is operationally and statistically feasible.

In April 2001, the NCHS developed a new Web-based data dissemination mechanism, the Early Release program, to quickly release the selected estimates from the

Box 3.5 continued

NHIS about six months after the end of data collection. The first release included seven health and health-care indicators such as a usual place to go for medical care, unmet needs for medical care due to cost, influenza vaccination, current smoking, excessive alcohol consumption, HIV testing, and general health status. As work continued and in response to changing data needs, new measures were added later, including obesity, leisure-time physical activities, pneumococcal vaccination, health insurance coverage, and personal care needs. In early 2002, another new measure, serious psychological distress, was added to monitor changes in mental health status of the United States' population after the 9/11/2001 terrorist attacks. For each selected health measure, a graph is presented showing the trend over time beginning in 1997 for the total population, followed by graphs and tables showing estimates by sex, age group, and race/ethnicity based on the NHIS data from the most recent year.

The data provided by the Early Release program can be used to measure progress toward national public health objectives and to monitor the health status of the United States population. For example, the program released quarterly estimates of influenza vaccination among adults aged 18 years and over, which showed a significant drop and rebound in the vaccination level for the 2000–2001 influenza season. The drop reflected the delay in the vaccine availability in the flu season and rebound reflected the effectiveness of the CDC's effort in dealing with the delay. Overall, the NHIS Early Release has had significant impact on federal, state, and local public health agency operations, because it provides timely data to measure progress toward national public health objectives.

survey to query a sample of households in the United States regarding diseases, injuries, disabilities, and impairments of household members. The goal of the surveillance system is to identify new trends in health status and in health care especially as those trends pertain to progress toward achieving the **national health goals** as set forth in ***Healthy People 2010 (HP 2010).*** The system has the potential for detecting emerging epidemics early in their onsets. With this system, prompt public health prevention and control activities can be initiated to abate these epidemics earlier in their progression than was possible in the past.

The national health goals and objectives of the United States are delineated in *HP 2010,* the disease- and injury-prevention agenda for the nation. *HP 2010* identifies the most important preventable threats to health in the United States and outlines prevention strategies and objectives to achieve the national goals by the year 2010. In addition, *HP 2010* identifies measurable health indicators to monitor progress toward reaching the national health goals and objectives. *HP 2010* is the third in a series of national prevention agendas, following the 1979 Surgeon General's report, *Healthy People,* and *Healthy People 2000: National Health Promotion and Disease Prevention Objectives.* As quoted from *HP 2010:*

Healthy People 2010 is designed to achieve two overarching goals:

- **Goal 1: Increase Quality and Years of Healthy Life**
  The first goal of Healthy People 2010 is to help individuals of all ages increase life expectancy [average age at death], *and* improve their quality of life.

- **Goal 2: Eliminate Health Disparities**
  The second goal of Healthy People 2010 is to eliminate health disparities among different segments of the population.

What Are the Leading Health Indicators?

The Leading Health Indicators will be used to measure the health of the Nation over the next ten years. Each of the ten Leading Health Indicators has one or more objectives from *Healthy People 2010* associated with it. As a group, the Leading Health Indicators reflect the major health concerns in the United States at the beginning of the 21st century. The Leading Health Indicators were selected on the basis of their ability to motivate action, the availability of data to measure progress, and their importance as public health issues.

The Leading Health Indicators are:

- Physical Activity
- Overweight and Obesity
- Tobacco Use
- Substance Abuse
- Responsible Sexual Behavior
- Mental Health
- Injury and Violence
- Environmental Quality
- Immunization
- Access to Health Care

Source: www.healthypeople.gov/LHI/.

SUMMARY

As with causal webs, the etiologies of epidemics are multifactorial and involve more than the presence of a potentially pathogenic or otherwise harmful agent. For example, although nearly one-third of the world's population harbors the bacillus that causes tuberculosis (TB), far fewer people have the active disease and fewer still, about 3 million people each year, die from TB. What factors account for the fact that some people become ill with TB while others remain symptom-free? Some of those factors have been identified. For example, increases in the numbers of immunocompromised individuals, particularly people infected with HIV, have led to increases in the numbers of people with active TB. In addition, some strains of TB have become resistant to drugs previously effective in treating the disease. Other reasons why some people have the TB bacillus but remain symptom-free remain elusive.

Other unanswered or only partially answered questions related to disease etiologies include the following:

- Why do some tobacco smokers develop lung cancers while other people develop other tobacco-related diseases and still others seem to be protected from serious tobacco-related illnesses?
- Why do some people infected with the West Nile virus develop full-blown encephalitis and other people recover after a mild, flulike ailment?
- Why do some cancers grow and kill rapidly, whereas others grow slowly and are found only during "routine" autopsies?
- What factors cause major structural birth defects such as certain heart diseases or cases of spina bifida, or cause metabolic defects such as Tay-Sachs disease, a fatal condition that affects the central nervous system, or phenylketonuria, a disease that affects how the body metabolizes the protein PKU?
- How do environmental factors and genetic factors interact to produce disease?
- Do people need to be exposed to disease-promoting or causative factors in a certain temporal sequence to develop disease, as is suspected for certain cancers and for dengue hemorrhagic fever (a mosquitoborne viral disease)?
- How can the "biologically important" amount and duration of a potentially harmful exposure best be quantified? What exposures have pathological thresholds of doses, below which no harmful effects occur? What factors modify any such thresholds?
- How can the quality and delivery of health services be improved by applying epidemiologic principles to health-care-management decision making and to the structure of health-care systems?
- What factors should routinely be monitored as sentinel predictors of an upcoming epidemic? How should the **public health system**—which comprises a diverse group of professionals including epidemiologists, clinicians, firefighters, and police officers, members of city and county boards of health, and state and federal agencies— respond to changes in sentinel predictors of epidemics or to the actual occurrence of an epidemic?
- How do members of the public health system know when an epidemic is "real" rather than, for example, a psychological response to fear, such as a false announcement of a bioterrorist event or a false announcement of contamination of drinking water or indoor air at a worksite?

Those questions are some of the medical and public health mysteries and practical dilemmas that epidemiology is solving or helping to solve. The next three chapters provide the fundamental, quantitative framework that epidemiologists use to evaluate possible answers to questions such as those asked above. Once again, as you read through these chapters, it is important to ask yourself what aspects of epidemiology you can use to help you become a more competent and successful public health professional.

REVIEW QUESTIONS

1. What is an "epidemic"? How is the occurrence of an epidemic determined?
2. What is an "epidemic curve"?
3. Define and provide several examples of an "attack rate." In an attack rate, how is the numerator determined? How is the denominator determined? What is a "category-specific" attack rate?
4. Define "population at risk."
5. What are "health indicators"?
6. What is *Healthy People 2010*? What are its goals, objectives, and leading health indicators?

REVIEW EXERCISES

1. Using the resources on the World Wide Web or other resources, list at least five factors that might affect the probability that a person who has a disease is diagnosed as having the disease. For example, one factor is a person's access to clinical health care because of his or her health insurance status. These factors are important not only because they affect which people receive medical treatment and preventive services but also because they affect the perceived magnitude of disease frequency among people having these factors.
2. Select one disease or injury. Then, outline the social, economic, and political systems and subsystems that affect the occurrence of that disease or injury. You may wish to refer to Figures 1.3 through 1.5 to gain a sense for how such systems and subsystems may be depicted.
3. How might social arrangements and relationships that affect disease and injury occurrence be quantified? For example, how might "marital (or partner) status" be quantified, taking into account factors such as current and former marital or partner status, duration of any relationship, and stability of a relationship?

■ SPECIAL CASE STUDY:

After-Action Report for the August 2003 Measles Investigation in Corvallis, Oregon

Charles Fautin, B.S.N., M.P.H., and Lora Jasman, M.D.

On 8/3/03 (Sunday), the index patient met 14 companions who were to travel from their home country in Asia to attend a program at Oregon State University (OSU) in Portland, Oregon. The index patient became ill with fever in the airport and was seen by an airport physician who ruled out SARS and measles and approved travel. The index case became increasingly ill during the flight and was attended to during the flight by a physician passenger who suspected measles but felt insecure in that diagnosis. Upon landing at San Francisco on 8/4/03 (Monday) the patient was transported by ambulance to a hospital emergency department. The ER physician did not think this was measles and performed no laboratory testing. The index case was released from the ER, immediately boarded a flight to Portland, and was lost to local health department follow-up.

Upon arrival at Portland the evening of 8/4/03 (Monday) the patient and 14 traveling companions were met by OSU program staff who noted that the index patient was visibly ill, had a rash, and "spots" on his hands. All were transported from Portland to Corvallis, the location of Oregon State University, via a charter bus. The following day the index patient was still ill and program staff began seeking medical advice.

On 8/5/03 (Tuesday) at 3:45 p.m., the Benton County Health Dept. (BCHD) Communicable Disease (CD) nurse on duty received a telephone call from a physician at the OSU Student Health Service (SHS). The physician had been in contact with OSU program staff who reported that an international visitor at OSU had developed symptoms which the physician recognized as consistent with measles. The ill person was not a registered student at OSU, and therefore not eligible for care at the Student Health Service clinic. Astutely recognizing the public health significance of this report, the OSU physician called the BCHD CD nurse for advice.

After notifying BCHD administration, the CD nurse contacted the OSU program the visitor was associated with and discussed how and where to obtain care. The CD nurse contacted Good Samaritan Regional Medical Center to advise them of the impending arrival of a possible measles case. The CD nurse then contacted the Oregon Department of Human Services (DHS) epidemiologist on-call and the BCHD Health Officer to report the case and initiated a contact investigation.

By Wednesday morning, 8/6/03, the BCHD was making arrangements to interview all of the patient's contacts to determine their ages, measles history, and vaccination status. Based upon the timing of rash onset, the original patient was no longer considered contagious. Following discharge from the hospital, care was arranged at the patient's residence.

Eighteen contacts were identified, located and interviewed. Fourteen contacts were traveling companions from Asia and had little or no facility in English, so utilization of translators was necessary. Many contacts were unaware of their medical history and immunization status, so arrangements were made for international telephone calls to elicit information from parents. Since disease/immunization information was incomplete from 16 contacts that were still within 72 hours of their initial contact, consent was obtained and those people were given Measles, Mumps, and Rubella (MMR) vaccine.

OSU staff in charge of housing and food services were contacted and arrangements for potential quarantine/isolation were discussed. Email and conference calls were utilized to coordinate information and give everyone the same information. This was extremely useful in assuring adequate patient care, clear communication, coordinated planning and consistent public information release.

By the morning of Thursday, 8/7/03, it had been determined that only one contact was unprotected by age, prior measles history, or vaccination. Arrangements were made for appropriate quarantine for that individual. Medical consultation with DHS (who had consulted the Centers for Disease Control and Prevention, CDC) determined that should this person become ill, the infectious period would not begin until Monday, 8/11/03. The contact was therefore allowed to move publicly through the weekend. The original patient continued to recover without sequelae. A news release and local Health Advisory were issued.

Lab confirmation of the initial case of measles was obtained on the morning of Saturday 8/9/03. Contact was maintained between OSU, BCHD, and DHS through the weekend. On Sunday afternoon at 7:00 p.m. the vulnerable contact voluntarily entered quarantine until 8/21/03.

On the morning of 8/11/03 (Monday), BCHD CD nurses began to monitor the vulnerable contact in quarantine. Just before noon the contact began to exhibit a low-grade fever and by 6:30 p.m. it was 102 degrees.

On 8/12/03 (Tuesday), this patient's temperature was 101 and exhibited coryza (symptoms of a "common cold") and conjunctivitis. On 8/13/02 (Wednesday), a presumptive diagnosis of measles was made based upon symptoms (rapid laboratory testing was not possible since the patient had received MMR vaccine on 8/6). A second media release was made at this time announcing a second presumed case of measles, and a local Health Update was issued to health providers.

Because of the earlier-than-expected onset of symptoms in the second case, investigation was begun to identify potential contacts during the previous weekend. Eleven possible contacts were identified in two counties. An additional group of low-risk potential exposures was sent letters explaining measles symptoms and urged to monitor themselves and report illnesses to their local health department.

The second patient became more acutely ill than the first, and it became clear that the patient needed trained, continual nursing care until recovery. OSU SHS physicians undertook medical consultation. This assistance was very important and prevented worsening of the patient's medical condition. Local home health-nursing was not trained to start and monitor gravity-drip IV therapy and their lead administrative staff was not available to facilitate the BCHD request for their staff immunization information. Medical and nursing care was undertaken by BCHD and OSU staffs. Since it was assumed this patient would recover fairly quickly after receiving IV fluids on 8/16/03, the length and severity of illness for the second patient was unexpected. Lay volunteers provided in-home care in consultation with BCHD nurses and an OSU physician. There were difficulties in communication however, and this resulted in one low-risk blood and body fluid exposure due to misunderstandings in communication with the volunteers. The second patient ultimately recovered without sequelae.

On the evening of 8/20/03 (Wednesday), another of the initial contacts (thought to have been fully immunized) began feeling ill and became febrile. But as symptoms occurred within the limits of the initial contact incubation period, this case was also assumed to be measles. The third patient was counseled, and voluntarily entered isolation. Since the patient had been at large in the community, another contact investigation was initiated.

The third patient continued to worsen through 8/23/03 (Saturday) with a fever of 101.9 and cough at 7:30 p.m., but without rash. Throughout that day (Saturday) twelve BCHD, OSU, and DHS staff investigated over 125 potential contacts in university offices, classrooms, and a cafeteria. Email advisories were sent to low-risk contacts that had been working or studying in the office building and flyers distributed in the cafeteria. Four BCHD, OSU SHS, and DHS nurses and one DHS health educator established an information and immunization desk at the cafeteria to assess potential contacts. University and personal health records were reviewed to determine immunization status. BCHD staff delivered ten doses of MMR.

On Sunday, 8/24, the third patient reported feeling substantially better and was afebrile all day. Consultation with DHS determined that isolation would be maintained through Monday with frequent status checks. On the morning of Tuesday, 8/26/03, the third patient was still afebrile and without any other symptoms, so measles was ruled out and the patient was released from isolation.

Identified Strengths

Planning: Between February and June, a task force of BCHD and OSU staff members met monthly to prepare for SARS. Discussions included plans for housing and feeding those in quarantine and isolation. These plans significantly facilitated a smooth and rapid response to the measles event. The existence of the task force meant that key players were acquainted, and the response could proceed even though some OSU staff were out of town and unreachable when initial action was required.—*Ongoing planning efforts must continue and new contingency plans made.*

Communication: Frequent emailing and especially conference calling enhanced understanding and cooperation of multiple agencies—this was important in coordinating patient care, limiting further exposure, and maintaining accurate supply of up-to-date information to the media. There was one person identified in each agency who had the complete information for that agency, or knew how to find it.—*Identify appropriate communication systems early and use them consistently.*

Media: Limiting each agency to one identified media spokes-person facilitated media information. Several reporters noted how much they appreciated knowing exactly whom to go to for primary information, and for follow-up. Plan and discuss your media information, what you will say and what is out of bounds, so all agencies are providing consistent information.—*Establish media-friendly and convenient points-of-contact; let the media know exactly whom to go to.*

Good Luck: Many serendipitous circumstances contributed to limiting this outbreak. Among these was that the initial case arrived in Corvallis, Oregon via a charter bus which was not used again for several days, was too ill on arrival to circulate publicly, and was quickly recognized as a possible measles case by both lay people and health professionals. Additionally, the Benton County Health Department was consulted immediately, all contacts were extremely cooperative, no serious medical complications occurred, agencies took public health information seriously, and the existing SARS response plan was implemented with minimal reservation.—*Hope but do not rely on having equally good fortune in other outbreak investigations.*

Identified Weaknesses

Lack of Perfect Information Control: Although this is impossible (and perhaps undesirable) to correct, it is important to recognize that the public, the media, and our own staff members will be receiving information outside of the channels we desire or approve. News media email and telephone hotlines, the internet, casual conversation, lack of appropriate confidentiality, and so forth will result in a proliferation of supplemental and sometimes inaccurate information. Perhaps naively, all media contacts in this case were surprised at the information reporters possessed beyond the agreed "talking points."—*Be aware that additional, and sometimes incorrect, information is a reality with which you will have to deal.*

Documenting Immunization Status: It is extremely difficult to reliably document the immunization status of campus students and associated visitors. This becomes even more difficult with foreign students and visitors, during summer session, and for programs whose students may not be subject to regular university requirements.—*Parents are great sources of information in every country.*

Differing International Immunization Practices: International vaccination and health care standards (including vaccination requirements, combination vaccines used, beliefs about vaccine effects, and so forth) differ significantly. This can lead to misunderstanding and miscommunication between American authorities and international students/families/health providers. Translation issues can further complicate these.—*Be sensitive to different health systems and health practices.*

Communicate with the Same People Consistently: When communicating with other agencies, utilize identified staff members from that agency who know the case.—*Do not expect others within the agency to know enough about what is going on to help or to provide reliable information.*

Home Health Nursing Limitations: When the second case needed IV therapy for rehydration, we contacted a local home-health service. The home-health RN determined that the agency did not have the capacity to start and maintain the IV on gravity drip or to provide ongoing assessment of a client with acute care needs. Therefore we were unable to utilize home-health services. Care for the second case was undertaken by lay volunteers overseen by BCHD and OSU staff members. Without any training in basic infection control and blood/body fluids precautions, these volunteers put themselves at greater risk than a trained person might have.—*A system needs to be identified to care for acutely ill Communicable Disease patients who are at home.*

Lessons Learned

Local Control: Ultimately it is the local health department and health providers who must deal with any communicable disease outbreak. While advice and consultation with state and federal authorities is necessary, every decision regarding CD control is made locally. Instituting quarantine earlier, as local personnel advocated, could have eliminated virtually all outside contacts to the second case. The additional contact investigation involved additional counties and could have led to a much larger outbreak. Decisions involving limitations on freedom of movement and freedom of choice can be counted upon to be contentious, even among co-professionals. There will probably be social, economic, and perhaps political pressure put on the health professionals depending upon the nature of the case.—*Remember that, ultimately, Communicable Disease outbreaks are a LOCAL public health issue and containment and control of the outbreak are the LOCAL health department's responsibility. We advise using the MOST CONSERVATIVE approach based upon medical expertise and literature.*

Translation: The commercial telephone translation line we used was fast, efficient, accurate, and worth its weight in gold every time.—*Establish an account and make sure your staff know how to access and use telephone language translation lines.*

Planning: The OSU/BCHD "SARS task force" meetings held between February and June 2003 resulted in most of the key players already being familiar with one another, trusting one another, and being on a first name basis. Although the plan was incomplete when implemented, and a lot of adaptation was necessary, the relationships were there and that facilitated things significantly.—*See the first strength (planning). Ongoing planning efforts should be continual and new contingency plans made based on your and others' experiences.*

Statistical Outliers and Coincidence: Early symptom onset and the occurrence of a coincidental infection significantly complicated this outbreak.—*Expect the unexpected and anomalous.*

Know How/Where to Find Your Team All the Time: All members of the extended team who are dealing with the situation should have others' home and cell phone numbers, and keep these numbers available at all times during an incident. Some of our most important work was done on weekends or evenings.—*Identify back-up personnel and make sure they are kept up-to-date.*

Determine the Limits of the Potential Outbreak: In this case, it worked well to assume that individuals who had been in contact with the persons with measles were adequately protected if they had received two prior measles vaccines (even if the second was within 72 hrs of exposure) or born before 1957 provided the contacts were otherwise healthy.—*Reaching this decision at the onset of the outbreak made it considerably easier to determine who was safe to remain at-large and who needed to be quarantined. This decision also helped to direct available resources toward contacts at higher risk of measles.*

Maintain a Firm Line with Patient Confidentiality: In our experience, news reporters understand when you tell them that you are under federal and state laws governing patient confidentiality.—*News reporters, nevertheless, still asked us questions we could not answer because of confidentiality concerns but they readily accepted our response that we could not answer these questions.*

BCHD Staff Utilization and Activities 8/5/03–9/1/03

- Total BCHD personnel involved: **13**
- Total BCHD staff hours: **262.95**
- Total # of confirmed measles cases (8/5–9/1): **2**
- Total # of possible contacts identified: **155**
- Total # of possible contacts actually contacted or notified: **141 (>90%)**
- Total # of MMR vaccinations delivered: **26**
- Total doses of Immunoglobulin (given to a person who was immunocompromised and therefore could not receive the live-virus vaccine) delivered: **1**

OSU and DHS Staff Utilization and Activities: Staff utilization and activities were not quantified but comprised as large or larger contributions of time and effort as the staff utilization and activities of the BCHD.

## CHAPTER 4

Measuring Disease Frequency: Incidence Rate

The three primary **measures of disease frequency** in epidemiology are the "incidence rate," "prevalence," and "cumulative incidence." Measures of disease frequency quantify the occurrence of disease and injury in populations. Of the three measures of disease frequency, the incidence rate is the most fundamental; each of the other two measures of disease frequency is a mathematical function of the incidence rate. This chapter focuses on the incidence rate; prevalence and cumulative incidence are covered in Chapters 5 and 6, respectively.

DEFINITION OF INCIDENCE RATE

The **incidence rate,** which is abbreviated IR, is defined as the number of new cases of disease divided by the amount of person-time during which the new cases arose. The IR summarizes how fast people in a certain population are changing from one state of health (often a state of no disease) to another state of health (often a diseased state). Notice that the IR is not a proportion; that is, it is not a quantity of the form ($a/(a + b)$). The IR is a true rate. Rates have the general form of being a change in one variable relative to the change in another variable of which it is a mathematical function. The speed of a car is a rate. How fast Newton's apple fell from the tree is a rate. How quickly cases of heart disease occur among Native American women aged 60–64 years is a rate. The range of possible values for an IR is 0 (no one develops disease) to infinity (everyone instantaneously develops disease).

RESTRICTION OF INCIDENCE RATES

All incidence rates, as in the IR example just presented for heart disease among Native American women, are restricted to people of a certain kind. The "kind" of person is defined by characteristics such as age, gender, geographic location, and/or exposure or "risk factor" status (for example, being a cigarette smoker or not). IRs also are restricted to a certain time frame. Thus, IRs always have an implicit or an explicit reference to the kind of person and time frame to which the IR pertains.

For example, an epidemiologist might ask:

- What is the IR of heart disease in the United States for the calendar year 1998?
- What is the IR of stroke during the first two years after a person's spouse dies?

Those two questions could be restricted further by more narrowly defining the type of person to whom the questions apply. For example, the first question might refer only to White men between the ages of 70 and 74 years, and the second question might refer only to women aged 60–69 years at the time of their husbands' deaths.

Notice that questions about IRs differ from questions such as "What *proportion* of people in the United States developed heart disease during the calendar year 1998?" and "What *proportion* of people have a stroke during the first two years after the death of a spouse?" These latter questions ask about the **cumulative incidence** (also known as **risk**) of developing a certain health outcome and not about the IR of developing the outcome. Cumulative incidence, abbreviated CI, is defined as the proportion of a population that develops a specific disease or injury over a specified period of time. CI is discussed in detail in Chapter 6.

Many publications in the epidemiologic and public health literature use the terms IRs and CIs interchangeably or express IRs differently. For example, it is common to find IRs reported as one of the following:

- "The number of new cases of disease per 100,000 person-years" (the expression for an IR used in this book)
- "The number of new cases of disease per 100,000 people per year
- "The incidence rate of disease per 100,000"

As mentioned in Chapter 3, the lack of a standard nomenclature and structure for expressing several of the fundamental concepts in epidemiology can be confusing. The essential point is to understand the *concept* of each epidemiologic term regardless of the different ways in which it is expressed.

COMPONENTS OF INCIDENCE RATES

An IR is comprised of two parts: the numerator (the number of new cases of disease or injury) and the denominator (the amount of person-time during which the number of new cases occurred). It is important to calculate each component of the IR correctly when estimating an IR.

The numerator should contain only *newly diagnosed* cases of disease or injury. The numerator should not contain **prevalent** (*previously diagnosed*) cases of disease or cases of disease other than the specific disease or injury category under study. An epidemiologist initially may rely on a computerized listing of clinicians' assignments of **International Classification of Diseases Codes** (ICD codes) to patients when identifying new cases of disease or injury. The ICD codes are a disease- and injury-categorization roster used worldwide to standardize disease and injury diagnoses. Though helpful, an ICD code assigned by a clinician may be incorrect; that is, a patient may have a disease or an injury that differs from the assigned code and so is **misclassified** (assigned a code that is wrong for the patient's actual health condition). For that reason, it often is necessary to review a patient's actual medical record to confirm the accuracy of the assigned ICD code.

Why is it important to include only newly diagnosed cases when calculating an IR? One reason is obvious: An incidence rate measures how fast (new) cases of disease or of injury are occurring. An IR does not measure, nor is it intended to measure, the frequency or presence of existing (previously diagnosed or previously diagnosed *plus* newly diagnosed) cases of disease or injury.

A second reason pertains to the use of IRs. Often, IRs are calculated for the purpose of mathematically relating an exposure, postulated to be a cause or a preventive of a disease or an injury, to the IR. If prevalent cases of disease or injury are included in the calculation of an IR, it is not possible to determine whether an exposure is related to the *occurrence* of the disease or the injury. Instead, the exposure may be related to the ability of cases to *survive* with the disease or the injury, and thus to continue to exist as cases (be **prevalent** cases).

Not all individuals who have a disease or an injury will be diagnosed and thus counted as new cases of disease or injury. Factors such as access to health services and health-care-seeking behaviors influence the chance that a person's disease will be identified. For example, until recently in the United States, African American women had considerably lower incidence rates of breast cancer but higher breast cancer **mortality rates** than White women. (A mortality rate, abbreviated MR, is an IR in which the new cases of disease or injury are newly *fatal* cases of disease or of injury rather than newly *diagnosed* cases.) This paradox resulted from the relative lack of access to health services for African American women compared with White women. The lack of access to health services meant that African American women were diagnosed for breast cancer later in the course of their disease (that is, at a later stage of cancer), and therefore had a higher **case fatality rate** (proportion of cases who die from their disease or injury) than did their White counterparts (Shapiro et al. 1982).

The second component of an IR is the denominator, the amount of person-time in which the new cases occurred. Typically, the unit of person-time used in expressing an IR is the "person-year."

What is a **person-year** (P-Y), and how is it calculated? Simply stated, one person-year is equal to one person who is followed for one year, during which time the person is at risk of becoming a new case of disease. Equivalently, one person-year is equal to two people, each of whom is followed for six months, during which time each person is at risk of becoming a new case of disease. Other combinations of numbers of people and periods of observation are possible. For example, one person followed for nine months plus one person followed for three months equals one person-year of observation.

Usually, the people who are contributing person-time to the denominator of an IR have certain characteristics, such as age, gender, and/or exposure status, in common. Implicit in the summation of person-years from different people is the idea that the people contributing person-time represent people of a certain kind (for example, women between the ages of 20 and 29 years) rather than being "unique individuals." It is not important whether some people contribute more person-time than do others, nor is it important how many people are contributing person-time. What is important is that the people who are contributing person-time have certain characteristics of interest in common (for example, being a woman between the ages of 20 and 29 years). Often, people who are participating in an epidemiologic study contribute person-time to more than one IR. For example, a person might contribute person-time to the IR of disease among men aged 60–64 years and then, upon that person's sixty-fifth birthday, contribute person-time to the IR for men aged 65–69 years.

Another point to appreciate when calculating IRs concerns the risk status of the people contributing person-time. The denominator of an IR must contain only those person-years (or some other measure of person-time) contributed by people who truly are "at risk" of contributing to the numerator, that is, of becoming a newly diagnosed case of disease. Thus, people who have been diagnosed with the disease of interest previously and people who are not susceptible to the disease of interest cannot contribute person-years to that particular IR. (These people are eligible to contribute person-time toward the calculation of an IR for a different disease.)

For instance, the gentleman referred to in a previous paragraph, who is contributing person-time in the age ranges of 60 to 64 years and then 65 to 69 years, no longer can contribute person-time if he is diagnosed with the disease of interest. For example, if he enters the study on his sixty-first birthday and is diagnosed with the disease of interest exactly 1.5 years later, he will contribute 1.5 person-years and one case to the age category 60–64 years, and no person-time or case to the age range 65–69 years. On the other hand, if he enters the study on his sixty-first birthday and is diagnosed with the disease of interest exactly 5 years later, he will contribute 4 person-years and no case to the age range 60–64 years, and one person-year and one case to the age range 65–69 years.

An excellent example of an error in calculating an IR is the IR for uterine cancer for women in the United States. Before about 1980, this IR was calculated by dividing the number of new cases of uterine cancer by the number of person-years contributed by all women, regardless of each woman's hysterectomy status. Calculating person-years in that manner is an error, because women who have had hysterectomies (approximately 20 million women in the United States) cannot develop uterine cancer.

Another approach for measuring person-years is to estimate the number of person-years during which a certain number of new cases of disease or injury arose by relying on census data. The United States government, as well as many states and localities, regularly counts the number of people living in a certain area. For instance, the United States Bureau of the Census conducts a national census every ten years. In the estimate of an IR for a calendar year, the denominator for the IR can be estimated by using the midyear population size listed in the census data. For example, if the midyear population size is 32,000 people, 602 of whom were involved in a motor vehicle injury, the estimated IR of motor vehicle injuries in this population would be 602/32,000 person-years, or, equivalently, 1.9/100 person-years. (By convention, IRs are expressed with denominators that are powers of 10. In this example, solving for x in the equation, $602/32,000 = x/100$ person-years, yields $x = 1.9$. It is easier to compare the magnitudes of a series of IRs with one another when each IR is expressed with the same power of 10 in the denominator.)

THE COHORT STUDY

The type of epidemiologic study in which person-time and the number of new cases of disease or injury are measured is called a **cohort study.** A **cohort** is a fixed group of people that is followed over time. In a cohort study, two or more cohorts of people are followed over time, and their durations of **follow-up** (the amount of person-time each person contributes to the study) and disease experiences are recorded and then compared with each other. One cohort, called the **exposed cohort** or **exposed group,** has some special exposure(s) in common. Examples of exposed cohorts are a group of smokers, a group of people who eat diets high in saturated fat, and a group of people who exercise on a regular basis. The exposure that defines the group is the **exposure of interest** in the study (the exposure an epidemiologist wishes to evaluate with respect to its causal or preventive relationship to a specific health outcome).

The other cohort that is included in a cohort study is the **unexposed cohort** or **unexposed group.** The unexposed cohort lacks the special exposure that defines the exposed cohort and serves as the comparison group with which the incidence rate of disease or injury in the exposed cohort is compared. Cohort studies are discussed in detail in Chapter 10. For now, it is important to appreciate only that cohort studies are the primary type of epidemiologic study that generates data from which IRs for cohorts having different exposures are calculated and compared.

CALCULATION OF INCIDENCE RATES

For illustrative purposes, the following simplified examples explain how to calculate IRs. Actual cohorts would contain more people.

EXAMPLE 1

Suppose there is a study in which three people are followed over time, and their periods of follow-up and disease experiences are counted.

- Person A is in the study for 2 years and develops the disease of interest exactly at the end of this 2-year period.
- Person B is in the study for 3 years and does not develop the disease of interest.
- Person C is in the study for 4 years and develops the disease of interest exactly at the end of this 4-year period.

What is the IR of disease in this cohort of three people? Remember that an IR has two components: a numerator (the number of new cases) and a denominator (the amount of person-time). In this example, the number of new cases of disease is 2 (Persons A and C each contribute one case). The total number of person-years is $2 + 3 + 4 = 9$. Thus, the IR = 2/(9 P-Y).

As stated previously, incidence rates are easier to interpret and to compare with other IRs when their denominators are a power of 10. For that reason, 2/9 P-Y should be expressed as 2.2/10 P-Y or 22/100 P-Y. (Solving for x, 2/9 P-Y = x/10 P-Y yields $x = 2.2$. Solving for x, 2/9 P-Y = x/100 P-Y yields $x = 22$.) The particular power of 10 used for the denominator typically is selected to yield a numerator that is between 1 and 10, or between 1 and 100.

EXAMPLE 2

- Person A is followed for w years and is diagnosed with the *disease of interest* exactly at the end of w years.
- Person B is followed for x years and then dies from a disease *other than the disease of interest* exactly at the end of x years.
- Person C is followed without mishap until the end of the study, y years.
- Person D is followed for z years and is **lost-to-follow-up** exactly at the end of z years.

"Lost-to-follow-up" means that a person removed himself or herself from the study and thus ended participation in the study prematurely. The person-times for subjects who leave a cohort study early must be included in the denominator of an IR up until the times of their self-removals from the study. For that reason, Person D's person-time is included in the denominator of the IR even though this person was lost-to-follow-up after z years. In Example 2, the IR is $1/(w + x + y + z)$ P-Y. Only one person (Person A) developed the disease of interest in $w + x + y + z$ person-years.

People who are lost-to-follow-up often have characteristics related to health status that differ from the characteristics of people who remain in studies. For example, people who are more "health conscious," such as nonsmokers, nonobese individuals, and non–alcohol abusers, may be more apt to remain in studies than are people who are less health conscious. The IR calculated for the cohort in Example 2 would be **biased** (invalid, or systematically in error) if Person D were lost-to-follow-up for reasons related to the disease of interest in the study. Specifically, if Person D were lost because she or he developed the disease of interest, the IR would have included all of Person D's years of follow-up but not the fact that Person D developed the disease of interest. Thus, the IR would be *underestimated* (smaller than the actual IR).

EXAMPLE 3

Suppose there are five people in a study. Two of these people are followed for 2 years, one for 3 years, and the remaining two for 2.5 years. Two of the five people develop the disease of interest. Given those data, what is the IR?

The answer is 2 (new cases of the disease of interest) divided by ((2 people times 2 person-years) + (1 person times 3 person-years) + (2 people times 2.5 person-years)), or 2/12 P-Y. The IR in this example would be reported as 2/12 P-Y, or, equivalently, 1.7/10P-Y.

EXAMPLE 4

In this example, the person-years and the numbers of cases by age group already have been counted and tabulated in the following table.

Table of Person-Years and Numbers of Cases by Age Category for Example 4

Age (years)	Number of Person-Years	Number of Cases
10–14	500	17
15–24	300	23
Total	800	40

Using the data in the table, calculate the **crude IR** and the **age-specific IRs.** The crude IR is the IR calculated by including the data for all subjects in the study. In this example, the crude IR is based on the data for both people aged 10–14 years and people aged 15–24 years. The crude IR equals 40/800 P-Y, which, expressed with a denominator in a power of 10, is equal to 5/100 P-Y. Age-specific IRs are IRs that pertain to a subset of the people in a study, based on age. In Example 4, the age-specific IRs are 17/500 P-Y for 10–14-year-olds and 23/300 P-Y for 15–24-year-olds. These IRs are equivalent to an IR of 3.4/100 P-Y for the younger people and an IR of 7.7/100 P-Y for the older people. (See Box 4.1 for an example of calculating IRs based on enumerations of new cases of dengue and dengue hemorrhagic fever and numbers of person-years.)

BOX 4.1

NATIONAL SITUATION OF DENGUE AND DENGUE HEMORRHAGIC FEVER IN THAILAND

SEEVIGA SAENGTHARATIP, PH.D.

MEDICAL ENTOMOLOGIST, OFFICE OF DENGUE HEMORRHAGIC FEVER CONTROL, DEPARTMENT OF COMMUNICABLE DISEASE CONTROL, BANGKOK, THAILAND

Surveillance Data

Dengue fever (a severe, flu-like illness) and the severe form, dengue hemorrhagic fever (DHF), have occurred in Thailand for several decades. DHF is a potentially fatal complication of dengue fever that is characterized by high fever, bleeding complications such as bleeding in the gastrointestinal tract and/or from gingiva, often enlargement of the liver, and in severe cases, circulatory failure. The number of dengue patients (dengue/DHF) has been rising steadily over the past forty-five years. Case surveillance, mainly on a clinical basis, has been conducted for years, with cases reported to the Bureau of Epidemiology. The epidemic pattern has changed from occurring in alternate years to an irregular pattern. Figure 4.1 shows the trend of dengue/DHF cases per 100,000 people in Thailand between 1958 and 2002. The largest number of cases

Box 4.1 continued

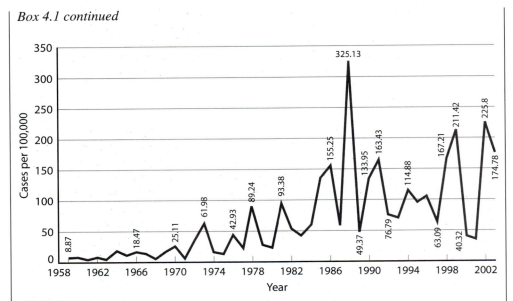

FIGURE 4.1
Dengue/DHF situation by year, Thailand, 1958–2002.

TABLE 4.1
Annual Summary of Dengue/DHF Cases, Deaths, Incidence and Mortality Rates,
and Case Fatality Rates (CFR) in Thailand between 1992 and 2002

Year	Cases	Deaths	Population at Risk (in 1,000s)	Incidence per 100,000 P-Y*	Mortality per 100,000 P-Y†	CFR‡(%)
1992	41,125	136	57,800	71.16	0.24	0.33
1993	67,017	222	58,330	114.89	0.38	0.33
1994	51,688	140	59,100	87.46	0.24	0.27
1995	60,330	166	59,250	101.82	0.28	0.28
1996	37,929	116	60,120	63.09	0.19	0.31
1997	101,689	253	60,820	167.20	0.42	0.25
1998	129,954	424	61,470	211.41	0.69	0.33
1999	24,826	56	61,470	40.39	0.09	0.23
2000	18,617	32	61,770	30.14	0.05	0.17
2001	139,725	244	61,880	225.80	0.39	0.17
2002	108,905	172	62,310	174.78	0.28	0.16

*(Number of cases/population at risk in 1,000s) × 100,000 person-years.
†(Number of deaths/population at risk in 1,000s) × 100,000 person-years.
‡(Number of deaths/number of cases) × 100.

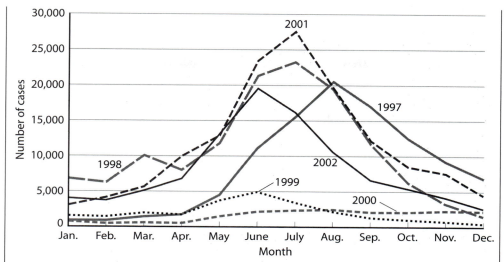

FIGURE 4.2
Dengue/DHF by month, Thailand, 1997–2002.

occurred in 1987 with 174,285 cases and 1,007 deaths; the incidence rate was 325.1 per 100,000 people while the mortality rate was 1.9 per 100,000 people. For that year, the case fatality rate (CFR) was 0.58%. Table 4.1 summarizes annual dengue/DHF cases, deaths, incidence and mortality rates per 100,000 people, and the CFRs in Thailand between 1992 and 2002.

Dengue/DHF cases have been reported from all four regions of the country, with the largest number of cases typically occurring among residents of the Southern Region. A descriptive analysis showed that approximately 65 percent of the reported cases occurred to children between the ages of 5 and 14 years. For the years 1997–2001, children between the ages of 5 and 9 years had the largest number of cases, followed by children ages 10–14 years, then by people ages 15 years and older, and finally by children aged 0–4 years. The overall ratio of male to female cases was 1.00:1.03.

The numbers of reported cases per month between 1997 and 2000 indicate that currently there is one peak of infection, which occurs during rainy months of May to October (Figure 4.2). The density of *Aedes* mosquitoes (the vector for dengue), as indicated by the House Index (percent of houses with larval mosquitoes) and the Container Index (percent of containers with larva mosquitoes), is higher during those months than in other months.

Serological Diagnosis

Serological diagnosis is important for confirmation of the etiological agent. Among patients first diagnosed with dengue/DHF based on clinical findings, 73.3 percent later were confirmed to have dengue infection based on serologic testing. Of the confirmed dengue cases, 82.8 percent experienced a **secondary infection** (an additional infection from a different agent during the course of infection from the primary agent).

Box 4.1 continued

Risk Factors Affecting Incidence and/or Mortality from Dengue/DHF

- Increasing urbanization
- Population movement
- Increased numbers and areas of mosquito breeding places
- Poor collection of garbage
- Rapid transportation systems
- Inadequate health education
- Lack of community participation in vector-source reduction
- Little sustainability in vector-source reduction
- Limited resources (including budget, manpower, equipment)
- Resistance of mosquitoes to insecticides
- Delays in the notification of dengue/DHF cases
- Inadequate clinical management in some hospitals

Surveillance System

Dengue/DHF is a **notifiable disease** (a disease whose reporting to a local, regional, or central health agency is required either by statute or by some other mandate). In some instances, suspected cases may be investigated by a team from the Epidemiology Division or from the Regional Epidemiology Center, emphasizing the need for cooperation among various agencies to enact an effective surveillance system. Even so, underdiagnosis of cases is possible if, for example, clinicians are not looking for the disease in patients over 15 years of age. Missed diagnoses are particularly likely during periods of low-level dengue transmission.

Clinical diagnosis of dengue/DHF should be confirmed serologically whenever possible. Laboratory confirmation has a significant function not only in improving the accuracy of clinical diagnosis but also in the planning and evaluating of vector-control programs and strategies.

MORTALITY RATES

As mentioned previously, a **mortality rate,** abbreviated MR, is an example of an IR in which the event of interest is death rather than a new case of disease or injury. (Death is regarded as a "new case of death.") The ten leading causes of death in the United States (all ages), based on preliminary data for 2002 (Table 4.2), show the dominance of the chronic diseases as major public health problems. The numbers of death and mortality rates by age category are available at the same source.

Sometimes, MRs are used as estimates of IRs. For example, the MR for lung cancer might be monitored over time in an attempt to assess whether the IR of lung cancer is changing over time. In general, an MR for a particular disease or injury is a good estimate of the corresponding IR if the disease or the injury has a high **case fatality rate** and is rapidly fatal. A case fatality rate, mentioned previously, is the proportion of

TABLE 4.2
Ten Leading Causes of Death in the United States, Preliminary Data for 2002

Rank	Cause of Death	Number of Deaths	Number of Deaths per 100,000 P-Y
	All causes	2,447,862	848.9
1	Diseases of the heart	695,754	241.3
2	Malignant neoplasms (cancers)	558,847	193.8
3	Cerebrovascular diseases	163,010	56.5
4	Chronic lower respiratory diseases	125,500	43.5
5	Accidents (unintentional injuries)	102,303 (44,572 were motor vehicle accidents)	35.5 (15.5 for motor vehicle accidents)
6	Diabetes mellitus	73,119	25.4
7	Influenza and pneumonia	65,984	22.9
8	Alzheimer's disease	58,785	20.4
9	Nephritis, nephrotic syndrome, and nephrosis	41,018	14.2
10	Septicemia	33,881	11.7
	All other causes	529,661	183.7

Source: Preliminary data for 2002 from National Center for Health Statistics, *National Vital Statistics Reports* 52, no. 13 (February 11, 2004): 27, Table 7. See also www.cdc.gov/epo/epo/pub_sw.htm.

people having a particular disease or injury who die from that disease or injury. MRs for diseases or injuries that are rapidly fatal (within a few years after diagnosis) most closely approximate their IRs.

Age-Adjusted Incidence and Mortality Rates

The numbers of deaths and the crude mortality rates for 1998, and **age-adjusted mortality rates** for 1998 and 1999, for the United States show the tremendous burden diseases of the heart and cancers, in particular, have on the health of people living in the United States. (See, for example, www.cdc.gov/nchs/ under the heading "Deaths: Leading Causes for 2000.") *Age-adjusted* IRs and MRs are different from *age-specific* IRs and MRs. Age-adjusted rates are IRs or MRs in which the age distributions of the populations for which IRs or MRs are being calculated are held constant. Age-adjusted IRs and MRs that have been adjusted to the same population age distribution can be compared with one another without concern that differences in age are affecting the comparison.

Why might differences in age affect a comparison of IRs or MRs? Age is a strong risk factor for disease, with both incidence and mortality rates generally increasing as age increases, so populations having different age distributions may have different *crude IRs or MRs* simply because one population has a proportionally greater number of older people than does the other population. The *crude IRs and MRs* may differ even if the *age-specific IRs or MRs* are similar. The following example illustrates the process of age-adjustment for two populations that have identical *age-specific IRs* but different *crude IRs*.

EXAMPLE: THE PROCESS OF AGE-ADJUSTMENT

Two Populations Having Identical Age-Specific IRs but Different Crude IRs

Age Category	POPULATION A			POPULATION B		
	# P-Y	# New Cases	IR	# P-Y	# New Cases	IR
Young	500	5	1/100 P-Y	1,500	15	1/100 P-Y
Old	1,500	75	5/100 P-Y	500	25	5/100 P-Y
Crude (young plus old)	2,000	80	4/100 P-Y	2,000	40	2/100 P-Y

The crude IR in Population A (4/100 P-Y) is two times the crude IR in Population B even though the age-specific IRs are the same in each population (1/100 P-Y for young people and 5/100 P-Y for old people). Interpreting the crude IRs to mean that there are favorable age-specific IRs in Population B compared with Population A would be an error. The difference in the crude IRs between these two populations is attributable entirely to the different distributions of person-years for young and for old people in these two populations.

One approach for calculating age-adjusted IRs would be to ask, "What would the age-adjusted IR be in Population B if the distribution of person-years for young and for old people in Population B were identical to the distribution of person-years in Population A?" The age-adjusted IR in Population B using the distribution of person-years in Population A is calculated as follows:

Age-adjusted $IR_{Population\ B}$

$= ((IR_{B\ Young} * P\text{-}Y_{A\ Young}) + (IR_{B\ Old} * P\text{-}Y_{A\ Old}))/(P\text{-}Y_{A\ Young} + P\text{-}Y_{A\ Old})$

$= ((15/1,500\ P\text{-}Y * 500\ P\text{-}Y) + (25/500\ P\text{-}Y * 1,500\ P\text{-}Y))/ (500\ P\text{-}Y + 1,500\ P\text{-}Y)$

$= (5 + 75)/2,000\ P\text{-}Y$

$= 80/2,000\ P\text{-}Y$

$= 4/100\ P\text{-}Y$

Adjusting the distribution of person-years for old and for young people in Population B to equal the age distribution in Population A results in the same crude IR in Population B as in Population A (4/100 P-Y). This identity is to be expected because the age-specific IRs are the same in the two populations. Comparing the age-adjusted IR for Population B with the crude IR in Population A resulted in a comparison that removed any effect of differences in the age distribution between the two populations. In epidemiologic parlance, age-adjustment removed **confounding** by age. For this example, confounding can be depicted in the following way:

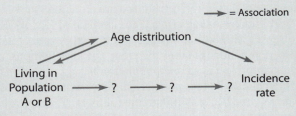

Pictorial representation of confounding.

In the depiction, age distribution is a confounding variable because (1) increased age is associated with an increase in the incidence rate of disease, and (2) age is associated with living in either Population A or Population B; specifically, Population A has proportionately more person-years for old people than has Population B.

In general, a confounding factor obscures the true size of association between an exposure and a health outcome because the confounding factor exerts an effect on the association that is "mixed in," to an unknown extent, with the true magnitude of association between the exposure and the health outcome. Confounding is discussed in more detail in Chapters 7 and 12.

What if the age distribution in Population A were adjusted to the age distribution in Population B? Would the age-adjusted overall IR in Population A equal the crude IR in Population B? The age-adjusted IR_A is calculated by applying the same distribution of person-years in age categories$_B$ to the age-specific IR_A and then divided by the total number of P-Y_B (a method called **weighting**). For that reason, using the age distribution in Population A to adjust the overall IR in Population A should yield the same IR (2/100 P-Y) because the age-specific IRs are identical in each population:

Age-adjusted $IR_{Population A}$

$= ((IR_{A\,Young} * P\text{-}Y_{B\,Young}) + (IR_{A\,Old} * P\text{-}Y_{B\,Old}))/(P\text{-}Y_{B\,Young} + P\text{-}Y_{B\,Old})$

$= ((5/500\ P\text{-}Y * 1{,}500\ P\text{-}Y) + (75/1{,}500\ P\text{-}Y * 500\ P\text{-}Y))/(1{,}500\ P\text{-}Y + 500\ P\text{-}Y)$

$= (15 + 25)/2{,}000\ P\text{-}Y$

$= 40/2{,}000\ P\text{-}Y$

$= 2/100\ P\text{-}Y$, the same as the crude IR in Population B

The phrase "age-specific rate" sometimes is confused with the phrase "age-adjusted rate." Category-specific rates refer to rates that pertain only to people who belong in a certain category, such as people in a particular age range or people having the same gender. For example, an age-specific IR for people between the ages of 50 and 59 years pertains only to people between the ages of 50 and 59 years. Likewise, a gender-specific IR pertains only to males or to females but not to both genders. A category-specific IR may also be specific to more than one variable, such as an IR for women between the ages of 50 and 59 years.

In contrast, a category-adjusted IR, such as an age- or gender-adjusted IR, is an overall IR that includes the data for all people in a study. In a category-adjusted IR, the distribution of person-years is changed (**adjusted**) to prevent confounding by the category that was adjusted. Note that the overall IR resulting from adjustment for one or more categories usually differs from a crude rate: A crude rate is calculated without adjusting for any categories, as is demonstrated in the numeric example on page 74.

Variation in Disease and Injury Frequency

A crude MR may mask substantial geographic or other variation in MRs. For example, within the United States, the age-adjusted heart-related MR for residents of the District of Columbia is approximately two times the age-adjusted heart-related MR for residents of Minnesota. Similarly, the age-adjusted stroke MR for residents of South Carolina is double the age-adjusted stroke MR for residents of New York. Table 4.3 lists additional examples of geographic variations in MRs by state.

TABLE 4.3
Examples of Geographic Variation in State-Specific Mortality Rates Within the United States, Preliminary Data for 2002*

Cause of Death, Year	Highest Age-Adjusted Mortality Rate[†] (State)	Lowest Age-Adjusted Mortality Rate[†] (State)
All causes, preliminary data for 2002	1,036.2/100,000 P-Y (Mississippi)	660.5/100,000 P-Y (Hawaii)
Heart-related, 2000	250/100,000 P-Y (District of Columbia)	122/100,000 P-Y (Minnesota)
Stroke, 2000	83/100,000 P-Y (South Carolina)	40/100,000 P-Y (New York)
Breast cancer in women, 2002	32.7/100,000 W-Y (Delaware)	22.4/100,000 W-Y (Nebraska)
Motor-vehicle-related, 2000	32.6/100,000 P-Y (Mississippi)	7.6/100,000 P-Y (Massachusetts)
Homicide, 2002[‡]	36.2/100,000 P-Y (District of Columbia)	2.0/100,000 P-Y (Massachusetts and Idaho)

Source: Preliminary data for 2002 from National Center for Health Statistics, State Health Profiles, *National Vital Statistics Reports* 52, no. 13 (February 11, 2004): 4–19. See also www.cdc.gov/epo/epo/pub_sw.htm.

*Year for which most recent data are available.

[†]Mortality rates adjusted to the United States population in 2000.

[‡]Data for six states were unavailable.

In addition to geographic variation, some diseases and injuries in the United States have marked **secular trends** (changes in disease or injury frequency over time). For example, lung cancer MRs for men and then later for women increased dramatically since 1930 before beginning to level off and then decline. MRs for stomach cancer, on the other hand, decreased markedly since about 1930, whereas MRs from heart diseases and from stroke decreased from about 1963 (in California first) and 1940, respectively. The reasons for the increases and decreases in disease-specific MRs have been elucidated only in part:

- Changes in tobacco smoking were pivotal in decreasing MRs associated with lung cancer.
- The reason(s) for the large decrease in mortality from stomach cancer, although less clearly identified, are postulated to be related to changes in dietary preferences and/or the processes used to store or prepare foods for consumption.
- The epidemiology of heart disease has become more clearly understood with the identification of new risk factors, including serum homocysteine (a sulfur-containing amino acid) levels and C-reactive proteins. (CRP is used to measure the presence and severity of bodily inflammation.) These two risk factors add to the list of previously known risk factors for heart disease, such as hypertension, overweight, serum cholesterol (especially low HDLs, and high LDLs and triglycerides), diabetes, and tobacco use.
- The striking decline in stroke mortality that became apparent about 1940 predates both the widespread development and use of antihypertension drugs and lifestyle changes such as reduced sodium intake (that is, "salt" [NaCl] added to foods) or

TABLE 4.4

Number of Deaths per 100,000 Infants Less than One Year of Age by Race and Gender in the United States, 2002

| | NUMBER OF DEATHS PER 100,000 INFANTS LESS THAN ONE YEAR OF AGE GENDER | |
Race*	Males	Females
Non-Hispanic White	644.8	506.0
Black	1,334.9	1,165.7
Non-Hispanic Black	1,353.6	1,181.6
American Indian	878.1	739.2
Asian or Pacific Islander	453.5	405.6
Hispanic	643.3	536.1

Source: Preliminary data for 2002 from National Center for Health Statistics, *National Vital Statistics Reports* 52, no. 13 (February 11, 2004): 9–14, Table 1. See also www.cdc.gov/epo/epo/pub_sw.htm.

*Note: The data for "race" should be interpreted with caution because of inconsistencies in how race is understood and reported.

increased exercise; thus, the decline in stroke mortality remains largely an epidemiologic mystery. The large secular *decrease* in stroke mortality occurred in spite of *increases* in tobacco smoking, and the interaction of tobacco smoking plus oral contraceptives, each of which causes strokes in some people.

Many causes of deaths and MRs vary by factors such as age, gender, and identification with a certain racial or ethnic heritage (Table 4.4). The terms "race" and "ethnicity" are difficult to define. The data presented in Table 4.4, which show number of deaths per 100,000 infants less than one year of age by race and gender in the United States for 2002, come from the National Center for Health Statistics (2004, February 11) with the notation that the data for "race" should be interpreted with caution because of inconsistencies in how race is understood and reported.

Large differences in MRs by "race" may occur in part because of an association of "race" with **median** family incomes. (A median, one statistical measure of central tendency for a distribution of numbers, is the number above which 50 percent of the distribution of numbers lie and below which 50 percent of the numbers lie.) Challenges associated with lower family incomes may include high stress, increased exposure to environmental and occupational hazards, and less effective health promotion campaigns. In addition, several studies have demonstrated that African Americans may have less access to health-care services and, when they have access, sometimes are not offered care that is comparable in quality to the care that is offered to White Americans (Bach et al. 1999; Canto et al. 2000).

Morbidity and Mortality Worldwide

Globally, child mortality (probability of death under five years of age) decreased from 147 per 1,000 live births in 1970 to approximately 80 per 1,000 live births in 2002. The largest reductions in child mortality occurred in regions in the eastern Mediterranean, Southeast Asia, and Latin America. The leading causes of childhood mortality in low-income countries (countries other than Australia, Canada, Japan, New Zealand, and the United States, and the countries of Europe and the former Soviet Union) mostly were infectious and parasitic diseases, partly as a result of the epidemic of HIV/AIDS. The five leading causes of death were perinatal conditions (typically the number of deaths per 1,000 infants of 28 weeks gestation plus infants weighing at least 1,000g at birth, plus the number of infants aged one week or less), lower respiratory infections, diarrheal diseases, malaria, and measles, accounting for 23.1, 18.1, 15.2, and 10.7, and 5.4 percent of deaths, respectively ("The World Health Report 2003," at www.who.int/whr/2003). Most of the perinatal conditions were deaths from infectious diseases; pregnancy-related complications such as placenta previa and abruptio placentae; delivery-related complications, including intrapartum asphyxia, birth trauma, and premature birth (Special Report: Reducing Perinatal and Neonatal Mortality, at www.reproline.jhu.edu/english/2mnh/perinatal.htm). Approximately 90 percent of all HIV/AIDS deaths and malaria deaths in low-income countries occurred in sub-Saharan Africa. Globally, child mortality is associated strongly with living in poverty ("The World Health Report 2003," at www.who.int/whr/2003).

Worldwide in 2002, approximately 75 percent of the deaths among adults (people aged 15 years or older) were caused by noninfectious diseases. An additional 10 percent of deaths were caused by injuries, and, among injuries, about 70 percent occurred to males. Many of the injury deaths to males were associated with traffic-related mishaps or with war or other forms of violence. (See for example, the special case study on public health in Afghanistan on pages 96–101.) The leading causes of death to adults worldwide are listed in Table 4.5. The data in Table 4.5 should be regarded as estimates, because even in countries having excellent health-related data systems, such as the United States, the actual cause of death listed on a death certificate or in a death registry

TABLE 4.5
Leading Causes of Death among Adults Worldwide, 2002, by Age Group*

ADULTS AGED 15–59 YEARS			ADULTS AGED 60 YEARS OR OLDER		
Rank	*Cause of Death*	*Percent[†]*	*Rank*	*Cause of Death*	*Percent[†]*
1	HIV/AIDS	27	1	Ischemic heart disease	32
2	Ischemic heart disease	16	2	Cerebrovascular disease	26
3	Tuberculosis	12	3	Chronic obstructive pulmonary disease	13
4	Road traffic injuries	10	4	Lower respiratory infections	8
5	Cerebrovascular disease	10	5	Trachea, bronchus, lung cancers	5
6	Self-inflicted injuries	8	6	Diabetes mellitus	4
7	Violence	6	7	Hypertensive heart disease	4
8	Cirrhosis of the liver	5	8	Stomach cancer	3
9	Lower respiratory infections	4	9	Tuberculosis	3
10	Chronic obstructive pulmonary disease	4	10	Colon and rectal cancers	3

Source: World Health Organization, "The World Health Report 2003," at www.who.int/whr/2003.

*The total number of deaths for both age categories combined account for approximately 60 percent of all deaths to adults.

[†]Approximate percent of deaths among ten leading causes.

may be in error. The reasons for errors globally include clerical oversights, disinterest in the actual cause of death (for example, for an old person or for an impoverished person) and failure to list a disease (such as HIV/AIDS or cholera) that is associated with a social stigma. In some regions of world, not only the *cause* of death may be unknown but even the *fact* of death may go unnoticed.

The leading causes of mortality for adults vary markedly by region. For example, about one-third of deaths in Africa were caused by noninfectious diseases, whereas almost 90 percent of deaths among people living in high-income regions were caused by noninfectious diseases.

Among the estimated 7.1 million cancer deaths in 2002, approximately 17 percent were attributed to cancer of the lung; among those cancers, 75 percent occurred among males. The number of lung cancer deaths increased about 30 percent between 1990 and 2000, mirroring the incidence of the epidemic of tobacco smoking in low- and middle-income countries (countries with per capita annual incomes less than $7,911 in United States currency).

Until recently, stomach cancer was the leading cause of cancer mortality worldwide. Mortality from stomach cancer now ranks second, behind lung cancer, as a leading cause of cancer mortality, followed by cancer of the liver and colon/rectal cancers, respectively. The leading cause of cancer mortality among women is breast cancer.

Causes of Death According to Exposure Status

Another approach for identifying the leading causes of death in the United States or elsewhere involves quantifying the health effects of the exposures that cause disease and injury rather than quantifying the types of diseases and injuries caused by those exposures. For example, in 2000, tobacco use was the cause of approximately 18.1 percent of, or 435,000, deaths among Americans. An additional 400,000 people (16.6 percent of all deaths) died from poor diet and physical inactivity leading to diseases related to obesity or being overweight (about 55 percent of American adults are overweight or obese), such as cardiovascular disease, diabetes, and certain cancers (see Box 4.2). In 2004, it was predicted that obesity soon will surpass tobacco use as the leading underlying cause of death in the United States (Mokdad et al. 2004).

Other leading causes of death in the United States in 2000 (Mokdad et al. 2004) include

- Alcohol consumption (85,000 deaths). Alcohol use and abuse cause approximately 38 percent of fatal traffic deaths, up to half of other injuries including burns, drownings, violence-related mishaps, and diseases such as liver cirrhosis and esophageal cancer (Drug Strategies 2000).
- Microbial agents (75,000 deaths).
- Toxic agents (55,000 deaths).
- Motor vehicle crashes (43,000 deaths).
- Incidents involving firearms (29,000 deaths).
- Sexual behaviors (20,000 deaths).
- Use of illicit drugs (17,000).

BOX 4.2

OBESITY AND THE SUPER-SIZED INDUSTRY

ADRIENNE McNAMARA, M.P.H.

The United States, like most other Western societies, is being plagued with fat: fat in regard to the content of our diets and, equally disturbing, fat in regard to our body compositions. According to the 1999–2000 **National Health and Nutrition Examination Survey (NHANES)** data, the age-adjusted prevalence of obesity in the United States is 30.5 percent, compared with 22.9 percent from the similar 1988–1994 survey. (NHANES is a health survey of the U.S. civilian, noninstitutionalized population between the ages of 1 and 74 years.) In addition, the prevalence of overweight has risen from 55.9 percent to 64.5 percent during the same time period. From a public health perspective, this increase is extremely disturbing. The World Health Organization (WHO) recognizes obesity as one of the top ten global health problems because of the disease's causal links to Type 2 diabetes, hypertension, and cardiovascular disease. When looking at the rising prevalence in obesity in Western society, health professionals and epidemiologists must consider the myriad of causes contributing to the epidemic.

Recent debates have centered specifically on the question of blame. Who should be held accountable for making us fat: we ourselves (the consumer) or big business?

The current trend in society appears to be the notion of "bigger is better." This trend applies to our houses, our income, our cars, and, unfortunately, our food consumption. Restaurants publicize their enormous portions and plate sizes. Advertisers convince us of the economic "good deal" of eating more through the increasingly prevalent message of "super-sizing." But is there fault with this practice? Essentially the answer is yes, because more food also means more calories and, typically, greater weight gain. A "small" portion of french fries contains about 210 calories, whereas a super-sized order of fast-food fries contains 610 calories, or approximately one-third of the average total number of calories required for an entire day. From a health standpoint, clearly bigger is not better.

In July 2002, an obese man sued the fast-food industry for causing his weight problems and the subsequent cardiovascular diseases from which he suffers. The plaintiff, Caesar Barber, stated that he ate fast food four to five times each week because it was "convenient and cheap." His claim was that four major fast-food chains failed to disclose the content of their products, along with any potential health risks. The claim was made notwithstanding the fact that the nutritional content of fast foods is available on the World Wide Web for people who have both access to the Web and an interest in finding out the content of fast foods. Another court recently dismissed a similar claim that one fast-food restaurant causes obesity in its customers. The court found that there was no sound causal evidence; an opportunity for future cases, however, was left open.

Box 4.2 continued

The question of "who is to blame" centers on two scenarios. Does the average citizen know the risks involved in eating fatty foods? If so, he or she would be participating voluntarily in an activity known to be dangerous, and consequently assuming the risks—much like participating in an extreme sport, say skydiving. The consumer chooses the product because of its attractiveness (taste) and convenience, and therefore would hold the primary responsibility should ill health effects occur. If, however, the average citizen does not know the risks, even after taking into account the media coverage surrounding health, should the fast-food companies issue a warning label, similar to the Surgeon General's warning on cigarettes? If warning labels need to be posted, then the industry could be held legally accountable for their advertising practices.

Like the alcohol and tobacco industries, the fast-food industry spends billions of dollars each year on advertisements depicting healthy people using unhealthy products—fast-food advertising usually centers on thin people eating fattening foods. The consequences of frequent consumption rarely are advertised, which could be considered unethical. In addition, children are socialized to accept the presence of certain brands of food through profitable (to the schools) school contracts. Approximately 30 percent of public schools in the United States receive funding through fast-food marketing and loyalties to companies wishing to win product allegiance from children and teenagers. Those agreements may be perceived as creating a conflict of interest with the teaching of proper nutrition in schools.

Although the fast-food industry is not promoting sound nutrition, the general consensus is that the responsibility lies equally (or more) with the consumer. It seems that Barber's reasoning for his diet of fast food is the key issue: It is more convenient and economical to buy fast foods than it is to purchase and cook healthy, low-fat food. Most major fast-food chains offer a variety of options for one dollar or less, which is appealing to youth and those with low incomes.

Wherever the "blame" lies, there most likely will be more cases like Barber's because of our culture's tendency to shift responsibility for individual actions to others. Residents of the United States will continue to grow in girth, however, unless substantial changes in food preferences and selections occur.

Note 1: In March 2004, the managers of one fast-food chain decided to phase-out its offerings on "super-sized" portions. The reason for the change was not disclosed.

Note 2: In July 2004, the federal Medicare program discarded its previous policy that obesity is not a "disease," thereby potentially opening the way for medical treatments for obesity, such as stomach surgery and diet regimens to be paid for with federal money under the Medicare program. Medicare is the national health insurance program for people aged 65 years or older, some people under age 65 with certain disabilities, and people with end-stage renal disease (permanent kidney failure requiring dialysis or a kidney transplant). (A.R.)

Dietary risk factors account for approximately one-third of all cancer deaths in the United States (American Cancer Society 2004, at www.cancer.org/).

Listing and emphasizing the leading causes of death by exposure/risk factors in addition to listing the causes of death by disease or injury is crucial from a public health programming and disease- and injury-prevention perspective. Many public health programs and preventive efforts seek to intervene on the root causes of morbidity and mortality and so require an accounting of which exposures/risk factors contribute most to ill health. Several of the models and data that help determine which exposures/risk factors contribute most to ill health are discussed in Chapter 8.

Obesity in the United States

The percentage of Americans who are obese, defined as a **body mass index (BMI)** greater than or equal to 30.0 (BMI equals a person's weight in kilograms divided by height in meters squared, w/h^2), rose from 11.6 percent in 1990 to 22.1 percent in 2002, according to the Centers for Disease Control and Prevention's **Behavioral Risk Factor Surveillance System (BRFSS)** (www.cdc.gov/brfss/). The BRFSS is a telephone survey that monitors health risks among a large sample of U.S. residents with the goal of improving the health of the American people. The percentage of Americans who are obese increased between 1990 and 2002 for people in each of four broad age categories (Table 4.6 and Figure 4.3). As noted previously, obesity now is an epidemic in the United States and may soon surpass tobacco use as the leading risk factor for morbidity and mortality.

TABLE 4.6
Obesity: By Body Mass Index*

Age (years)	18–34		35–49		50–64		≥65	
Year	Median %	# States	Median %	# States	Median %	# States	Median %	# States
1990	7.4	45	13.6	45	15.8	45	12.1	45
1991	8.2	48	14.7	48	16.9	48	12.7	48
1992	8.5	49	15.2	49	17.5	49	12.7	49
1993	9.4	50	15.8	50	18.9	50	13.1	50
1994	10.5	50	16.5	50	19.9	50	14.2	50
1995	11.3	50	17.6	50	21.4	50	14.7	50
1996	12.2	52	18.9	52	21.1	52	14.9	52
1997	12.8	52	18.9	52	21.8	52	16.3	52
1998	13.1	52	20.2	52	23.8	52	16.6	52
1999	14.2	52	20.9	52	25.0	52	18.6	52
2000	15.8	52	22.0	52	26.7	52	18.2	52
2001	16.0	54	23.5	54	27.1	54	19.8	54
2002	16.5	54	23.5	54	27.9	54	19.4	54

Source: National Center for Chronic Disease Prevention and Health Promotion, Behavioral Risk Factor Surveillance System, Trends data, Obesity: By Body Mass Index, Nationwide—Grouped by Age, at www.cdc.gov/brfss/.

*All respondents 18 and older who report that their body mass index (BMI) is 30.0 or more. Denominator includes all survey respondents except those with missing, don't know, and refused answers.

Note: # of states includes District of Columbia, Guam, Puerto Rico, and the U.S. Virgin Islands in applicable years.

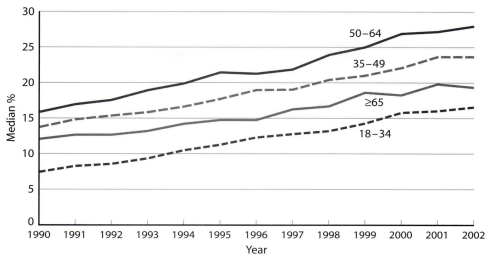

FIGURE 4.3
Obesity: By body mass index nationwide—grouped by age.
Source: National Center for Chronic Disease Prevention and Health Promotion, Behavioral Risk Factor Surveillance System, Trends data, Obesity: By Body Mass Index, Nationwide—Grouped by Age, at www.cdc.gov/brfss/.
Note: Age categories are in years.

Other Leading Causes of Death

As noted previously, decisions regarding the approach used to categorize the leading causes of disease or injury (that is, either by exposure or by disease/injury) affect the priorities targeted for prevention. In addition, exposures that lead to ill health cannot be targeted for prevention unless the exposures have been identified and their contributions to ill health quantified. Identifying and quantifying the health effects of existing or new exposures is a primary objective of many epidemiologic studies. Sometimes the exposures discovered to be harmful are surprising. For example, medical errors are estimated to cause between 44,000 and 98,000 deaths each year in the United States (Kohn, Corrigan, and Donaldson 2000), although some people believe that those estimates are too high (Blendon et al. 2002). Prescription-drug effects result in an estimated 2 million hospitalizations and 100,000 deaths in the United States annually. If true, prescription-drug effects would rank as the third leading cause of death in the United States. **Nosocomial infections** (infections transferred from patient to patient within a hospital, either through the hands of health-care workers or through the contamination of inanimate objects such as clothing and equipment) affect approximately 2 million patients in the United States each year and cause 90,000 deaths. Nosocomial infections might be viewed as the fourth leading cause of death, although it can be difficult to separate the effects of the infection from the effects of disease or injury that brought the patient to the hospital. Between 5 and 10 percent of patients admitted into acute-care hospitals in the United States each year acquire one or more nosocomial infections (Burke 2003).

Worldwide, tobacco use, lack of access to potable water, poor road conditions, violence, poor nutritional status and/or famine, alcohol use, lack of education, lack of empowerment for girls and women, and unprotected sexual encounters are among the primary contributors to the global burden of disease, injury, and disability. Foremost among the underlying causes of ill health globally is poverty and its associated exposures (see Box 4.3).

BOX 4.3

ETHICS MATTERS: DO TROPICAL DISEASES CAUSE POVERTY, OR DOES POVERTY CAUSE TROPICAL DISEASES?

PHILIPPE A. ROSSIGNOL, PH.D.

PROFESSOR, DEPARTMENT OF FISHERIES AND WILDLIFE, OREGON STATE UNIVERSITY

An argument often is put forward that tropical diseases cause economic underdevelopment. In temperate regions of the world, economic development and its consequent affluence bring about an improvement in health because the conditions favorable to the transmission of microbial diseases are eliminated. Tropical or parasitic diseases that are vector-borne and require a permissive environment are of minor importance. In tropical regions, economic development can bring about similar improvements, but associated disturbances of the environment, particularly in drainage, provide increased breeding grounds for vectors and parasites. Benefits to health due to economic development may be negated by tropical diseases.

A two-month stay in Tamil Nadu, India, has led me to reject this outlook. In this area, where poverty is immense, tropical diseases are caused by poverty, and not so much the reverse. Filariasis is a case in point. This mosquito-borne parasite is one of the most obvious of tropical diseases because one of its consequences, **elephantiasis** [extreme enlargement of the legs, scrotum, and sometimes other parts of the body due to the obstruction of lymph channels], is visible, permanent and an indication of high endemicity (10–20% prevalence). One solution to filariasis is painfully obvious and requires little scientific insight. Any decent habitat with screened windows and a solid bed with a bednet will solve this problem, even in an **endemic** area. [A disease that is endemic is present constantly in a population. In the example of the vector-borne tropical diseases, endemic means that the disease-causing agent is transmitted year-round.]

I had great difficulty, however, in purchasing bednets in a town of three million inhabitants because their high price, approximately US$25, created no demand in an area where most inhabitants make less than US$2 per day and sleep under a thatched palm lean-to, if not on the street. If such simple tools are economically unrealistic in poor areas, how can the expensive products of scientific research be of consequence to the vast masses in tropical regions?

Box 4.3 continued

The argument that tropical diseases cause underdevelopment addresses human health indirectly, focusing on the parasite rather than its host. The approach is zoological rather than epidemiological. My outlook has changed, and I now consider economic development as an important step in reducing the tropical disease burden. Long-term economic intervention, in the form of women's education, family planning and development incentives, reduces disease of any type because it attacks the root cause. Economics and social sciences, and not the contributions of "scientific" research, must be seen as the predominant tools of public health. A full and rigorous integration of those fields, particularly of their quantitative and analytic models, into our approach to tropical disease epidemiology is long overdue.

Source: P. A. Rossignol, "Do Tropical Diseases Cause Poverty, or Does Poverty Cause Tropical Diseases?" Reprinted with permission from the *EpiMonitor* 19:9. Copyright © 1994 Roger H. Bernier.

EPIDEMIOLOGY IN ACTION: DISEASE ERADICATION

One of the major public health triumphs of the last century was the worldwide eradication of smallpox. On May 8, 1980, the World Health Assembly officially certified smallpox as having been eradicated. This terrifying disease killed an estimated 400,000 people annually in Europe at the end of the eighteenth century and accounted for approximately one-third of the cases of blindness. Included among the dead during the eighteenth century were five ruling European monarchs. The case fatality rate associated with smallpox typically was 20 percent or higher.

Part of the success of the smallpox eradication campaign can be attributed to the characteristics of the disease. For example, smallpox has no animal reservoirs and no human carrier states. In addition, the manifestations of the disease (skin pox) are easily recognizable and leave residual marks on the skin. Those characteristics coupled with the availability of an effective, heat-stable vaccine made global eradication a realistic goal. In contrast, the worldwide effort to eradicate malaria, discussed in Box 4.4, failed in part because of the complex life cycle of the malaria parasite and the lack of an effective vaccine.

Given the success of the smallpox eradication campaign in preventing this disease for millions of people worldwide, it is especially troubling to ponder its possible reintroduction as a bioterrorist weapon of "mass destruction." In addition, administration of the smallpox vaccine, historically given to young children, now is associated with death from heart failure when administered to otherwise healthy adults.

What other diseases are candidates for eradication? Within the United States, tuberculosis has been targeted as a disease for which eradication may be possible. The practical and ethical considerations of achieving that goal are discussed in Box 4.5.

BOX 4.4

GLOBAL PROGRAM TO ERADICATE MALARIA

PHILIPPE A. ROSSIGNOL, PH.D.

PROFESSOR, DEPARTMENT OF FISHERIES AND WILDLIFE, OREGON STATE UNIVERSITY

The history of malaria control and other vector-borne diseases as well may hold some important lessons for public health and epidemiology. Those lessons, however, remain to be generalized. Were malaria control a building that collapsed during construction, engineers would have spent considerable effort in elucidating the reasons for the disaster. Indeed, specialists in the field of disaster reconstruction exist. The same unfortunately is not true in worldwide health campaigns.

There, however, was some, albeit incomplete, evaluation of the malaria eradication campaign. Indeed, it is clear that the campaign did fail and that several specific, direct reasons for the failure, such as drug and insecticide resistance, were ascertained. What is not clear is whether any basic, underlying assumptions in the design of the malaria campaign were at fault.

A rapid review of history is warranted. Malaria control as such started with the name itself, which is from the Italian for "bad air" and reflects the disease's strong link to the environment. Soon after the Spanish conquest of the Andes, quinine, an antimalarial moiety in the plant of the chichona tree, became an effective drug for the treatment of malaria. Its use in public health, however, was highly restricted. There were never any campaigns to use quinine on a large scale to control the health of populations. Rather, quinine was used initially to treat nobility in Europe, where malaria was rampant, and then used to provide relief to colonials in their outposts. Its effectiveness was dubious, because even Ronald Ross, the discoverer of the malaria life cycle, acquired malaria in India during the late nineteenth century while a student there.

The great campaigns against vector-borne diseases, targeting **vectors** [an animal, often an insect, that is part of the life cycle of an organism that causes disease in humans], started in earnest with the attack on yellow fever in the Americas, first in Cuba, then in Panama, and finally in the Americas more generally. Fred Soper of the Rockefeller Foundation led the campaign against the disease in the Americas and, between the world wars, developed the organizational foundation for such campaigns. The Second World War, and the years just preceding and soon following, brought about an extraordinary convergence of events that made a malaria eradication campaign seem within reach:

- DDT was found to have **residual insecticidal activity** (the lasting ability to kill targeted insects after the time of DDT application). DDT was the first modern insecticide; moreover, it was inexpensive, relatively safe to humans, and had residual and long-lasting effects on mosquito vectors of malaria.
- Chloroquine, a synthetic and far more effective substitute for quinine, was discovered.

Box 4.4 continued

- The United Nations was founded, and the World Health Organization (WHO) became an organizational and coordinating center or "command post" for worldwide health campaigns.
- The great practical theoreticians, notably C. Garrett-Jones and George Macdonald, designed specific targets of attack and evaluation plans for worldwide heath campaigns.

By the 1950s, plans had been made and actions taken to launch great eradication campaigns against old foes, notably smallpox, polio, and malaria. The campaign against smallpox succeeded, the campaign against polio may soon succeed, and the campaign against malaria failed miserably. In fact, the malaria eradication program can be labeled a major defeat for public health. By 1972, WHO realized the futility of its Global Eradication of Malaria Program and terminated it.

The malaria eradication campaign consisted of a highly effective, paramilitary design with coordinated organizations in each country that laid out each geographical area, identified human habitations, assessed parasite levels and transmission parameters, delivered insecticides, evaluated the campaign's local efficiency, and of course routed resources, dispensed information, and trained workers. The United States contributed well over a billion dollars in support of the campaign.

A number of strategic questions must be answered before a second malaria eradication campaign—be it with vaccines, drugs, or genetically modified vectors—is attempted.

- First, not only did the first campaign fail, but also there is evidence that the campaign made malaria-related morbidity and mortality substantially worse, not only in resurgence, but also in resurgence of malaria that now is resistant to drug-based and insecticidal controls.
- Second, the pathogenic potential and attributes of the malaria parasite are important and require a more rational and realistic incorporation into an eradication program. For example, malaria, despite popular perception, is not a killer or a crippler on the same scales as were smallpox and polio. The vast majority of individuals living in malaria-endemic areas suffer little from malaria, even from the so-called malignant species of malaria such as *P. falciparum.* Individuals in epidemic areas, or exposed through travel, whether as tourists, war refugees, or internally displaced persons, tend to suffer the most from malaria. Yet, the eradication campaign targeted all people indiscriminately.
- Third, malaria detection can be difficult, at both the individual and the population levels, requiring sophisticated and therefore expensive training and the always unpopular drawing of blood. The character of human immunity to malaria also is unusual, at least compared with smallpox. Humans do not develop significant, long-term protection against reacquisition of malaria, yet maternal milk (from an infected mother) and constant exposure to the parasite clearly protect against morbidity. The malaria campaign paradoxically, and tragically, removed both of those benefits.
- Fourth, mosquitoes rarely are pests (major annoyances because of their bites) in malarial areas, making their control suspect to local populations.

Box 4.4 continued

- Finally, the goal of the campaign—namely, eradication of malaria based on the control of a zoological target of another organism (that is, the mosquito vectors)—raises serious concerns. Any attempt to bring about a major disequilibrium in an ecological system must be approached with grave skepticism. Even the simplest mathematical models for biologic systems will exhibit rebound and oscillations following a perturbation. Sexual and highly heterogeneous organisms, such as mosquitoes and malaria, can exhibit rapid selection of resistance to insecticides and anti-malarial drugs, as indeed occurred soon after the malaria campaign started. Most important, the ethics and public health benefits of evaluating the effectiveness of campaigns against human diseases using zoological indices, such as mosquito longevity and the **parasite index** (the proportion of individuals in a population in whose blood malaria parasites are detected), rather than indices based on human morbidity and mortality, require serious examination.

BOX 4.5

PRACTICAL EPIDEMIOLOGY IN A PUBLIC HEALTH SETTING: ETHICAL CONSIDERATIONS AND TUBERCULOSIS ELIMINATION

SUE ETKIND, R.N., M.S.

DIRECTOR OF TUBERCULOSIS PREVENTION AND CONTROL,
MASSACHUSETTS DEPARTMENT OF PUBLIC HEALTH

When the incidence and the prevalence of a disease in a given location decline to historically low levels, it is not unusual for discussions about disease elimination to intensify. The remaining cases often are among hard-to-reach portions of the population. A renewed commitment to existing and new strategies often is needed to meet the new challenges of the evolving epidemiology of the disease. Such is the situation with tuberculosis (TB) in the United States in the beginning of the twenty-first century. An example of each strategy, and ethical considerations that are essential to the success of both, will be discussed.

Involuntary Detention of TB Cases

Prolonged treatment schedules, such as those typical of but not restricted to tuberculosis, pose challenges to ensuring that medications are taken according to schedule for the required period of time. Successful adherence to treatment regimens is essential to the success of not only treating the individual but also sustaining a programmatic commitment to disease elimination. The risks of nonadherence include the recurrence of

Box 4.5 continued

active disease (a danger to the infected individual as well as increasing the risk of airborne transmission to others) and development of microbial resistance to the antibiotics. The ramifications extend beyond the individual's health and pose dangers to the well-being of the community, so there are legal precedents for a public health response. One of the adherence measures available is involuntary detention of the individual to ensure adequate treatment. Involuntary detention should be the final step in a range of responses to ensure adherence. Thus, there should be a series of increasingly restrictive steps to follow to ensure that the least restrictive measures necessary are used first before involuntary detention. Due process should be honored throughout, and the individual's constitutional rights must be protected. Detention should be in a medical setting. Putting nonadherent people in jails is stigmatizing and places them in a situation where their medical problem is secondary to the mission of the institution. A medical institution offers the social and psychological services that will deal with the root(s) of the patient- or system-related factors that facilitated a lack of adherence.

Latent TB Infection (LTBI)

Eliminating tuberculosis in the United States will require an extension of the current strategy of identifying and treating people with active disease to include identifying and treating people with latent infections (inactive infections) who are not infectious and pose no risk to others. This raises significant ethical issues. It is abundantly clear from experience that targeted testing among those at greater risk of the condition in question is the most efficient strategy. For TB, that means giving a tuberculin skin test and, if that is positive, following up with additional diagnostic testing. A number of issues are raised, however, when considering strategies for preventing TB disease through approaches concerning LTBI.

- Can testing be conducted in a way that avoids stigmatizing the individuals and communities at risk?
- Should there be mandatory reporting of LTBI?
- Should there be mandatory reporting of selected high-risk groups, such as children under five years of age? This would be a sentinel surveillance system, because children that young who develop TB are likely to do so only if they are a close contact to a person with (possibly unrecognized) TB disease.
- Should testing be voluntary or mandatory? One might be able to argue for mandatory screening of contacts because they are at highest risk of infection and subsequent progression to TB disease. Public health authorities currently retain a registry of all close contacts of TB cases and conduct a contact investigation for all infectious TB cases. This investigation identifies all persons as contacts; skin testing and follow-up of contacts, however, are not mandatory in most states. This is a sentinel system for identifying when or if a person with LTBI develops disease.
- Finally, how should treatment decisions be made for those found to have latent infections? Chest x-rays are the next diagnostic measure for persons with a positive skin test and are the only means of ruling out TB disease. Should chest x-rays be mandatory for all persons with LTBI to evaluate for disease? Should there be mandatory

Box 4.5 continued

treatment of all found to have LTBI or for those (somehow) deemed to be at highest risk of progression to disease? Treatment means medications or antibiotics (with the possibility of adverse reactions) and is a process that will disrupt daily life for a prolonged period of time (usually six to nine months of multiple visits to a clinic and/or visits from a public health nurse or outreach worker to verify adherence to the treatment protocol). All of this is proposed because there is a *possibility* of disease at some time in the future. Thus, a public health intervention is proposed on the basis of a measurable statistical level of risk of developing disease derived from population-based epidemiological data. No predictive or diagnostic test or data to define the actual risk of subsequent disease for an individual exists.

There are no clear answers to this particular work in progress. What is clear is that the issue of latent infections needs to be addressed if we are to successfully achieve TB elimination in the United States. Answers will have to come from active collaborations between public health professionals and the communities at greater risk for latent infections to ensure that a balance can be reached between public health police powers and values such as informed consent and autonomy.

Within the Americas, the ministers of health from the Region of the Americas, working with the Pan American Health Organization (PAHO) in 1994 targeted measles for eradication in the Western Hemisphere by 2000. Although that goal was not achieved, the eradication program nonetheless resulted in a dramatic decrease in the numbers of measles cases. In 1996, only 2,109 measles cases were reported, and in spite of an outbreak of 20,000 cases in Brazil in 1997, the campaign to make the Western Hemisphere measles-free still is deemed an achievable goal (www.cdc.gov). Part of the reason for this optimistic appraisal for measles eradication resides in the characteristics of the disease, which, like smallpox, normally infects only humans (some primates can become infected) and does not survive on its own in the environment.

Globally, the polio eradication campaign, initiated in 1988, set a goal of eradicating polio by 2005. As of December 3, 2002, 1,461 cases of polio were identified compared with only 483 cases in 2001. These numbers of cases compare favorably with the more than 50,000 cases reported to the World Health Organization (WHO) in the early 1980s. The increase in polio cases between 2001 and 2002 largely was a result of a fivefold increase in the number of cases reported from northern India and Nigeria. Over 85 percent of the cases in 2002 occurred in just nine states in India, and in Nigeria and Pakistan. It was estimated that by the end of 2002, polio cases would be restricted to no more than seven countries compared with ten countries in 2001 (www.polioeradication.org).

Communities, such as certain religious groups that prefer not to have their children immunized, are at risk of developing and transmitting a poliovirus (either a **wild type virus** [not from a vaccine that contains a live, modified poliovirus] or a vaccine-derived, live poliovirus). These communities may serve as a reservoir, in which a poliovirus can live and replicate, potentially leading to disease outbreaks among other community members or unvaccinated visitors.

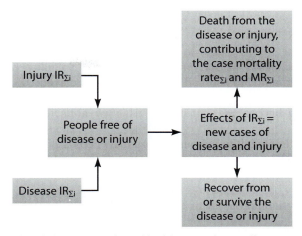

Pictorial representation of incidence and mortality rates.

As a case in point, in October 2005 four cases of polio occurred among a largely unvaccinated Amish community in Minnesota. The **index case** (first case) occurred among an unvaccinated, immunocompromised infant girl aged seven months. The stools from thirty-two family members and close associates revealed three additional cases in unvaccinated siblings living in one household (not the index case's household). In each case the poliovirus was identified as a vaccine-derived virus from a Sabin vaccine. As a result of laboratory findings, it was estimated that the virus had been replicating in human populations for approximately two years. The most likely source of the virus was from an international visitor, because the specific strain of poliovirus identified had not been used in the polio vaccine in the United States since 2000 or in Canada since 1997. (www.cdc.gov/mmwr/mmwr_wk.html)

Whether the polio eradication campaign ultimately will be successful depends on a variety of factors, including the ability to interrupt transmission in countries, such as Egypt, India, and Nigeria, in which gaps in immunization coverage still occur and local sentiments about the safety of the polio vaccine may hinder compliance with the campaign (see, for example, Raufu 2004). A "Polio Endgame" plan has been developed as part of the Global Eradication Initiative. The Polio Endgame plan calls for **polio containment** (minimizing the risk of an accidental or intentional reintroduction of wild-type polioviruses into the environment), **certification** (the official verification that the poliovirus has been interrupted in a WHO region), and the development of a **postcertification immunization policy** (deciding whether and how immunization against polio can be stopped).

SUMMARY

Incidence rates are the most fundamental measures of disease and injury frequency in epidemiology. Mortality rates, companion measures, are incidence rates in which the health outcome of interest is death rather than a new case of disease or injury. For that reason, knowledge of mortality rates also is basic to understanding the dynamics of health and disease in human populations.

Disease and injury incidence and mortality rates can be viewed as forces that press on a population to move members of the population from one state of health to another. The *effects* of those rates acting on a population are to move people from a state of good health to a state of injury or disease (incidence rates) or to remove people from the population (mortality rates). Related to those rates are the concepts of case fatality, case recovery or cure, and surviving with a disease or an injury (being a **prevalent case** of disease or injury, as discussed in Chapter 5).

The dynamics of incidence and mortality rates (IRs and MRs) may be depicted pictorially as follows. The subscript ($_{\Sigma i}$) for the IR and MR refers to the IR or MR for each disease or injury that is pressing on a population.

The magnitude of IRs and MRs may vary considerably according to variables such as age; gender; environmental exposures, including nonpotable water, toxicants, polluted air, and weather patterns; occupation; nutrition; tobacco use; alcoholic beverage use; level of physical fitness; genetic makeup; exposure to and age of exposure to infectious agents or to human parasites; and access to health care, including the availability of vaccines. Diseases and, often, injuries occur as a result of a combination of exposures acting together in individuals. An example is tuberculosis in which infection by the tuberculin bacillus does not invariably result in active disease (see, for example, Box 4.5). Another example is smoking tobacco and the incidence of any of the numerous tobacco-related diseases (lung cancer, emphysema, bladder cancer, and oral cancer among others): Why do some tobacco smokers live long lives but others succumb to a tobacco-related disease at a young age? For some diseases, such as certain sites and cell-types of cancers, exposures may result in disease only when the exposures occur in specific temporal patterns in which one or more exposures initiate the process of cancer development, whereas other, later exposures promote the process.

As you read through the subsequent chapters, remember that diseases and injuries occur within causal webs that include not only suspected causes and preventives of disease or injury but also other educational, cultural, social, economic, legal, and political factors that may influence the probability of good or ill health. Recall also that physical boundaries that used to lessen the transmission of pathogens (such as West Nile virus, and the etiologic agents for SARS and for dengue fever) and other factors (such as hazardous wastes, the sale of cigarettes, availability of "infant" formula, pharmaceuticals, mad-cow-infected beef, "fast food" products, and pesticide residues on foods) from one geographic area to another no longer function as major obstacles to disease transmission. Epidemiologists now must consider the effects of international trade agreements on the import and export of potentially harmful consumer and industrial products, the increase in the rapid movement of potentially ill people by airplanes, and the migration or displacement of ill people from one geographic area to another in their attempts to understand the health statuses of populations.

REVIEW QUESTIONS

1. Define "incidence rate (IR)." What are the two components of an IR, and how is each component measured?

2. What is meant by "restricting an IR" to people of a certain kind? Why is restriction a useful idea in reference to an IR?
3. Define "International Classification of Diseases Code (ICD code)."
4. Why is it important to include only newly diagnosed cases of disease when calculating an IR?
5. Define "person-time." How is person-time measured?
6. Define "cohort study."
7. What is meant by "lost-to-follow-up"?
8. What are the differences among "crude IR," "category-specific IR," and "age-adjusted IR"?
9. Define "mortality rate (MR)." How does an MR differ from an IR? When is an MR a good estimate of the corresponding IR?
10. How does an MR differ from a "case fatality rate"?
11. Compare the leading causes of death in the United States with the leading causes of death worldwide. What factors might account for any differences among these mortality rates? Do mortality rates differ among geographic regions within the United States?
12. Why was the global smallpox eradication program successful? Why is it likely that the global polio eradication program will be successful? Why did the global malaria program fail?
13. List the advantages and the disadvantages of listing causes of death by disease/injury and/or according to causal exposure statuses.

REVIEW EXERCISES

1. The data below come from a study of an outbreak of aseptic meningitis associated with a mass vaccination campaign with an urabe-containing measles-mumps-rubella vaccine in Brazil (Dourado et al. 2000). (Urabe AM9 is the strain of mumps used in the vaccine.) The campaign was conducted among children ages 1 through 11 years. Using these data, calculate the crude and age-specific precampaign and postcampaign incidence rates of aseptic meningitis in this population. Notice that the unit for person-time is *person-months* rather than *person-years*.

Age Group (years)	23 Weeks Pre-Campaign			10 Weeks Post-Campaign		
	Cases of Aseptic Meningitis	Person-Months	Incidence Rate ?	Cases of Aseptic Meningitis	Person-Months	Incidence Rate ?
1–3	9	2,658,294		15	462,312	
4–8	12	4,531,920		37	788,160	
9–11	8	3,282,698		6	570,904	
Total	29	10,472,912		58	1,821,376	

2. In epidemiology, incidence rates that are similar in magnitude often are combined, allowing the data to be presented in fewer categories of, for example, age or gender. With that idea in mind, calculate the ten age-specific incidence rates for the following data. Then, combine the data for adjacent ages for which the incidence rates are

similar, and recalculate the incidence rates. How many age-specific incidence rates do you need to accurately reflect the differences in incidence rates according to age in this population? Is the magnitude of the incidence rate modified by age?

Age (years)	Number of Cases	Number of Person-Years	Incidence Rate ?
1	45	1,000	
2	150	3,500	
3	175	2,500	
4	270	4,000	
5	72	1,000	
6	210	2,000	
7	470	4,500	
8	360	3,500	
9	265	2,000	
10	465	3,500	

3. The following data come from a study of animal bites to people in Benton County, Oregon (Sherburne, Rossignol, and Wilson 1997). In which age categories are the animal bite *rates* the highest? In which age categories are the animal bite *rates* the lowest? Can you think of environmental or behavioral explanations for this variation in animal bite rates? In which age categories are the *numbers* of animal bites the largest? In which age categories are the *numbers* of animal bites the smallest? Are there enough data provided to answer these questions? Why or why not?

Age Category (years)	# Animal Bites per 100,000 Person-Years
0–4	363
5–9	284
10–14	264
15–17	200
18–19	57
20–24	69
25–29	89
30–34	128
35–39	123
40–44	105
45–49	157
50–59	115
60 and older	68

4. The following are hypothetical data from a (small) cohort study with person-time denominators. Each subject was followed for seven years unless indicated otherwise. The outcome of interest is coronary heart disease (CHD). Using these data, calculate the CHD IR and MR. ("DX" means "is diagnosed.")

Person	Length of Follow-Up	Outcome
1	3 years	Lost-to-follow-up
2	7 years	End of the study
3	4 years to CHD DX; 7 years total follow-up	DX with CHD; still alive at the end of the study
4	5 years to CHD DX; 6 years total follow-up	DX with CHD; dies from CHD one year later
5	2 years	DX with CHD in ER; dies in the ER from CHD
6	6 years	Lost-to-follow-up
7	7 years	End of the study
8	7 years	End of the study; develops CHD one year later

5. Using the following data, calculate and compare (a) the crude incidence rates for Populations A and B, (b) the gender-adjusted incidence rates for Populations A and B using the distribution of person-years in Population A as the weights, and (c) the gender-adjusted incidence rates for Populations A and B using the distribution of person-years in Population B as the weights. What effect(s), if any, does the distribution of person-years for males and for females in each population have on the crude and gender-adjusted incidence rates?

	Population A				Population B		
	Males	Females	Both Genders		Males	Females	Both Genders
Number of new cases	600	100	700	Number of new cases	150	800	950
Number of person-years	4,000	1,000	5,000	Number of person-years	3,000	4,000	7,000

See selected answers for exercises 1–5 on page A-1.

■ **SPECIAL CASE STUDY:**

Public Health in Afghanistan

John S. Monro, D.V.M., M.S.

The technology of modern warfare has reduced Afghanistan to a premodern level of existence. The Afghan war consisted of two phases: the Soviet conflict (1979–1992), which ended with the withdrawal of Soviet forces, but which was then transformed into the second phase, civil conflict (1992–2001) between rival Mujahideen groups and militias that could never settle on an acceptable power-sharing agreement. Civil war finally ended with the victory of American-supported Northern Alliance forces over the Taliban (whose organizational roots sprang from Islamic religious schools [madrasahs] based in rural Pakistan and Afghanistan) and the al-Qaeda forces loyal to Osama bin Laden.

The Afghan war was one of the deadliest and most persistent conflicts of the second half of the twentieth century. Nearly 2 million Afghans were killed, and 600,000 to 2 million more were wounded. Over 6 million fled to Pakistan and Iran, and at least 2 million more were internally displaced. At least 50 percent of the Afghan indigenous population, now estimated to be 22 million, became casualties—killed, wounded, or made homeless by war. Half of Afghanistan's 24,000 villages were destroyed, cities were reduced to rubble, and roads were destroyed and farms made unsafe as a result of antipersonnel mines. Social and political institutions were destroyed or irrevocably altered, especially government institutions, armed forces, political organizations, and universities (Goodson 2001).

Over two decades of war, four years of drought, extreme poverty, and a lack of any kind of civil cohesiveness have destroyed Afghanistan's public health infrastructure. War and drought have decimated agriculture. Fifty percent of the population is at risk of malnutrition and micronutrient deficiency, exacerbating susceptibility to endemic infectious diseases. Acute and chronic malnutrition in children are estimated at 10 and 50 percent, respectively. Micronutrient deficiencies such as scurvy and night blindness have become serious problems due to diets deficient in vitamins C and A (Ahmad 2002). Less than 12 percent of the population has access to potable water. Vaccination programs have largely been abandoned or interrupted, and controllable and preventable infectious diseases threaten to explode to epidemic proportions.

Not surprisingly, Afghanistan has some of the worst developmental indicators in the world. Average life expectancy has fallen to less than 46 years, nearly 20 years less than in economically developed countries. Child mortality of 252/249 (male/female) per 1,000 children and infant mortality of 165 per 1,000 live births are the highest in the world. Annual per capita income has declined to $717. Sixty-five percent of Afghans have no access to health services, and the annual average per capita total health expenditure is only $11 (World Health Organization 2002a).

Afghanistan's professional and intellectual classes and educational system suffered tremendously during the war. Under Taliban control, many doctors and nurses were executed, left the country, or were expelled from their profession and sent to work in the fields (Piedagnei 2002). A 1997 WHO estimate of health personnel in Afghanistan lists 11 physicians and 18 nurses per 100,000 people. Those numbers are in sharp contrast to the physician/nurse proportions of 279/972, 164/497, and 303/497 found in high-income countries such as the United States, the United Kingdom, and France, respectively. Those numbers also pale significantly in comparison with those of neighboring countries (48/45, 57/34, 85/259, 201/484, and 309/1011 reported for India, Pakistan, Iran, Tajikistan, and Uzbekistan, respectively) (World Health Organization 2002c).

Men and women requiring hospitalization were segregated into separate facilities that were usually lacking in basic requirements for health care. The prohibition against female employment prevented thousands of female doctors, nurses, and pharmacists from providing health care even in segregated facilities (Goodson 2001), and because male doctors were not allowed to see them, female patients died from simple wounds. The overall outcome of those policies has been to deny women and many children health care for many years. Even after the defeat of the Taliban, hospitals remain desperate for supplies and funds. Medicines, electricity, and potable water are in demand (Associated Press 2002a).

Lack of adequate emergency care has resulted in Afghanistan having one of the highest maternal mortality rates in the world, at 1,700 deaths per 100,000 live births. Fewer than 6 percent of births are attended by trained medical personnel (Ahmad 2001). An Afghan woman still dies in childbirth every twenty minutes, and three-quarters of babies born to mothers who die in childbirth will themselves die within the first year of life—mostly from malnutrition due to lack of breast milk (UNICEF) (Associated Press 2002b). One-fourth of Afghan children do not survive past their fourth year.

Dilapidated water and sewage systems and lack of clean drinking water, overcrowding and mass population movements associated with refugee-camp conditions, poor personal hygiene, inclement weather, and collapse of vaccination programs have led to high morbidity and mortality from infectious disease (Wallace, Hale, Utz, et al. 2002). Inadequate laboratory facilities and disease-reporting measures limit diagnostic capabilities, and many diseases remain undefined and/or underreported. Nevertheless, available data indicate that infectious diseases are taxing heavily the health of the Afghan populace.

Epidemic cholera reemerged in Afghanistan in 1988, and cholera and cholera-like illnesses have been intermittently widespread in Afghanistan ever since (Wallace, Hale, Utz, et al. 2002). Enterotoxigenic *Escherichia coli* (ETEC), *Shigella, Salmonella,* and *Campylobacter* also are presumed significant bacterial etiologic agents of enteric disease. Over 90 percent of five-year-olds have been infected with hepatitis A.

Acute respiratory disease is a major cause of morbidity and mortality in Afghanistan. Lower-respiratory-tract infections are one of the leading causes of death in children under five years of ages. Adenovirus, influenza virus, *Streptococcus pneumoniae, Mycoplasma pneumoniae,* and *Bordatella pertussis* traditionally have been implicated as causative agents. The level of *Mycobacterium tuberculosis* transmission has always been one of the best mirrors of socioeconomic conditions of a society (Wallace, Hale, Utz, et al. 2002). In 2001, the estimated annual incidence of active tuberculosis in Afghanistan was 325 per 100,000 people, approximately 50 times the year 2000 United States tuberculosis incidence of 5.8/100,000 person-years. Mortality approaches 15,000 deaths per year (Khan and Laaser 2002). The annual risk of infection of Afghan school children between five and nine years of age is 13.7 percent. Bacille Calmette-Guerin (BCG) vaccination may be effective in preventing severe manifestations of tuberculosis in children such as tuberculosis meningitis, but for more than a decade, Afghanistan has had only an intermittent, frequently interrupted tuberculosis control program, and prophylactic BCG programs have been discontinued in almost all health-care centers.

Rabies is responsible for hundreds of human deaths annually in Afghanistan, primarily from the bites of rabid dogs. Packs of wild dogs are common, and there are essentially no vaccination programs or public health controls. From March 1 to April 30, 2001, rabid dogs in the capital city of Kabul attacked more than eighty people. Postexposure human rabies vaccine has typically been unavailable in recent years in Afghanistan (Wallace, Hale, Utz, et al. 2002).

Polio remains a major problem in Afghanistan and regionally is the leading cause of disability among those under fifteen years of age (Wallace, Hale, Utz, et al. 2002). Polio is prevented by vaccination and has been eradicated from most of the world. In Afghanistan, however, it is estimated that only 3–13 percent of children have received their complete set of polio vaccinations (Lambert, Francois, Salort, et al. 1997). Measles, uncommon in most industrialized countries, is responsible for considerable morbidity and mortality in Afghanistan. It has been reported as causing 15.7 percent of all deaths and as one of the top two causes of death in children less under ten years old in Afghanistan's Kohistan district and is a leading cause of blindness among children. A measles epidemic claimed at least 2,000 lives in April of 2000 in Afghanistan. Diphtheria, traditionally a disease of children under fifteen years of age, occurs in any unvaccinated population, and in Afghanistan, case fatality rates are estimated at between 4 and 20 percent. Several hundred cases of tetanus are reported yearly, and that number probably reflects only a small percentage of the true number. Neonatal tetanus, resulting from umbilical contamination within the setting of poor sanitation and low maternal vaccination rates, accounts for a large proportion of deaths, with case fatality rates approaching 90 percent (Wallace, Hale, Utz, et al. 2002).

Cutaneous leishmaniasis (an intracellular parasitic disease transmitted by the bite of some species of sand flies that occurs either in a cutaneous [skin] or in a visceral [internal organ] form) has reached epidemic proportions in refugee camps as well as in the capital city of Afghanistan, Kabul (World Health Organization 2002b). Of the estimated 230,000 Afghans with active disease, more than 90 percent have no access to anti-leishmaniasis drugs because of their high cost (Wallace, Hale, Utz, et al. 2002). Despite its widespread emergence, leishmaniasis remains a neglected disease in Afghanistan. Compared with diseases that have high mortality rates, leishmaniasis has been considered a "cosmetic disease" and of lower priority. Though rarely fatal, the disease frequently results in permanent scarring, a stigma that may be associated with social exclusion, further marginalizing Afghan women, and with long-term disability.

Key to impacting these negative public health indicators is the development of a successful public health infrastructure that is dependent upon the emergence of a functioning Afghan state. Deep and multifaceted cleavages in the Afghan populace challenge the existence and eventual rebuilding of the Afghan nation. Afghanistan exists not as a homogeneous populace but as a collection of disparate groups divided along ethnic, linguistic, religious, and racial lines. Ethnicity, based on language and self-identity, is the most important factor in shaping Afghanistan. There are more than twenty-five distinct groups in Afghanistan. This Afghan ethnic mixture traditionally has shown a high propensity for violence, often between ethnic groups, subtribes, and even cousins. Only outside threats seem to unite Afghans, and those alliances are temporary and limited. When the threat is eliminated or reduced, people typically return to regular patterns of warfare (Goodson 2001). But, for lasting change, a semblance of national unity must occur and policies that revitalize economic and social life must be implemented by a legitimate central government.

Most of Afghanistan's domestic economic production had centered on subsistence agriculture, which was severely disrupted by war. Almost two-thirds of Afghanistan's people live off the land, and the success of the harvest is fundamental to the recovery and stability of the nation. Approximately 30 million antipersonnel mines were scattered around the Afghanistan countryside by the Soviet Army and the Afghan Communist government, and subsistence economies were deliberately destroyed. Although mine clearing has been under way for over a decade, there still are an estimated 10 million mines throughout Afghanistan, making resettlement of some areas and resumption of traditional economic activities there still dangerous. Indeed, nearly 300 Afghans lose their lives or limbs each month as a result of mine incidents. The prevalence of land-mine-caused disabilities to men older than fifteen years has been estimated at 9.5 per 1,000 men (Andersson, da Sousa, and Paredes 1995; Lambert, Francois, Salort, et al. 1997). It may cost as little as $3 to produce a land mine. It costs $300–$1,000 to remove one. Approximately half of the irrigation canals were destroyed or abandoned during the war.

Four consecutive years of drought have dried up many rivers used for irrigation as well. The success of "high yield" crops such as wheat and barley, dependent upon irrigation for water, has been curtailed. Seeds for landrace crops, which rely on rainfall for water and which have adapted to survive in locally harsh environments, have seemingly been lost for future harvests. The war and the drought have decimated many of the agricultural areas where landrace crop-seed, fundamental to the recovery of Afghanistan agriculture, was grown. Famine has been so severe that starving refugees have eaten the surplus stored seed (Charles 2002; McDowell 2002).

Destruction of the traditional agricultural economy opened the door to the growth of a narcotics subsector that has become increasingly important (Goodson 2001). In the 1980s and 1990s, farmers switched from a wheat-based agriculture to growing opium, which proved to be a more lucrative crop. (Afghanistan produced more that 75 percent of the estimated 1999 global output of 6,000 metric tons.) Opium poppies require less irrigation than wheat, the residue provides fuel for the winter, it has medicinal value, the oil is used for cooking and oil cake for winter fodder, and the opium resin commands large profits and is easily transportable. It is doubtful that farmers could be persuaded to switch back to wheat farming, given the advantages of poppy production over other crops (Goodhand 2002).

The destruction/dispersion of an already small educated/professional group has left Afghanistan among the five lowest-ranked countries in literacy. Less than one-third of the total adult population can read and write. Women have literacy rates of approximately 15 percent (Goodson 2001).

There are few young engineers, physicians, and scientists to provide the technical and scientific leadership that this ravaged country needs. Afghanistan also has been deprived of most of its finest administrative and technical talent, which could have assisted the country in its recovery. A huge, long-term commitment by international lenders to rebuilding the institutions and infrastructure that make up civil society will be required to create lasting change (Starr 2002).

To restore Afghanistan's public health infrastructure, long-term commitments are necessary to rebuild potable water, irrigation, and sewage programs; transportation systems; agricultural self-reliance; medical facilities; and schools and educational programs to train the indigenous population to become physicians, nurses, and various other public health personnel. Donors have tended to fund shorter-term, relief-oriented activities, such as food aid, mine clearance, refugee return, and short-term health care. The longer-term work, such as improvements in livelihood, education, agriculture and animal husbandry, and water and sanitation, however, has received very limited funds. For donors, large-scale developmental assistance with national orientation has become conditional upon durable peace (which is unlikely to occur) and palatable human rights practices rather than upon humanitarian need (Atmar 2001; Macrae and Leader 2001).

Following the Soviet withdrawal in 1989, the perception of Afghanistan in the West changed from heroic freedom fighters to brutal, sexist bandits, even though the individuals remain largely unchanged. In addition, with the rise of the Taliban, large-scale developmental assistance was withheld because of the Taliban's discriminatory practices, specifically in regard to basic rights for women, and continued conflict.

Afghanistan now is caught in an era of "ethical foreign policy" linked to protection and advancement of human rights, where the principle of impartiality has systematically fallen victim to the political considerations of donor states (Atmar 2001). Although the Taliban have been defeated and have retreated to their villages, conditions in Afghanistan are not so different now from those that fostered the Taliban's rise to power. Violence and lawlessness, government abuse and corruption, unemployment, hunger, poverty, and regional fighting between competing warlords accurately describes Afghanistan's current situation.

Militant Islamic schools in Pakistan, from which the Taliban movement arose, still operate. Gender-equality issues that resulted in aid conditionalities and withdrawal of aid during Taliban rule predate the Taliban and, even now, girls' schools located outside the capital have been rocketed and attacked (Associated Press, September 14, 2002). What may be required for Afghanistan's survival is an acceptance from the international donor community "that it is possible to negotiate principled goals from 'unprincipled people' or those who have different principles" (Macrae and Leader 2001).

REFERENCES

1. Ahmad, K. 2002. Scurvy outbreak in Afghanistan prompts food aid concerns. *Lancet* 359 (9311): 1044.

2. _____. 2001. WHO and humanitarian aid groups take first steps to rebuild Afghanistan. *Lancet* 358 (9296): 1884.

3. Andersson, N., C. P. da Sousa and S. Paredes. 1995. Social cost of land mines in four countries: Afghanistan, Bosnia, Cambodia, and Mozambique. *British Medical Journal* 311: 718–21.

4. Associated Press. 2002. *Eugene (OR) Register-Guard.* September 14.

5. Atmar, M. H. 2001. Politicisation of humanitarian aid and its consequences for Afghans. *Disasters* 25 (4): 321–30.

6. Charles, D. 2002. Agriculture: Reseeding project offers aid to strapped Afghani farmers. *Science* 295 (5563): 2200.

7. Goodhand, J. 2002. From holy war to opium war? A case study of the opium economy in north-eastern Afghanistan. *Disasters* 24 (2): 87–102.

8. Goodson, L. P. 2001. *Afghanistan's endless war: State failure, regional politics, and the rise of the Taliban.* Seattle: University of Washington Press.

9. Khan, I. M., and U. Laaser. 2002. Burden of tuberculosis in Afghanistan: Update on a war-stricken country. *Croatian Medical Journal* 43 (2): 245–47.

10. Lambert, M. L., I. Francois, C. Salort, et al. 1997. Household survey of locomotor disability caused by poliomyelitis and landmines in Afghanistan. *British Medical Journal* 315: 1424–1425.

11. Macrae, J. and N. Leader. 2001. Apples, pears and porridge: The origins and impact of the search for "coherence" between humanitarian and political responses to chronic political emergencies. *Disasters* 25 (4): 290–307.

12. McDowell, N. 2002. Seed imports raise hopes of Afghan recovery. *Nature* 417 (6884): 7.

13. Piedagnei, J. M. 2002. Separating humanitarian aid from politics. *British Medical Journal* 324 (7333): 319.

14. Starr, K. 2002. Ending the cycle-turning crisis into opportunity in Afghanistan. *Western Journal of Medicine* 176:6–7.

15. Wallace, M. R., B. R. Hale, G. C. Utz, et al. 2002. Endemic infectious diseases of Afghanistan. *Clinical Infections Diseases* 34 (Suppl. no. 5): S171–207.

16. World Health Organization. 2002a. Afghanistan. www.who.int/country/afg/en/ (accessed December 24, 2002).

17. _____. 2002b. Communicable Disease Surveillance and Response (CSR): Leishmaniasis in Afghanistan—Update. www.who.int/disease-outbreak-news/n2002/june/28bjune2002.html (accessed June 28, 2002).

18. _____. 2002c. WHO estimates of health personnel. www3.who.int/whosis/health_personnel/health_personnel.cfm (accessed August 30, 2002).

## CHAPTER 5

Prevalence and Its Application to Screening Programs

The second measure of disease frequency is **prevalence,** which is abbreviated P. Some epidemiologists prefer to use the phrase "**prevalence rate,**" rather than "prevalence." The two terms refer to the same measure of disease frequency.

Prevalence is defined as the proportion of a population that has a particular disease, injury, or risk factor at a specific point in time. For example, the estimated global prevalences of HIV/AIDS among adults in 2001 or 2003 (the most recent data available) ranged from almost 0 in some countries, including Afghanistan (0.01%), Qatar (0.09%), Saudi Arabia (0.01%), Svalbard (0%), Syria (less than 0.01%), and Tunisia (less than 0.01%), to over 30% in Botswana (37.3%) and Swaziland (38.8%). The prevalence of HIV/AIDS among adults in the United States in 2001 was 0.6% (World Factbook 2006).

Prevalence refers to existing cases of disease or injury and not to newly diagnosed cases, as does the IR. Because prevalence is a proportion, of the form $a/(a + b)$, this measure of disease frequency does not have units associated with it. In that respect, P differs from the IR, which always has the unit of (1/time). In the formula $a/(a + b)$, a is the number of existing cases of disease or injury in the population of interest, and b is the number of people not having the disease or injury in the population of interest.

Because prevalence is a proportion, the range of possible values for prevalence extends from 0 (no one in the population has the disease or injury) to 1 (everyone in the population has the disease or injury). Prevalence usually is expressed as a percentage ranging from 0% (no one in the population has the disease or injury) to 100% (everyone in the population has the disease or injury).

Sometimes, rather than measuring the proportion of a population that has a certain disease or injury at a specific point in time, prevalence is used to refer to the proportion of a population that has a certain risk factor for disease or injury. For example, the prevalence of tobacco smoking, unsafe sexual practices, low levels of physical activity, or obesity in a population may be measured to aid in planning programs to reduce the prevalence of those risk factors, thereby reducing the future incidence of diseases and/or injuries associated with those factors.

Prevalence can be measured and calculated using either of two approaches, depending upon what data are avail-

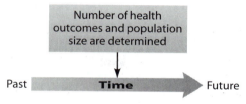

FIGURE 5.1
Cross-sectional survey for measuring prevalence.

able. In the first approach, a **cross-sectional survey** of a population is taken. In a cross-sectional survey, a tally of disease, injury cases, and/or risk factors is taken of people in a certain population at a specific point in time. The number of cases of disease or injury, or the number of persons having a certain risk factor, and the size of the population are recorded, and then P is estimated as P = number of existing cases or people having a risk factor divided by the size of the population (Figure 5.1).

As an example of calculating P from a cross-sectional survey, the estimated **crude prevalence** (overall prevalence for all people in a certain population) of diabetes in the United States in 2002, based on a cross-sectional survey, was 6.3% and increasing rapidly (http://www.cdc.gov/diabetes/pubs/factsheet.htm). The **age-specific prevalences** of diabetes in the United States were 0.25%, 8.7%, and 18.4% for people under the age of 20 years, people aged 20 to 64 years, and people aged 65 years or older, respectively.

As another example of estimating prevalence using a cross-sectional survey, in 2001, the U.S. prevalence of **low-birth-weight babies** (infants weighing less than 2,500 grams at birth) was 7.7% of all live births (U.S. Department of Health and Human Services 2003). The prevalence of low-birth-weight infants is of public health importance because low birth weight is a risk factor for the occurrence of congenital malformations and for conditions of the mother such as poor nutrition, tobacco use, or drug use during pregnancy.

Box 5.1 discusses several of the ethical challenges associated with the medical treatment of infants having **extremely low birth weight (ELBW).** ELBW infants are newborns weighing 1,000 grams or less, or born at 27 weeks' gestation or earlier. A related topic, assessing the cost-effectiveness of intensive neonatal care, sometimes is expressed in terms of **quality-adjusted life years (QALYs).** QALYs measure not only the average length of life but also the quality of the remaining years of life. There are a number of different approaches to estimating the "quality" of remaining years of life. Many of those approaches are based on a person's ability to perform certain tasks, such as walking, and conducting usual activities, such as going to work or school, and on a person's level of pain/discomfort and emotional state. For additional information about QALYs, see www.evidence-based-medicine.co.uk.

The second approach for measuring P takes advantage of the fact that P is a mathematical function of the IR of disease or injury and of D, the average duration of the disease or injury. Specifically, $P = (IR * D)/(1 + (IR * D))$. This approach shows the explicit mathematical relationship between P, IR, and D. Specifically, the formula

BOX 5.1

ETHICS MATTERS: BABY DOE REGULATIONS AND THE CARE OF PREMATURE INFANTS

KATHY BLAUSTEIN, M.P.H.

"Gandhi once wrote that the greatness of a nation and its moral progress can be judged by the way its animals are treated. I would also add, by the way its children are treated" (Mother Hildegard George).

In 1982, a baby was born to a family in Bloomington, Indiana. The baby suffered from esophageal defects, a heart defect, and Down syndrome. After consulting with attending physicians, the parents were told that their baby would likely suffer severe mental retardation. The parents of Baby Doe, so named to protect the family's privacy, declined surgery to correct the medical defects. Their decision to have the baby sedated, while withholding nutrition and hydration, was challenged in court by some of the hospital staff. The Indiana State Court upheld the parents' decision, but it was appealed to the United States Supreme Court. While awaiting a decision and six days after life support was withheld, Baby Doe died.

In 1984, Congress passed the Child Abuse and Treatment Act, the revised Baby Doe regulations, which defined the withholding of "medically indicated" treatment as child abuse and neglect. The act allows for treatment to be withheld only when (1) the infant is chronically and irreversibly comatose, (2) treatment would be "futile" and "merely prolong dying," or (3) treatment would be both "virtually futile in terms of survival of the infant" and "inhumane." The terms *futile, virtually futile,* and *inhumane* were not clearly defined, making the act difficult to interpret in a clinical setting. The result is that the majority of infants born extremely prematurely receive maximal life-prolonging treatment.

Today's technological and medical advances give neonatologists the ability to prolong life for even extremely-low-birth-weight (ELBW) babies, defined as having a birth weight of 1,000 grams (2.2 pounds) or less or born at 27 weeks of gestation or earlier. Babies weighing between 500 and 750 grams at birth have only a 54 percent probability of survival. Of babies weighing 751–1,000 grams, 86 percent survive. Although gains in neonatal and perinatal care continue to improve survival rates of these tiny babies, there appears to be no improvement in the neurodevelopmental problems they experience. ELBW babies who survive infancy go on to develop a multitude of physical, behavioral, and mental problems that reduce the quality of their lives and require intensive and continuing medical and financial support (Frader 2000; LEND Fellows 2002).

The Baby Doe regulations have created an ethical dilemma for physicians, families of ELBW babies, and society at large. The rights of ELBW babies to have access

Box 5.1 continued

to the best medical care our society can offer them (what kind of care is ethical in this situation?) must be weighed against the rights of their families and physicians to make informed decisions based on the medical facts unique to each case, the ability and desire of the family to make the necessary financial and emotional commitment to care for a seriously disabled child, and the ethics involved in prolonging life when the quality of life may be poor. Both the Canadian Pediatric Society and the American Academy of Pediatrics have issued statements encouraging the involvement of parents in decision making. Both societies support the primacy of parental decisions for all infants who are at the threshold of viability.

An assessment of the cost-effectiveness of intensive neonatal care can be expressed in terms of **quality-adjusted life years (QALYs),** which measure an increase in length of life by quality-adjusted life gained. If an expensive medical procedure results in improved survival but many survivors suffer major disability, the QALY will be reduced. QALYs are similar to DALYs, disability-adjusted life years, in the sense that both measures are used in determining the global burden of disease. This type of assessment should be included when determining the financial and emotional costs of treatment.

Many would argue that the debate over providing medical care for ELBW babies diverts attention and money from the larger problem of preventing premature births. Nearly 12 percent of all births are premature, occurring before 37 weeks' gestation. Each year more than 400,000 infants are born prematurely in the United States. A complicated premature birth can cost from $20,000 to $400,000 per infant, compared with $6,400 for an uncomplicated delivery. Follow-up care for mother and child adds significantly to the cost.

The risk factors and risk indicators for having a pregnancy end with a premature birth in the United States are fairly well documented. Those factors/indicators include poverty, low economic status, low educational levels, minority status, stress, lack of prenatal care, tobacco smoking or other substance abuse during pregnancy, and maternal age less than 18 years. Those same conditions contribute to the development of a multitude of medical and social problems. Working toward eliminating those conditions will help to provide a healthy start for all babies and improve the quality of life for their families.

REFERENCES

Frader, Joel E. 2000. Baby Doe binders. *MS JAMA On-Line* 284 (September 6): 1143. http://www.ama-assn.org/sci-pubs/msjama/articles/vol_284/no_9/jms00020.htm.

LEND Fellows. 2002. Tiny children, tough choices. *Leadership Perspectives in Developmental Disability* 2 (2). http://www.mnip-net.org/ddlead.nsf/TrimTOC/TinyChildren,ToughCh.

shows that to be a prevalent case of disease, not only must a person's disease have occurred (that is the "IR" part) but also the disease must have lasted long enough to be an existing case when the estimate of disease prevalence is made (that is the "D" part).

Sometimes, the relationship between P, IR, and D is expressed as P is approximately equal to (IR * D). This expression for P yields approximately the same value for P when P is less than about 0.10 (10%).

The prevalence formula based on the IR and D should be used only when the estimates of IR and of D are appropriate for the point in time to which the P refers. For example, estimating the prevalence of influenza in January by using the IR of influenza in July will not yield the correct estimate for P because of the marked **seasonal variation** in the IR of influenza. Seasonal variation means that the IR of disease or injury varies in magnitude from one month to the next around the calendar year, as is typical for many types of injuries and infectious diseases. In this example, the IR of influenza in July is considerably lower (usually 0) than is the IR of influenza in the months of December, January, and February.

More generally, the formula P = (IR * D)/(1 + (IR * D)) is appropriate to use when the disease of interest is in a **steady state.** When a disease is in a steady state, the *prevalent **number** of cases of the disease* (the number of existing cases) remains constant over a period of time equal to the longest duration of any single case of the disease. Another way to think about the meaning of "a disease being in a steady state" is to realize that for the prevalent *number* of cases to remain constant, every time a new case of the disease occurs, a prevalent case of the disease terminates through either cure, death, or moving away from the population for which the prevalence of disease is being calculated (Figure 5.2). The rate at which prevalent cases cease to be cases is called the **termination rate.**

A final important point related to the prevalence formula pertains to the meaning of D. Recall that the "D" in the prevalence formula is the *average* duration of disease. In actuality, some cases of the disease have durations that are shorter, and some cases have durations that are longer, than is the average duration of disease. Thus, the dura-

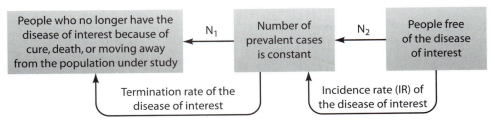

Number of people who no longer have disease *equals* the number of people who develop disease ($N_1 = N_2$)

| People who no longer have the disease of interest because of cure, death, or moving away from the population under study | N_1 | Number of prevalent cases is constant | N_2 | People free of the disease of interest |

Termination rate of the disease of interest

Incidence rate (IR) of the disease of interest

FIGURE 5.2
Depiction of a disease in a steady state.

tions of disease for different cases form a distribution. Understanding that the durations of a disease follow an often predictable distribution is helpful in visualizing the dynamic nature of disease in a population.

EXAMPLES ILLUSTRATING HOW TO CALCULATE PREVALENCE

EXAMPLE 1

In May 1995, a tent-to-tent, cross-sectional smoking health risk survey was conducted in one of the Cuban migrant camps at the Guantanamo Bay Naval Base (GTMO) in Cuba (Bonnlander and Rossignol 1998). One of the objectives of the survey was to estimate the prevalence of smoking and of self-reported chronic respiratory illness among the camp's inhabitants aged 15 years and older. The survey yielded the following data.

Gender	Number of Smokers	Number of Nonsmokers	Total Number of People Surveyed
Males	237	218	455
Females	42	69	111
Total	279	287	566

Based on those data, what are the crude and gender-specific prevalences of smoking in this population? The first approach for estimating prevalence should be used, because the data give the number of existing smokers in the population and the sizes of the populations surveyed. Using the formula P = number of existing cases divided by the size of the population surveyed, we determine that the crude prevalence of smoking in the population is P = (279/566) = 0.49, or 49%. The gender-specific prevalence estimates are P = (237/455) = 0.52, or 52%, for males, and P = (42/111) = 0.38, or 38%, for females.

In the study, 53 of the smokers reported having a chronic respiratory problem such as asthma, **dyspnea** (shortness of breath), or bronchitis. Among nonsmokers, 40 reported having a chronic respiratory problem. Thus, the prevalence of chronic respiratory problems among smokers is P = (53/279) = 0.19, or 19%. The corresponding prevalence for nonsmokers is P = (40/287) = 0.139, or 13.9%.

EXAMPLE 2

Hypothetical data: Suppose that the IR of heart disease in a particular population is (2/100 P-Y), and the average duration of having heart disease is 5 years. What is the P of heart disease in this population? Because data on the IR and D of disease (rather than on the number of existing cases and the size of the population) are given, the appropriate prevalence formula to use is the formula that calculates P from the IR and D. Using P = (IR * D)/(1 + (IR * D)), P = ((2/100 P-Y) * 5 Years)/(1 + ((2/100 P-Y) * 5 Years)) = 0.091, or 9.1%.

If prevalence had been calculated using the approximate formula for P, (P = IR * D), the calculation would have yielded a P equal to 0.1, or 10% (2/100 P-Y * 5 years), compared with 0.091, or 9.1%. Thus, the approximate formula for P gave an estimate that was about 10% higher than the actual prevalence. Table 5.1 illustrates how changes in the magnitude of an IR or in D affect the prevalence estimates based on either the full formula or the approximate formula.

TABLE 5.1
Comparison of Prevalence Estimates Based on the Full or Approximate Formula

IR	D	P Based on Full Formula $(P = IR * D)/(1 + (IR * D))$	P Based on Approximate Formula $(P = IR * D)$
2/100 P-Y*	5 years	0.091 (9.1%)	0.10 (10%)
2/10 P-Y	5 years	0.50 (50%)	1.00 (100%)
2/100 P-Y	20 years	0.29 (29%)	0.40 (40%)
2/10 P-Y	20 years	0.80 (80%)	4.00 (400%)[†]

*Data from Example 2.
[†]Prevalence exceeds the upper bound for the range of possible values for P (range = 0 to 1, or, equivalently, 0% to 100%).

The accuracy of a prevalence estimate depends on the collection or availability of high-quality data either on the number of existing cases or number of people having a certain risk factor *and* the size of the population, or on the incidence rate *and* the average duration of disease or injury. Factors that may affect the quality of the data used in the prevalence formulae include the following:

- Errors in diagnosing new or existing cases
- Inability to identify ill people who lack access to health services
- Under- or overestimating the size of the population or numbers of person-time from whom the existing or new cases arose
- Refusal of some people to participate in a cross-sectional prevalence survey
- Lack of information on the average duration of disease or injury
- Lack of information on *changes* in the IR or D of disease or injury due to effective prevention programs or to improved medical treatments

For that reason, prevalence estimates, like estimates of incidence and mortality rates, should be evaluated critically with the understanding that all data collected from human populations are subject to error from a variety of sources. It is a responsibility of an epidemiologist to assess "how much error may have occurred" and to interpret estimates of disease frequency, and other data on human populations, cautiously.

SCREENING PROGRAMS

A topic related to prevalence as a measure of disease frequency is screening for **preclinical disease,** overt disease, or risk factors for disease or injury. "Preclinical disease" refers to stages in the progression of a disease that occur before the time that a clinician ordinarily would diagnose the disease based on a person's health-related signs and symptoms. Examples of a preclinical disease include small cancers whose symptoms, if any, would not compel a person to seek medical care, high blood pressure (although high blood pressure may be viewed as a risk factor for disease as well as a disease in itself), and **colon polyps** (growths projecting from the lining of the large intestine or rectum that may become cancerous).

The objective of screening *programs* is to identify people who may benefit from early intervention with respect to the disease or the risk factor that was the target of the screening program. Thus, screening *tests* identify prevalent (existing) cases of preclinical disease and include Papanicolaou Smears (PAP smears) to identify cervical cancer and tests to identify risk factors for disease or injury, such as intraocular hypertension for glaucoma. Screening may be conducted either in a clinical setting or in a nonclinical setting such as a school, a community setting, or a mobile medical van. Screening in nonclinical settings often targets populations who are at increased risk of the condition that is the object of the screening program. Some screening tests, such as mammograms, may be conducted either in a clinical setting or in a mobile van. The vans typically try to reach women who may otherwise lack access to preventive health services such as screening tests. Like the prevalence of overt disease, preclinical disease stages also may be in a steady state and may have a predictable distribution of durations. Knowledge of those attributes of a preclinical disease offer excellent opportunities to develop screening programs that are efficient in identifying preclinical disease. For example, knowledge of the preclinical distributions of small breast cancers that are either fast-growing or slow-growing offers the opportunity to design mammography programs that incorporate an appropriate frequency of screening to identify breast cancers early in their clinical progression. Box 5.2 describes an innovative screening program targeting elementary-school children in Wisconsin and also discusses the public health importance of oral health as an integral component of overall health.

The characteristics of a "good" *disease or risk factor* for which to screen differ from the characteristics of a "good" *screening test* and from the attributes of a "good" *screening program.* Each of these aspects of screening will be discussed in turn.

BOX 5.2

PRACTICAL EPIDEMIOLOGY IN A PUBLIC HEALTH SETTING: WISCONSIN'S ORAL-HEALTH SCREENING PROGRAM

PAUL BOLLINGER, M.P.H.

Dental caries (tooth decay) is the number one chronic disease among children aged 5 to 17 years old; it is five times more common than asthma (Centers for Disease Control and Prevention 2000). Dental caries left untreated in children can lead to interference with chewing, difficulty speaking, and significant pain as well as the potential for serious medical problems (U.S. Department of Health and Human Services 2000). It has been estimated that 51 million school hours are lost per year in the United States because of dental-related illness alone (Gift 1997).

The Association of State and Territorial Dental Directors (ASTDD) in its 1998 position paper on "Building Partnerships to Improve Children's Access to Medicaid Oral Health Services" addressed the challenge of improving oral health by writing that "the prevalence and severity of dental disease and the risk factors for dental disease, and the

Box 5.2 continued

myriad obstacles impeding access to oral health care for certain populations, have created a public health crisis in this country. What appears to be lacking, in the macro view, is the political will on both the federal and state levels to engage the problems in any meaningful manner."

In 2001, using the survey methods outlined in the *1999 Basic Screening Surveys: An Approach to Monitoring Community Oral Health* from the ASTDD, the Wisconsin Division of Public Health (DPH) conducted its first oral-health screening called "Make Your Smile Count," a statewide screening of third-grade children in each of the five DPH regions (northern, northeastern, southern, southeastern, and western) of the state. Ninety elementary schools participated in the screening. All third graders in each selected school were eligible to participate. Depending on the preference of the school and school district, **active consent** (permission to screen form is signed by a child's parent or guardian) or **passive consent** (school sends notification to parents and guardians; those not wishing their child to participate in the screening return a form to the school indicating that choice) was used for student participation. A total of 3,307 children (67 percent response rate) were surveyed and received an oral-health screening. Five regional Oral Health Data Collection Consultants (dental hygienists) provided the oral-health screenings.

Recruitment Strategies

The Wisconsin Division of Public Health sent a packet of information to each school's district superintendent and principal inviting schools to participate in the survey. Close consultation with Department of Public Information (DPI) personnel helped to facilitate the dissemination of superintendent and principal information packets throughout the state. Each packet included a cover letter explaining the program, an incentive gift (an oral-health curriculum called FUNDAMENTALS), program permission letters, an Oral Health and Learning Fact Sheet, a letter of support from the DPI Assistant Superintendent and Chief Dental Officer, and a "please fax back" form to confirm participation.

Once school participation was confirmed and a contact person designated, the Data Collection Consultants arranged an appointment with the school, established the number of children and the number of Hmong- and Spanish-translated forms required, and active or passive permission forms. That information was provided to the State Oral Health Consultant, and a packet was sent to the schools in advance of the appointment for distribution of the forms.

Training and Calibration

The Chief Dental Officer and the State Epidemiologist facilitated the training and calibration session for each screening team. Each screening team included a dental hygienist (Oral Health Data Collection Consultant) serving as a survey examiner and a dental assistant (Oral Health Data Collection Assistant). The calibration was a formal session consisting of an evening of orientation, followed by a morning of program operation (including occupational safety, health protocol, and survey protocol), and an

Box 5.2 continued

afternoon of actual practice of the screening. The calibration of the Oral Health Data Collection Consultants and Assistants was conducted on ten children, with the Chief Dental Officer serving as the standard for screening. Differences in the standard were reconciled immediately. Fifty additional children were screened to familiarize the teams with the protocol.

Survey Findings

- *Survey Sample:* Ninety elementary schools participated in the survey. A total of 3,307 (67% response rate) third-grade children received oral-health screenings during a three-month period of data collection in 2001.
- *Statewide Oral Health Needs:* Of the children participating, 39.9% were caries-free, 60.1% had a history of caries, 30.8% had untreated caries, 47% had at least one permanent molar with a dental sealant, 31.1% needed restorative care, 27.1% were in need of early dental care, and 4% were in need of urgent care. (The sum of the percentages is greater than 100% because children could be in more than one category.) Because radiographs were not taken, these findings were assumed to be an underestimation of the dental care that was needed.
- *Racial/Ethnic Disparities:* Compared with White children, a significantly higher proportion of minority children had experienced caries and untreated decay. Of the White children screened, 25% had untreated decay compared with 50% of the African American, 45% of the Asian, and 64% of the American Indian children. More than 11% of the African American and 13% of the Asian children were in need of urgent dental care. Compared with White non-Hispanic children, a significantly higher proportion of Hispanic children had caries experience and untreated decay.
- *Regional Findings:* Of the children screened in the northern region (rural section of the state), 46% had untreated decay, significantly higher than in other regions (36% in the southeastern region, 32% in the northeastern region, 19% in the southern region, and 15% in the western region).
- *Lower-Income Schools:* Children attending lower-income schools had significantly more untreated decay (45%) than did to children in both middle- (32%) and higher-income schools (17%). Eight percent of the children in lower-income schools were in need of urgent dental care.

Lessons Learned and Plans for Improvement

- The Oral Health Data Collection Consultants were subcontracted by DPH to conduct screenings in each of the five DHFS regions. The Consultants were Registered Dental Hygienists with certificates in Community Dental Health or with a master of science in public health. Having highly qualified Data Collection Consultants facilitated the screenings because the Consultants understood the core public health functions and already were familiar with survey methods. The State Oral Health Consultant administered the program through the DPH Central Office. That aspect of the study protocol helped to facilitate necessary follow-up with schools and management of program staff.

Box 5.2 continued

- The Chief Dental Officer and State Epidemiologist suggested that the "please fax back" form for school participation have only a "yes" answer so that nonresponding schools could be contacted directly to request participation. Ninety schools agreed to participate, achieving 100% of the targeted number.
- Difficulties were encountered in determining race and ethnicity for the children screened. Because the Data Collection Consultants were not trained to determine race and ethnicity, it was decided that school rosters would be used to record those data; methods used by different schools to collect and record those data, however, were inconsistent. Race and ethnicity sometimes were recorded together (for example, "Hispanic" identified as race rather than ethnicity). There is a need to include better methods in the collection plan for race/ethnicity data from school records.
- Hourly compensation for the dental hygienists serving as examiners should reflect the state average salary.

The success of Wisconsin's first oral-health screening was made possible by a variety of community and governmental partnerships. The survey provided baseline data and will serve as a catalyst for oral-health program planning, funding, MCH Block grant reporting, education, and advocacy. You cannot be healthy without oral health!

REFERENCES

Centers for Disease Control and Prevention. 2000. Preventing chronic disease: Investing wisely in health preventing dental caries. Available from: cdcinfo@cdc.gov.

Gift, H. C. 1997. Oral health outcomes research—Challenges and opportunities. *Measuring Oral Health and Quality of Life.* Chapel Hill: University of North Carolina, Department of Oral Ecology.

U.S. Department of Health and Human Services. 2000. *Oral Health in America: A Report of the Surgeon General.* Rockville, MD: National Institute of Dental and Craniofacial Research.

Source: The data included in this report were provided by the Wisconsin Department of Health and Family Services, Division of Public Health, Office of Public Health Improvement, Oral Health Program.

CHARACTERISTICS OF A GOOD DISEASE OR RISK FACTOR FOR WHICH TO SCREEN

The characteristics of a good disease or risk factor for which to screen include the following: First, the disease must be able to cause significant morbidity or even death, and that aspect of the disease must be known among members of the population targeted for screening. If a risk factor is the object of the screening, then the risk factor should be a strong predictor of a serious disease. As an example, screening for colon polyps as an indication of an increased risk of colon cancer makes sense because colon cancer is a disease with serious, often fatal, consequences. Screening for the presence of hangnails would not make sense. Members of a population targeted for colon-polyp screening must be aware of the relationship between colon polyps and colon cancer *and* feel personally vulnerable to colon cancer if participation in the screening program is to achieve acceptable levels. In the United States, where colon cancer is a leading cause of cancer mortality, screening for colon polyps is recommended for all people beginning at age 50 years.

Second, the preclinical form of the disease or the risk factor usually must have a high prevalence among the population targeted for screening. If the prevalence of the factor is too low, the screening test will find few cases, resulting in an inefficient (not cost-effective) screening program. How prevalent a factor must be depends somewhat on the seriousness of the disease and the societal and personal costs of failing to identify cases early. For example, all newborns in the United States are screened for phenylketonuria (PKU). Newborns with PKU disease are unable to metabolize phenylalanine. As a result, these children develop brain damage and subsequent mental retardation unless the disease is found early. With early identification, these children can be given a diet that is low in phenylalanine, thereby usually preventing brain damage. Thus, although the prevalence of PKU disease is relatively low—approximately 1 in every 10,000 to 20,000 White newborns and considerably lower among Black newborns—the potential seriousness of the disease makes PKU a good condition for which to screen.

On the other hand, screening for the mutated gene that causes **Tay-Sachs disease** (a fatal genetic disorder in which harmful quantities of a fatty substance accumulate in the nerve cells in the brain) should be targeted at specific risk groups because the genetic mutation that causes Tay-Sachs disease has been found only in certain populations. Those populations include Ashkenazi Jews, French Canadians of southeastern Quebec, and the Cajuns of southwest Louisiana. Patients and carriers of Tay-Sachs disease can be identified by screening for a specific substance in their blood. In the case of Tay-Sachs disease, it may be a couple contemplating having a child that are screened. Both members of the couple must be **carriers** (have the mutated gene) for their child to develop the disease. When both parents have the genetic mutation, the probability is 25 percent with each pregnancy that their child will be affected. At this time, there is no treatment for Tay-Sachs, and most affected children die before age 5 years.

The first time a population is screened essentially is a prevalence survey of preclinical disease or risk factor in the targeted population. The second and later screens of the population probably will find a lower prevalence of preclinical disease, and perhaps of the risk factor if it is able to be modified, because of the large numbers of cases found during the initial screening.

Third, a good disease or risk factor for which to screen must have a "good" screening test available. (The characteristics of a good screening test are discussed in the next section of this chapter.) Fourth, the screening test must be able to identify a preclinical form of the disease at a time when early treatment results in an improved health outcome or to identify a risk factor whose alteration or monitoring results in a lower probability of developing disease.

An example of a controversial screening test is the PSA test for prostate cancer, which uses an increased level of prostate-specific antigen (PSA) to identify the disease. The United States Preventive Services Task Force (USPSTF) concluded that PSA testing is able to identify prostate cancer in its early stages. The task force, however, also concluded that evidence was inconclusive regarding an improved health outcome following early detection and treatment for prostate cancer. In the task force's own words, "Screening is associated with important harms, including frequent false-positive results and unnecessary anxiety, biopsies, and potential complications of treatment of some cancers that may never have affected a patient's health. The USPSTF concludes that evidence is insufficient to determine whether the benefits outweigh the harms for a screened population" (www.ahcpr.gov/, link to PSA, accessed December 17, 2002). In the task force's statement, the phrase **false-positive results** refers to a man's PSA test categorized as positive for prostate cancer when in fact the man did not have prostate cancer. One recent study found that 15 percent of men who consistently screened negative for prostate cancer (had low levels of PSA) were found by biopsy to have prostate cancer, and thus were **false-negatives** (Thompson et al. 2004). In another recent study, an *annual increase* in PSA of 2.0 nanograms per milliliter or greater was a better predictor of death from prostate cancer than was a *one-time, cross-sectional* PSA value (D'Amico 2004).

CHARACTERISTICS OF A GOOD SCREENING TEST

A good screening test has at least five attributes. The test must have a high **sensitivity,** have a high **specificity,** be low in cost and inconvenience, cause few adverse health effects, and be acceptable to the target population. Sensitivity is defined as the proportion of screened people who have the factor that is the object of the screening test who are correctly categorized as having this factor by the test. Specificity is defined as the proportion of screened people who do *not* have the factor that is the object of the screening test who are correctly categorized as *not* having the factor by the test. Sensitivity and specificity are defined symbolically in Table 5.2. In the table, the letters *a, b, c,* and *d* represent the number of people in each **cell** (division) of the table. For example, *a* is the number of people who are positive for the factor in the "real world" and who are categorized as positive for the factor by the screening test.

A good screening test will correctly categorize people as either having or not having the preclinical disease or factor that is the object of the screening test. In a perfect test, all screened people who *have* the factor would appear in the *a* cell in Table 5.2, and all screened people who in *do not have* the factor would appear in the *d* cell.

TABLE 5.2
Definitions of Sensitivity and Specificity

		TRUE ("REAL WORLD") SITUATION	
		Positive for Factor	*Negative for Factor*
SCREENING TEST RESULTS	*Positive for Factor*	a	b
	Negative for Factor	c	d

Sensitivity = $a/(a + c)$.
Specificity = $d/(b + d)$.

For some screening tests, such as the PSA test for prostate cancer, a decision must be made regarding which values of the test will be regarded as "positive" and which values as "negative." In other words, the test does not provide for a dichotomous outcome but rather a continuum of values ranging from "clearly positive" to "clearly negative" and all the values in between. For such a test, the decision regarding where to place the **cutoff point** (test value that divides positive results from negative results) depends in part upon how serious the error of failing to identify a case might be. Will missing a case result in a high probability of serious, adverse health consequences to the person whose result incorrectly was categorized as negative? If the answer to that question is yes, perhaps the cutoff point for the test needs to be more conservative than if the answer is no. Referring to Table 5.2, a more conservative test would result in more people categorized by the screening test as being positive and thus more people in the *a* and *b* cells.

On the other hand, there is a trade-off regarding the percentages of screened people who are categorized as "positive" or as "negative," depending upon the placement of a screening test's cutoff point. For example, a conservative cutoff point, as mentioned previously, probably will result in more screened people categorized as "positive" who in reality do not have the factor that was the object of the screening test. These people, incorrectly categorized into the *b* cell in Table 5.2, may be subjected to extensive, costly, and even potentially harmful follow-up procedures, such as a biopsy, that were not necessary and also may have caused undo anxiety.

The example of PSA for prostate cancer again provides an illustrative example. PSA screening using 4.0 ng/dl as the cutoff point between a positive and a negative test identifies 80–90 percent of prostate cancers. Using a lower cutoff point would detect a greater percentage of cancers but also result in more false-positives and follow-up procedures such as biopsies. This idea is illustrated in Figure 5.3. In this figure, the shaded areas, using a cutoff test value of "A," and in the lighter shading only, using a cutoff test value of "B," denote tests that are considered "positive."

If the test value denoted as "A" is used as the cutoff point for a positive test, the test will correctly classify most of the people *who have* the preclinical disease or risk factor that is the object of the screening test but also will **misclassify** (place a person into an incorrect category) a substantial proportion of people who *do not have* the preclinical disease or risk factor. If the cutoff point for being test-positive is moved to the value denoted as "B," the test will misclassify a larger portion of people who *have* the preclinical disease or risk factor but will correctly classify a larger proportion of people who *do not have* the preclinical disease or risk factor.

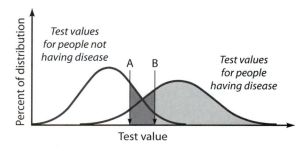

FIGURE 5.3

Effects of changing the cutoff point between a positive and a negative screening-test value.

CHARACTERISTICS OF A GOOD SCREENING PROGRAM

The primary characteristics of a good screening program include a high **predictive value positive,** a high **predictive value negative,** and an improved health outcome for people found by the screening test to have the preclinical disease or risk factor that is the object of the screening program. In Table 5.2, predictive value positive (PVP) is defined as $a/(a + b)$. In other words, PVP is the proportion of people screened positive for the preclinical disease who in fact *do have* the preclinical disease that was the object of the screening program. Predictive value negative (PVN) is defined as $d/(c + d)$. In other words, PVN is the proportion of people screened negative for the preclinical disease who in reality *do not have* the preclinical disease.

Four factors affect the magnitude of the PVP:

- The prevalence of the preclinical disease or risk factor among the population screened
- The specificity of the screening test
- The sensitivity of the screening test
- The "cutoff point" between tests categorized as positive or as negative, as discussed previously

The first factor, the prevalence of the disease or risk factor among the population screened, helps to determine which populations to screen. Often, the goal is to offer a screening program to populations who have an increased prevalence of the condition that is the object of the screening program. Targeting high-risk populations increases the efficiency of the screening program, because the screening test will identify a proportionately larger number of people who screen positive on the test and who have the condition of interest. In addition, populations who knowingly are at an increased risk of the targeted disease may be more agreeable to participating in the screening program, because the disease will be viewed as a serious personal possibility.

The second characteristic of a good screening program, specificity of the test, usually is more influential in determining the PVP than is sensitivity. The importance of specificity can be appreciated by referring to Table 5.2 and Figure 5.3. PVP is determined by the relative sizes of the numbers in the *a* cell and in the *b* cell. In most screened populations, the numbers of people without the screened condition far outnumber the people with the condition. For that reason, even a small downward change in the specificity of a test results in a large increase in the number of people categorized into the *b* cell even though they do not have the condition that was the object of the screening test. A large number of **false-positives** (individuals who screen positive on the test but do not have the preclinical disease or risk factor that is the target of the screening program) can result in a substantial decrease in the magnitude of the PVP. In other words, when the number in the *b* cell is substantially larger than is the number in the *a* cell, most of the people who screened positive for the disease *do not have* the disease in question.

In contrast, a downward change in the sensitivity of the screening test results in fewer people categorized into the *a* cell and more people categorized into the *c* cell. This change usually has little effect on the magnitude of the PVP. This lack of effect occurs because the number of people in the screened population who have the targeted preclinical disease or risk factor typically is substantially smaller than is the number of people in the screened population who are free of this condition.

For a screening program to have an adequately high PVP, the sensitivity of a screening test normally should be at least 90 percent. The specificity of the screening test should be at least 98 percent. A hypothetical numerical example (Box 5.3) illustrates how changes in the specificity and sensitively affect the magnitude of the PVP.

BOX 5.3

NUMERICAL EXAMPLE DEMONSTRATING THE IMPORTANCE OF SPECIFICITY IN DETERMINING THE PREDICTIVE VALUE POSITIVE OF A SCREENING PROGRAM

The hypothetical data in Table A generate the following metrics:

Sensitivity = 90% (900/1,000).

Specificity = 99% (48,510/49,000).

PVP = 65% (900/1,390).

Notice that, in the true situation, 1,000 people have the disease in question, whereas considerably more people (49,000) do not have this disease. In an actual screening program, an overabundance of people in the target population who do not have the disease in question is the usual situation.

TABLE A

		TRUE ("REAL WORLD") SITUATION		
		Positive for Factor	*Negative for Factor*	*Total*
TEST	*Positive for Factor*	900	490	1,390
RESULTS	*Negative for Factor*	100	48,510	48,610
	Total	1,000	49,000	50,000

In Table B, the sensitivity of the screening test remains at 90%, but the specificity of the test is decreased from 99% to 90%, generating the following metrics:

Sensitivity = 90% (900/1,000).

Specificity = 90% (44,100/49,000).

PVP = 16% (900/5,800).

Notice that the change in the specificity of the test resulted in an unacceptably low predictive value positive associated with the screening program.

TABLE B

		TRUE ("REAL WORLD") SITUATION		
		Positive for Factor	*Negative for Factor*	*Total*
TEST	*Positive for Factor*	900	4,900	5,800
RESULTS	*Negative for Factor*	100	44,100	44,200
	Total	1,000	49,000	50,000

Box 5.3 continued

In the final table, Table C, the specificity of the screening test remains at 90%, the same specificity as in Table B, although the sensitivity of the screening test is increased to 99%, yielding the following metrics:

Sensitivity = 99% (990/1,000).

Specificity = 90% (44,100/49,000).

PVP = 17% (990/5,890).

Thus, increasing the sensitivity of the screening test resulted in only a marginal improvement in the size of the predictive value positive, demonstrating that the magnitude of the PVP is determined largely by the specificity of the screening test and not by its sensitivity.

TABLE C

		TRUE ("REAL WORLD") SITUATION		
		Positive for Factor	*Negative for Factor*	*Total*
TEST	*Positive for Factor*	990	4,900	5,890
RESULTS	*Negative for Factor*	10	44,100	44,110
	Total	1,000	49,000	50,000

Why should an epidemiologist be concerned about the magnitude of the PVP? Individuals who screen positive on a test may well undergo expensive, perhaps invasive (for example, a biopsy) medical tests to determine the actual presence or absence of disease. If the PVP associated with a screening program is low, most of the individuals undergoing these additional tests will be found not to have disease. Health-care dollars will be wasted, and the people inaccurately screened positive may suffer physically and psychologically from the follow-up testing.

Of additional concern are individuals who screened negative on the test but who in fact do have the disease that was the object of the screening program. In other words, a low predictive value negative (PVN) also has health consequences. These individuals may be lulled into a false sense of security believing that they are free of the disease in question. Such individuals may ignore early symptoms of the disease, thereby losing the opportunity to undergo early treatment associated with an improved health outcome.

False-negatives (people who screened negative for the disease who in fact *have* the targeted condition) have received less attention in the epidemiologic literature and elsewhere than have individuals who were false-positives. A "good" screening pro-

TABLE 5.3

Estimating Sensitivity and Specificity from People with and without Overt Disease

		Have Overt Disease	*Do Not Have Overt Disease*
SCREENING TEST RESULTS	*Positive for Disease*	*a*	*b*
	Negative for Disease	*c*	*d*

Sensitivity $= a/(a + c)$.
Specificity $= d/(b + d)$.

gram, however, needs not only to identify people who have disease and whose prognosis improves with early detection but also to provide accurate information to people whose tests are negative to help ensure realistic interpretations of their test results.

How are the sensitivity and the specificity of a screening test determined? Originally, these metrics were estimated by applying the screening test to people with overt disease; that is, the test was given to people who already had been clinically diagnosed with the disease the screening test was designed to identify early. The test also was applied to people who had not been clinically diagnosed with the disease in question. Both the sensitivity and the specificity of the test were estimated from the test results for the diseased and nondiseased individuals, as illustrated in Table 5.3.

This approach for estimating the sensitivity and the specificity of a screening test is problematic. A screening test should be designed to identify *early, preclinical disease* and may well function differently for people with overt disease than it does for people having preclinical disease.

A better approach for estimating the sensitivity and the specificity of a screening test is to apply the test to a population that then is followed over time to identify the true health status of each individual at the time the screening test was applied. In that way, referring to Table 5.2, the true health status of all people screening positive for the disease (the $a + b$ people) and the true health status of the people screened negative for the disease (the $c + d$ people) will be known from the results of the follow-up study. From those data, the number for each cell in the table can be entered and, from those numbers, the sensitivity and the specificity of the screening test can be estimated.

As an example, suppose a cohort of 10,000 people is enrolled in a study. At the start of the study, using the screening test whose sensitivity and specificity are being estimated, 1,000 people screen positive for preclinical disease ($a + b$ people). Of these 1,000 people, 100 are diagnosed with the disease during the follow-up period (a people). Of the 9,000 cohort members who screened negative for preclinical disease at the start of the study ($c + d$ people), 150 subsequently are found to have the disease (c people). The sensitivity and the specificity of the screening test can be estimated as follows (Table 5.4):

TABLE 5.4
Numeric Example Estimating the Sensitivity and the Specificity of a Screening Test Using a Cohort Approach

		CLINICAL DIAGNOSIS OF DISEASE DURING THE PERIOD OF FOLLOW-UP		
		Have Disease	*Does Not Have Disease*	*Total*
TEST RESULTS AT THE	*Positive for Disease*	$a = 100$	$b = (1,000 - 100) = 900$	1,000
START OF THE PERIOD	*Negative for Disease*	$c = 150$	$d = (9,000 - 150) = 8,850$	9,000
OF FOLLOW-UP	*Total*	250	$9,750 = (10,000 - 250)$	10,000

Based on those data, the sensitivity of the screening test is 40% (100/250), and the specificity is 91% (8,850/9,750). The PVP is 10% (100/1,000); the PVN is 98% (8,850/9,000).

LEAD TIME

Lead time is defined as the length of time between the date a preclinical disease is identified by a screening test and the date the disease would have been diagnosed by a clinician if the screening test had not found the disease, as depicted in Figure 5.4. Lead time for a particular disease and screening test cannot be determined for any one individual. In other words, if a person's preclinical disease is identified by a screening test, then it is unknown when a clinician would have diagnosed the disease for that particular person. For that reason, lead times are estimated by comparing the distributions of severity, stage, or other pathogenic phases of the disease when identified by a screening test with the distributions of these disease states when the disease is diagnosed by clinicians. The differences between these distributions provide an estimate of how much earlier in the disease process the disease was identified by the screening test compared to the time a clinician would have taken to diagnosed the disease.

Theoretically, the longer the lead time, the greater the opportunity to treat a person at a point in the disease process that increases the probability of an improved health outcome, such as reduced morbidity or mortality. Several early assessments of the degree of improved outcome associated with identifying a disease using a screening test were not valid. Colon cancer screening provides of good example of this point. The error in several of the early assessments of the value of colon cancer screening arose from comparing time to mortality between screened and unscreened populations. A

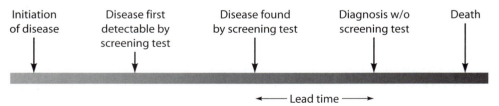

FIGURE 5.4
Depiction of lead time.

presumed benefit of colon cancer screening was made on the basis of a longer time between disease diagnosis and death for screened than for unscreened populations. Reference to Figure 5.4 aids in understanding the error made in this kind of comparison.

As an example, suppose Person A's colon cancer was identified by a screening test when the person was aged 55 years. This person subsequently died from colon cancer at the age of 64 years. Thus, the time between diagnosis and death was ten years. Person B's colon cancer was diagnosed by a clinician when the person was aged 62 years. This person subsequently died from colon cancer at 64 years of age, yielding a time between diagnosis and death of two years.

In this example, did Person A fare better than did Person B? The time between diagnosis and death was ten years for Person A and only two years for Person B, and yet both people died at the age of 64 years. There was no gain in age at death associated with having colon cancer detected by the screening test. In fact, Person A probably underwent a colostomy (a surgical procedure that gives the content of the large bowel an opening through the abdominal wall) and suffered anxiety related to knowing of his or her illness throughout the ten-year interval between diagnosis initiated by the screening test and death. If so, all the screening test provided for Person A was eight more years of morbidity and no additional years of life.

A preferred approach for evaluating the effectiveness of a screening program, in terms of improved health outcomes associated with identification of an early phase of disease, is to compare the age-specific mortality rates for screened and unscreened populations. This comparison answers the question, Did the screening program reduce age-specific mortality rates and increase life expectancy? Other health indicators, including measures of morbidity and quality of life, might be developed to aid in evaluating whether the screening program resulted in a public health benefit.

Weighing the potential risks against the potential benefits of screening programs can be challenging. Examples of those challenges for mammography as part of a screening program for breast cancer in women and prostate-specific antigen (PSA) as part of a screening program for prostrate cancer are discussed in Box 5.4.

FINAL COMMENT REGARDING SCREENING PROGRAMS

Having a screening test available for a population is not synonymous with having a screening program. All true screening programs have provisions for following up on people who screen positive for the preclinical disease condition or risk factor of interest. Offering a screening test to a population will not improve health outcomes without provisions for providing definitive diagnostic tests and, if necessary, medical treatment to people who have the health condition of interest. A positive test with no follow-up may produce adverse health effects if the test result causes anxiety, stress, or other psychological symptoms related to the knowledge of having a disease that is not being treated.

Numerous sites on the World Wide Web, including www.savebabies.org/diseasedescriptions.php and www.cancerindex.org/clinks4p.htm, provide examples of screening tests and screening programs. In addition, books such as *Screening in*

BOX 5.4

WEIGHING THE RISKS AND THE BENEFITS OF SCREENING PROGRAMS

RACHEL WOODS, M.P.H.

Screening programs have long provided the medical community with the means to detect preclinical disease. Some of these programs are beneficial, allowing individuals to improve their medical outcomes and quality of life. It is important, however, to weigh the risks of screening for a particular program against the potential benefits when considering whether to be screened or to refer an individual to a screening program. Consider the cases of screening programs for breast and prostate cancer.

Breast Cancer Screening

Mammography for the early detection of breast cancer has been used widely for years and has proven to be an effective way to find cancer in its early stages, before it invades other parts of the body. Early detection allows for better treatment outcomes and improves quality of life for thousands of women each year. There has been controversy, however, over which women should be screened for breast cancer and the risks of screening women who are not at high risk for the disease.

Breast cancer incidence is highest in women between the ages of 50 and 64 years, and it has been documented clearly that women in this age group benefit tremendously from an annual screening mammography. However, many physicians and health-care organizations recommend also that women between the ages of 40 and 49 years have an annual mammogram. Only 15 percent of breast cancers are found in women under the age of 50 years. Further, evidence shows that to prevent one cancer among women aged 40 to 49 years, up to 2,500 women must undergo screening mammography.

Mammograms miss approximately 20 percent of the breast cancers that are present at the time of screening and generate false-positive results in women aged 40 to 49 years at a proportion of up to 30 percent. Evidence shows that many women, particularly women in the younger age groups, suffer ongoing psychological distress caused by anxiety while false positive results are being evaluated. Many thousands of mammograms are needed to prevent one cancer death, and for each woman who derives a direct benefit in terms of a prevented breast cancer death, hundreds of women suffer the anxiety of a false-positive screening mammography.

Prostate Cancer Screening

Prostate cancer is second only to lung cancer as a contributor to cancer deaths among men in the United States. Prostate cancer is characterized by a wide variability in the rates of disease progression and often by long preclinical, nonsymptomatic disease phases. Many men die with prostate cancer, not because of it.

Box 5.4 continued

One of the principal screening tests for prostate cancer is the prostate-specific antigen, or PSA, test. PSA screening can detect 80 to 85 percent of prostate cancers but has a high false-positive rate. The positive predictive value of the PSA test is only 28–35 percent. In addition, there are potential harms associated with the screening test, including the morbidity associated with evaluating abnormal results and complications from additional diagnostic testing and treatment. Such complications include impotence and incontinence.

Scientists have compared prostate cancer screening to breast cancer screening, implying that prostate cancer screening similarly should reduce cancer mortality. There is no definitive evidence, however, that early detection of prostate cancer reduces morbidity or mortality. Screening does detect prostate cancer at an earlier stage, but it is unproven whether this early detection improves survival or overall quality of life. In addition, screening may detect cancers that would have never caused morbidity or mortality. Thus, the balance between the benefits and the harms of prostate cancer screening remains uncertain in the absence of better evidence.

The appropriateness of screening depends in part on the burden of suffering from the disease, and on the effectiveness, potential harms, and costs of screening. Prostate cancer clearly satisfies the first requirement, but lack of data makes the relationship among its benefits, harms, and costs uncertain. Similarly, breast cancer screening meets many of the qualities of a good screening program, but the benefits and harms associated with screening women under the age of 50 years remain controversial.

Screening programs may burden large numbers of men and women with both psychological and physical complications that may offset potential benefits. Because the best option depends in part on personal preferences, it is important to help individuals understand the pros and cons of screening, to assist them in clarifying their own values, and to encourage them to consider the preferred options with their medical provider.

Additional information concerning breast cancer screening may be found at www.acpm.org/breast.htm and on prostate cancer screening at www.acpm.org/pol_practice.htm, as well as on the Web pages of the American Cancer Society.

Chronic Disease (Alan S. Morrison, Oxford University Press, 1992) and *Psychosocial Effects of Screening for Disease Prevention and Detection* (Robert T. Croyle, Editor, Oxford University Press, 1995) as well as articles in the professional literature are available for more detailed discussion of screening with respect to specific diseases and risk factors for disease.

SUMMARY

Prevalence, like the incidence rate, is a basic measure of disease frequency in epidemiology. Unlike the incidence rate, however, prevalence refers to existing cases of disease or injury rather than to new cases of disease or injury. Whereas the incidence rate measures how fast disease or injury is occurring in a population, prevalence reflects not only how fast cases of disease or injury are occurring but also how rapidly those cases are removed from a population. Cases may be removed from a population by either cure, remission, death, or relocation out of the target population. When prevalence refers to existing cases of *preclinical* disease, as in a screening program, cases may be removed from a target population by being identified as cases by the screening test, by being diagnosed by a clinician (apart from the screening program), or by relocating out of the target population.

Because prevalence is based on two variables, the incidence rate of disease or injury and the average duration of disease or injury, and on factors that affect the magnitude of the incidence rate or average duration, interpreting prevalence estimates among entire populations can be challenging. Do prevalence estimates among populations or among subgroups of the same population differ because of dissimilarities in their incidence rates and/or because of dissimilarities in the factors that affect their average durations of disease? If the prevalence estimates are similar, is the similarity due to comparably sized incidence rates and average durations of disease or injury or to the "balancing out" of the incidence rates and average durations of disease, yielding prevalence estimates that are equivalent? For example, the prevalence estimate would be the same (0.17) in a population having an incidence rate equal to 5/100 P-Y and an average duration of disease equal to four years and in a population having an incidence rate equal to 10/100 P-Y and an average duration of disease equal to two years.

An additional challenge occurs in interpreting prevalence estimates because prevalence is based on the incidence rate and *average* duration of disease or injury. The incidence rates and the average durations of disease or injury may be similar among populations even when the *distributions* of durations of disease or injury are different. For example, an anatomic site of cancer in one population may comprise two subtypes of cancer: one subtype that is fast-growing and rapidly fatal and another that is slow-growing and fatal only after a long period of time. The same anatomic site of cancer in a second population may have no subtypes, and the cancer may grow at a moderate pace and be fatal after a moderate period of time. The average duration of the cancer in these two populations may be comparable even though the distributions of the durations of the cancer differ. This concept is illustrated in Figure 5.5 for two populations. The first population, Population A, has a distribution of clinically diagnosed disease that is skewed to the right, whereas the second population, Population B, has a distribution that is symmetrical.

With respect to screening programs, information regarding the distribution of durations of preclinical disease or of a preclinical form of a disease, aids in determining potential lead times. For example, assuming use of the same screening test, the possible lead times for rapidly growing cancers would be shorter than the possible lead times for slow-growing cancers. Determining the durations of preclinical forms of a disease may be pivotal in designing a screening program. That knowledge may aid in deciding when a screening test first should be offered to a population and how often the screening test should be offered in order to prevent mortality, for example, from rapidly growing cancers or from other rapidly developing but treatable "if-detected-early" diseases.

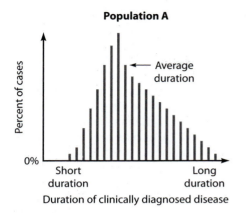

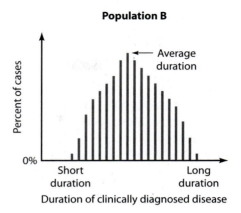

FIGURE 5.5
Illustration of two populations having the same average duration of a clinically diagnosed disease in the absence of a screening program but having different distributions of disease durations.

REVIEW QUESTIONS

1. Define "prevalence." How does prevalence differ from an incidence rate?
2. What is the range of possible values for prevalence? Often, prevalence is expressed as a percentage. What is the range of possible values for prevalence when prevalence is expressed as a percentage?
3. Explain the two approaches used to estimate prevalence. When is each approach appropriate to use?
4. Sometimes the formula $P = (IR * D)$ is used to estimate prevalence. Explain when this formula can be used.
5. What is the primary objective of a screening program?
6. List the characteristics of a good disease (or risk factor) for which to screen.
7. List the characteristics of a good screening test.
8. Define "sensitivity" and "specificity."
9. List the characteristics of a good screening program.
10. Define "predictive value positive" and "predictive value negative."
11. Why are the characteristics of a good screening test different from the characteristics of a good screening program?
12. Why is specificity usually more important than sensitivity in determining the predictive value positive of a screening program?
13. Define "false-negative" and "false-positive."
14. Define "lead time." Why is lead time an important consideration when designing a screening program?

REVIEW EXERCISES

1. The following (somewhat modified) data come from a cross-sectional study of existing musculoskeletal symptoms reported by clerical workers who used personal computers at work in the mid-1980s, before the ergonomic challenges posed by the long-term, almost-daily use of computers were well understood (Rossignol, et al. 1987). Widespread use of personal computers at work was relatively new at that time. Musculoskeletal symptoms included pain or inflammation of the hands, wrists, elbows, shoulder, or back, or the presence of **carpal tunnel syndrome** (compression of the medial nerve at the wrist leading to numbness, weakness, and/or pain, especially in the fingers).

Industry	Daily Personal Computer Use (hours)	Total # Workers	# Workers with Symptoms	Prevalence ?
Both categories of industries				
	0	366	62	
	0.5–3	417	63	
	4–6	250	50	
	7 or more	414	128	
Computer and data processing; public utilities				
	0	188	28	
	0.5–3	183	31	
	4–6	151	29	
	7 or more	321	103	
Banking, communications, and hospitals				
	0	178	36	
	0.5–3	234	33	
	4–6	99	23	
	7 or more	93	25	

a. Using these data, estimate the prevalence of musculoskeletal symptoms for each industry, for each category of daily personal computer use.

b. What is the interpretation of the prevalences that you calculated?

c. Is there a consistent increase or decrease in the magnitude of the prevalence as the number of daily personal computer use (hours) increases? Why, or why not?

d. Prevalence is a function of the IR and the average duration of disease or injury. Using the data for personal computer use, can you determine whether the prevalence estimates vary by industry and/or by daily computer use because of differences in the IRs of musculoskeletal problems or because of differences in the average durations of having musculoskeletal problems? Why, or why not?

e. Do you think the prevalences of musculoskeletal symptoms associated with personal computer use at work, at home, or in both locations have changed since the 1980s? How might you locate data to support or refute your answer to this question?

2. a. Calculate the prevalence of disease, using the (hypothetical) data in the following table.

Age	Incidence Rate	Average Duration of Disease	Prevalence?
Young	2.3/(100 P-Y)	7 years	
Middle-aged	2.9/(100 P-Y)	2 years	
Older	5.1/(100 P-Y)	1 year	
Oldest	5.4/(100 P-Y)	4 *months*	

  b. Are the age-specific prevalences a good indication of the relative magnitudes of the age-specific IRs? Why, or why not?

  c. In general, if data on the prevalence of disease, but not on the IR of disease, are available, what if anything can you conclude about the IR of disease?

3. If the prevalence of a preclinical stage of cancer is 10 percent, and the average duration of the preclinical stage is 3 years, what is the IR of the preclinical stage?

4. The following data come from a study of health problems among teenage smokers in Norway. Based on these data, estimate the prevalence of smoking for boys and for girls.

Question and Respondent's Age (years)	Boys			Girls		
	Total #	# Smokers	Prevalence of Smoking ?	Total #	# Smokers	Prevalence of Smoking ?
Ever Tried Smoking						
13–14	1,311	516		1,303	559	
15–16	1,395	818		1,391	837	
17–18	1,237	819		1,212	849	
Current Smoking (daily and occasionally)						
13–14	1,282	108		1,289	133	
15–16	1,351	278		1,366	335	
17–18	1,201	323		1,191	405	
Daily Smoking						
13–14	1,282	58		1,289	41	
15–16	1,351	132		1,366	159	
17–18	1,201	182		1,191	246	

Source: Turid L. Holmen, Elizabeth Barrett-Connor, Jostein Holmen, and Leif Bjermer, "Health Problems in Teenage Daily Smokers versus Nonsmokers, Norway, 1995–1997: The Nord-Trondelag Health Study," *American Journal of Epidemiology* 151, no. 2 (2000): 148–55.

5. The following data come from the Centers for Disease Control and Prevention, National Center for Health Statistics, National Health Interview Survey, as reported in a subset of the data from Table 80, page 2, of *Health, United States, 2003*. Data from the National Health Interview Survey come from household interviews of a sample of the civilian, noninstitutionalized population. What is your interpretation of these data?

Use of Mammography for Women 40 Years of Age and over according to Selected Characteristics: United States, Selected Years 1987–2000

Characteristic	1987	1990	1991	1993	1998	2000
Age and Education	*Percent of Women Having a Mammogram within the Past Two Years*					
40–49 Years						
No HS* diploma or GED[†]	15.1	38.5	40.8	43.6	47.3	46.9
HS diploma or GED	32.6	53.1	52.0	56.6	59.1	59.0
Some college or more	39.2	62.3	63.7	66.1	68.3	70.5
50–64 Years						
No HS* diploma or GED[†]	21.2	41.0	43.6	51.4	58.8	66.3
HS diploma or GED	33.8	56.5	60.8	62.4	73.3	76.6
Some college or more	40.5	68.0	72.7	78.5	79.8	84.1
65 Years and Older						
No HS* diploma or GED[†]	16.5	33.0	37.7	44.2	54.7	57.5
HS diploma or GED	25.9	47.5	54.0	57.4	66.8	72.0
Some college or more	32.3	56.7	57.9	64.8	71.3	74.1

*HS = high school.

[†]GED = General Educational Development high school equivalency diploma.

6. Using the following data, estimate the sensitivity and the specificity of the screening test and the predictive value positive and predictive value negative of the screening program. On the basis of your results, what might you conclude about the merits and demerits of the screening test and program? What other factors might affect your assessment of the merits and demerits of the test and the program?

		TRUE ("REAL WORLD") SITUATION	
		Positive for Factor	*Negative for Factor*
SCREENING TEST RESULTS	*Positive for Factor*	180	1,000
	Negative for Factor	20	4,000

7. You, as a professional in health services, are asked to conduct a cost-savings analysis for a new screening program. You are asked to calculate the cost of lives saved versus the cost of the program, and to provide a comparison of future health-care costs (in the absence of the new screening program) versus the costs of the program. In addition, you are asked to indicate in which target populations (defined by age, gender, racial and ethnic backgrounds, and health risk factors) the program should be implemented, and at what time intervals the screening test should be applied, to achieve an acceptable ratio of program costs to benefits.

   What epidemiologic data would you need to answer these questions? How would you find these data, or would you need to collect these data yourself? What factors might affect the screening program's effectiveness in different populations?

8. You work for a major insurance company or for a managed care organization. You are asked to design and evaluate a program to increase prescription-medication compliance among patients having a variety of diseases or at-risk health conditions (for example, patients having diabetes, high blood pressure, or high serum cholesterol). Your preliminary data suggest that full compliance with the medication protocols at baseline is about 20 percent (a typical percentage). You know that raising full compliance to 50 percent would save your organization many millions of dollars each year in reduced medical costs. In addition, at this time, the only routinely collected data you have available to you on which to design and evaluate the program are billing charges and costs to your organization for people being treated for the diseases and at-risk health conditions of interest. These data identify charges and costs per month per medical encounter but do not identify charges and costs for individual patients' encounters for any month, or from one month to the next (the usual situation).

   What steps might you take to design and evaluate an effective medication compliance program? Do you think that health-care costs, in general, can be reduced through effective preventive and intervention programs without sacrificing the quality and extent of needed health care? Why, or why not?

See selected answers for exercises 1–4 and 6 on page A–3.

## CHAPTER 6

Cumulative Incidence (Risk)

The third measure of disease frequency is **cumulative incidence,** which is known also as **risk.** Cumulative incidence is abbreviated CI. ("CI" is used also as an abbreviation for "confidence interval"; thus, care should be taken not to confuse the two terms.) Cumulative incidence is defined as the number of new cases of disease or injury that occurs in a population over a specified period of time divided by the initial size of the population. Thus, cumulative incidence, like prevalence, is a proportion. Because cumulative incidence is a proportion, CI, like prevalence and unlike the incidence rate, has no units. Also like P and unlike IR, cumulative incidence has a range of possible values that extends from 0 to 1. When cumulative incidence is expressed as a percentage, its range of possible values is 0% to 100%.

A "new case" of disease or injury can mean "a new case of death." Thus, the CI can refer to the proportion of people in a population who develop disease or injury over a specified period of time, or the CI can refer to the proportion of a population who die from a particular disease or injury over a specified period of time.

FIRST APPROACH FOR ESTIMATING CUMULATIVE INCIDENCE

As with prevalence, there are two approaches for estimating CI, depending upon what data are available. In the first approach, a **cohort of people** (a set group of people followed over time) is followed over a specified period of time, and the number of new cases of disease or injury of interest is enumerated. This number of new cases of disease or injury is divided by the initial size of the cohort to yield the CI. Thus, CI = $(a/(a + b))$, where a = the number people in the cohort who develop the disease or injury of interest over the specified period of time, and b = number of people in the cohort who *do not* develop the disease or injury over the specified period of time.

It is important to appreciate that the people who make up the cohort initially are free of the particular disease or injury of interest. For example, in estimating the CI of heart disease over a two-year period, any person who previously had been diagnosed with heart disease would be ineligible for the study. This person already is "a case of heart disease" and thus cannot be a "new" case of heart disease.

The phrase "over a specified period of time" is an important part of the concept of CI. Every CI is associated with a specific period of time over which the new cases occurred. That time period should be stated explicitly every time a CI is calculated or mentioned. The longer a cohort of people is followed over time, the larger the proportion of the cohort who develop disease or injury will be, as long as the IR of disease acting on the cohort is larger than 0 (that is, the IR is not equal to 0). Thus, if a cohort was followed for one year, with 25 percent of the cohort developing the disease or injury of interest, the appropriate phrase to report the CI is the "one-year CI was 25 percent." If instead the cohort was followed for ten years during which 25 percent of the population developed the disease or injury of interest, then the appropriate phrase is "the ten-year CI was 25 percent." It is helpful to state the length of the time period over which a cohort was followed each time a CI is reported.

When the period of time over which the disease or injury of interest occurs is short (a few months or shorter), CI often is called an **attack rate.** Attack rates were discussed in Chapter 3. Typically, the term "attack rate" is used in reference to acute outbreaks of infectious diseases or toxic events in which the exposure occurs approximately as a **point exposure** (all people are exposed at approximately the same point in time) and the time interval between exposure and disease is short.

Examples Using the First Approach

An example of how to calculate a CI using the first approach, which is based on following a cohort of people over time, is provided by the following historical example. The watch-dial painters who worked during the early part of the twentieth century used fine-tipped brushes to paint numbers on watches. The paint contained radium, enabling the numbers to glow; thus, the numbers could be read in the dark, a novel feature at that time and a selling point. The watch-dial painters, all of whom were women, had the habit of placing the brush tips in their mouths to keep the tips pointed, thus facilitating the painting of high-quality numbers on the watches. Placing the brush tips containing radioactive paint in their mouths resulted, of course, in the women swallowing some of the paint. The women also inhaled a considerable amount of radioactive material, because part of the radium from the paint became airborne. Many of the watch-dial painters developed cancers as a result of those exposures.

Using somewhat modified, although realistic, data from studies of the watch-dial painters, it is possible to estimate their seven-year CI of bone sarcoma. Eight hundred painters were followed for seven years beginning in 1917. Over the seven-year period, fourty-eight cases of bone sarcoma were diagnosed, eighteen of which were fatal.

Based on those data, the estimated 7y-CI of developing bone sarcoma in this cohort was 48/800, or 0.060 (= 6.0%). The 7y-CI of dying from bone sarcoma was 18/800, or 0.0225 (= 2.3%).

As another historical example, it is possible to estimate the five-year CI of death for boys who worked as chimney sweeps in London during the seventeenth through the ninteenth centuries. The somewhat modified, although realistic, data show that eighty-nine deaths occurred among four hundred chimney sweeps over a five-year period. Thus, the 5y-CI was 89/400, or 0.223 (= 22.3%). There are numerous other examples of diseases caused by employment in certain occupations. (See Boxes 6.1 and 6.2.)

BOX 6.1

ETHICS MATTERS: BUSINESS AND ENGAGED EPIDEMIOLOGY

The ethical stature of large corporations matters to epidemiologists. Literally hundreds of occupational and/or environmental diseases have been named after specific occupations, or first identified in specific occupational groups, because the association between ill health and working in those occupations was so obvious. These diseases include boilermakers' deafness, neighborhood berylliosis, matchmakers' phossy jaw, coal miners' pneumoconiosis (black lung), cotton millers' byssinosis (brown lung), plastic makers' angiosarcoma, glassblowers' cataract, and rubber workers' aplastic anemia.

As a case example, the following paragraph, taken from Rosner and Markowitz (1985), portray the strong link between disease and occupational and environmental exposure to tetraethyl lead during the 1920s and thereafter, during the rush to use leaded gasoline in motor vehicles in the United States to increase power.

> The industry's assurances of the safety of leaded gasoline were undermined by a horrifying disaster that occurred in the Standard Oil Company's experimental laboratories in Elizabeth, New Jersey. Between October 26 and October 30, 1924, five workers died and 35 others experienced severe palsies, tremors, hallucinations, and other serious neurological symptoms of organic lead poisoning. Thus, of the 49 workers in the tetraethyl lead processing plant, over 80 percent died or were severely poisoned. On the first day, the *New York Times* quoted the company doctor who suggested that "nothing ought to be said about this matter in the public interest," and one of the supervisors at the Bayway facility who said "these men probably went insane because they worked too hard." The father of the dead man, however, "was bitter in denunciation of conditions of the plant" and told reporters that "Ernest was told by doctors at the plant that working in the laboratory wouldn't hurt him. Otherwise he would have quit. They said he would have to get used to it."*

And, later in the same manuscript, Rosner and Markowitz write, "The symptoms of lead accumulation due to exhaust emissions would be unlike anything they had previously encountered in industrial populations. In the long run, those most affected would not be adults, but children, slowly accumulating lead. . . ."

---

*Quotations from the *New York Times,* October 27, 1924, pp. 1, 6.

Box 6.1 continued

The exact number of children in the United States who suffered permanent cognitive deficits because of exposure to inorganic lead from motor vehicle emissions (tetraethyl lead is emitted as inorganic lead) is not known. Estimates of between 1 million and 2 million have been made. The majority of these children lived in inner cities and thus faced multiple environmental challenges to their health statuses.

Perhaps there needs to be a new concept, **engaged epidemiology,** that emphasizes the creative, dynamic application of epidemiology in identifying and solving public health problems and that challenges the people, agencies, and corporations whose innovations, new technologies, and practices may contribute to the public's health. In many respects, epidemiologists are uniquely educated to serve in this capacity, serving as the sentinel professionals safeguarding population health and safety.

REFERENCE

Rosner, David, and Gerald Markowitz. 1985. A "gift of God"? The public health controversy over leaded gasoline during the 1920s. *American Journal of Public Health* 75 (4): 344–52.

SECOND APPROACH FOR ESTIMATING CUMULATIVE INCIDENCE

The second approach for calculating CI depends on the fact that CI is a mathematical function of the IR of the disease or injury of interest and the period of time over which the cohort of interest is followed. Explicitly, $CI = 1 - e^{-(IR\Delta t)}$. "$\Delta t$" is a shorthand notation that means "change in time"; as used here, Δt means the "period of time over which the cohort is followed." Time can be measured as age (that is, the time or number of years from one age to another), time after exposure to a putative cause or preventive of disease or injury, or calendar time. In the formula, "e," or exponential, is the inverse of the natural log function; e is approximately equal to 2.72. When CI pertains to new cases of death, MR is substituted for IR in the formula. Thus, in the following discussion of CI, MR can be substituted for IR when the rate of interest is a mortality rate instead of an incidence rate.

The formula for calculating the CI from the IR can be modified to take into account changes in the magnitude of the IR over Δt. The IR might change, for instance, if Δt extends over a wide range of age. Many IRs increase with age; thus, within a wide Δt, there may be young people whose IR is quite different from the IR for older people. To accommodate changes in the IR, the CI formula can be modified to $CI = 1 - e^{-\Sigma(IR\Delta t)}$. In words, this formula states that to calculate the CI, each IR is multiplied by the period of time for which the IR applies, and these products are added together (this is what "Σ," the summation sign, means); "e" is raised to the power equal to the summation of the IRs times their Δts; and the result is subtracted from "1."

It is important to appreciate that the summation (the $\Sigma IR\Delta t$) is taken over each segment of Δt for which the IR varies substantially from the IR in the preceding and

BOX 6.2

THEORETICAL WEB OF CAUSATION FOR ERGONOMIC-RELATED DISABILITY

Another problem related to the ethical challenges seemingly engulfing some businesses and the way in which those businesses manufacture and market consumer products is depicted in a web of causation (Figure 6.1) pertaining to ergonomic and other hazards that may cause occupational disabilities. The web emphasizes not only decisions made by business managers but also the lack of adequate federal and/or state regulations, engineering and educational controls to prevent certain work-related disabilities.

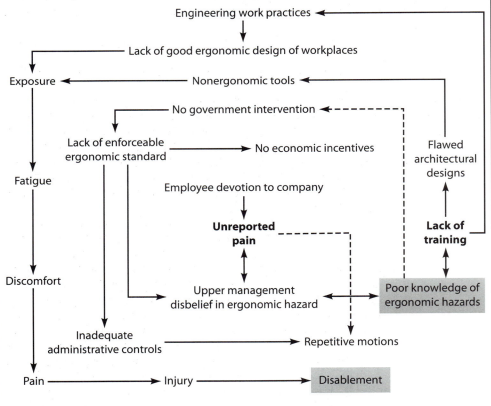

FIGURE 6.1

Theoretical web of causation for ergonomic-related disability.

Source: Levi Herman

following segments of Δt. Almost always, the segments of time are intervals of age. As noted previously, however, sometimes the intervals are times after exposure to a putative cause or preventive of disease or injury, especially if the cause or preventive occurred as a point exposure, or calendar time.

It often is not easy to determine the appropriate boundaries for the segments of time. An "appropriate" segment of Δt is an interval of time during which the IR or the MR is relatively constant but differs substantially from the IR or the MR in the adjacent segments of Δt. Sometimes, the segments of time are determined by looking at the study data at hand and noticing when the IR seems to change. In those situations, often investigators decide which segments of Δt to use on the basis of criteria such as the amount of data available in the current study (for example, more data mean there are enough data to divide the data into more and narrower segments of Δt) and/or convention (for example, using uniform, ten-year age intervals). Ideally, however, when feasible, the segments should be determined a priori, before the current study is undertaken, based on published results from the epidemiologic literature or on some other criterion. From a theoretical, biostatistical perspective, the segments should be formed a priori if statistical tests are to be performed with the data, because these segments are part of the hypothesis that is being tested.

Why is $e^{-\Sigma(IR\Delta t)}$ subtracted from the number 1? $e^{-\Sigma(IR\Delta t)}$ is equal to the proportion of the cohort that is free of the disease or injury of interest after Δt. Thus, 1 minus this proportion is the proportion of the cohort that developed the disease or injury of interest over Δt. Recalling that the range of possible values for CI extends from 0 to 1 (0% to 100%), the "1" in the CI formulae represents 100% of the cohort under study.

There are a number of implicit assumptions that underlie the CI formulae based on the IR(s). These assumptions include the following:

1. Individuals in the cohort under study must be free of the disease or injury of interest at the start of Δt.
2. The outcome of interest (disease or injury) can occur at most once to any person in the cohort under study.
3. There can be no **competing causes of lost to follow-up;** that is, the only way in which a person can be removed from the study is by developing the outcome of interest or reaching the end of the study period.
4. The IR (or MR) must be constant throughout each segment of Δt.

Note that when the CI formula based on the IR is used, an actual cohort of people is not followed over time, as occurs when the first approach for calculating CI is used. In this second approach, typically, age-specific, and often gender- and race-specific, IRs are calculated from one study population and then used in the CI calculation of interest. For example, in estimating the lifetime CI of developing lung cancer for male smokers in the United States aged 25 years in the year 2000, the age-specific lung cancer IRs for smoking males, calculated from current data, are used in the CI formula. Thus, current IRs are assumed to apply in the future, as these 25-year-old smoking males age. That assumption may or may not be valid.

Examples Using the Second Approach

The following examples demonstrate how to use the CI based on the IR(s) formulae.

EXAMPLE 1

The first example compares the first approach for calculating CI (the approach in which a cohort of people is followed over time and the number of people who develop the disease or injury of interest is calculated) with the second approach (the approach based on the IRs and Δts). In this hypothetical example, 5,000 women who use oral contraceptives (OCs) and who smoke cigarettes are followed for five years starting with the date of their thirty-fifth birthdays. Over this five-year interval, 18 of the 5,000 women die from a stroke. (These data, while hypothetical, are realistic for OC plus tobacco use in the 1970s in the United States.) Using these data, calculate the 5y-CI of stroke mortality (starting at age 35 years) for this population: The 5-year CI beginning at age 35 years is 18/5,000, or 0.0036 (= about 0.4%).

Now, calculate the CI for these data using the second approach for calculating CI, that is using the CI formula that is based on the MR. Before doing so, you will have to estimate the MR of stroke for this cohort of women. For an exact calculation of the MR, it would be necessary to know precisely how long each woman in the study was followed. That information is not known. The number of person-years, however, can be estimated as follows:

Which Women?	*Number of Years of Follow-Up*
Survivors; that is, the (5,000 − 18) or 4,982 women who did not die from a stroke over the five-year follow-up period	4,982 * 5 years, or 24,910 P-Y
Nonsurvivors; that is, the 18 women who died from a stroke over the five-year follow-up period were followed *on average* for half of the total five-year period of follow-up	18 * (5/2) years, or 45 P-Y
Total = All women; that is, both survivors and nonsurvivors	(24,910 P-Y) + (45 P-Y) = 24,955 P-Y

Why is (5/2) years used as the length of follow-up for the 18 women who died from stroke over the five-year period of follow-up? An assumption was made. It was assumed that these 18 women died **uniformly** throughout the five-year follow-up period. In other words, although some of these 18 women died early in the follow-up period (for example, after six months) and some of the 18 women died late in the follow-up period (for example, after 4.5 years), on average the 18 women survived for half of the interval, or (5/2 years) = 2.5 years. Basing the estimate of the number of person-years of observation on that assumption might result in an error. With only 18 of the 5,000 study subjects' person-years based on that assumption, however, the error will be small.

Having estimated the number of person-years of observation for the study women, it now is possible to calculate the 5y-CI of stroke mortality in this population. The MR = (number of deaths/number of person-years) = (18/24,955 P-Y). Using this MR in the CI formula, the 5y-CI $= 1 - e^{-((18/24,955 \text{ P-Y}) * (5 \text{ Y}))}$, or 0.0036 (= about 0.4%).

The following table shows the calculation step-by-step.

Order of Steps in Calculating Cumulative Incidence

Step 1	Multiply the IR by Δt: $(18/24,955$ P-Y$) * (5$ Y$) = 0.0036$.
Step 2	Take the negative of IRΔt: $-(0.0036)$.
Step 3	Raise e (about 2.72) to the $(-0.0036$ power): $2.72^{-0.0036} = 0.9964$.
Step 4	Subtract the result from step 3 from 1: $(1 - 0.9964) = 0.0036$ ($\approx 0.4\%$)

The fact that the numerical result using the first approach for calculating the CI is identical to the result obtained using the second approach is not a coincidence. Either approach will yield the same or nearly the same numerical result because each is an appropriate approach for estimating the CI. Remember that the number of deaths, used in the CI formula in the first approach, occurred as a result of the MR acting on the study cohort. Thus, the effect of the MR is observed (that is, a certain number of deaths occurred) even though the MR itself is not measured.

Suppose the number of cases had been 1,800 instead of 18. Would the two approaches still yield similar results? Using the first approach, the 5-y CI = $(1,800/5,000)$, or 0.36 (= 36%). The MR = $(1,800/((5,000 - 1,800) * 5$ years + $(1,800 * 5/2$ years$))) = (1,800/(16,000$ years + 4,500 years$)) = (0.0878/$P-Y$)$. Using this IR and the formula for the second approach, the 5-y CI = $1 - e^{-(0.0878/\text{P-Y}) * 5 \text{ years}} = 0.355$ (= 35.5%). Thus, the calculated 5-y CI is nearly identical using either approach.

If the two approaches for calculating CI yield the same result, why "bother" using the second approach, given that the first approach is so easy to use? The answer to that question was provided earlier in the discussion of CI: For situations in which the IR (or MR) changes over the Δt and especially if Δt is wide, the second approach often is the only realistic approach for calculating CI. The first approach would require an impractically long period of follow-up, such as thirty, forty, or even fifty years or more.

As an example, the lifetime CI of dying from a specific disease in a certain population is a common point of interest. Such risks are estimated using the second approach for calculating CI. Current, age-specific IRs are inserted into the CI formula (along with the appropriate Δt to which each IR applies), and the lifetime CI is calculated. Thus, the need to follow a large cohort of people many years from birth until old age and death is avoided. As mentioned previously, when age-specific IRs for the current calendar year are used in the CI formula, the assumption is being made that those IRs will be similar in magnitude to the age-specific IRs in the future, when the cohort is older. As stated previously, that assumption may or may not be valid.

As an aside, people quite commonly ascribe CIs to themselves. For example, because about 23 percent of people in the United States die from some type of cancer, many people in the United States interpret that statistic to mean that one's individual probability of dying from cancer is 23 percent. That interpretation, although alluring, is not correct. Each individual person's probability of dying from cancer is either 0 (does not die from cancer) or 1 (does die from cancer). The lifetime CI of 23 percent is the *average* of all the individual CIs of "0" and "1."

EXAMPLE 2

The second CI example uses the CI formula in which more than one IR and segment of Δt is appropriate because the IR changes over Δt. The data for this example are as follows:

Age Category	Number of Deaths	Number of Person-Years	Mortality Rate (MR)	MRs Expressed with a Common Denominator
10–19 years	10	1,500	10/1,500 P-Y	6.67/1,000 P-Y
20–24 years	14	4,000	14/4,000 P-Y	3.50/1,000 P-Y
Total	24	5,500	24/5,500 P-Y	4.36/1,000 P-Y

Notice that the MR for people between the ages of 10 and 19 years is almost twice as high as the MR for people between the ages of 20 and 24 years. Thus, it is necessary to calculate the 15-year CI taking the different age-specific MRs into account. Notice also that the segments of Δt are not the same width; the CI formula does not require the segments of Δt to be the same width. One segment of Δt is ten years wide, whereas the other is five years wide. The calculation is as follows: $15Y\ CI = 1 - e^{-(((10/1500\ P\text{-}Y)) * 10\ \text{Years}) + ((14/4,000\ P\text{-}Y) * 5\ \text{Years})))} = 0.081$, or 8.1% The interpretation of this CI is as follows: 8.1% of the cohort will die over the 15-year interval beginning at age 10 years.

The following box provides a step-by-step explanation of the calculation.

Step 1	Calculate each MRΔt:
	• For the 10–19-year-olds, MRΔt = ((10/1,500 P-Y) * 10 Years) = 0.06667.
	• For the 20–24-year-olds, MRΔt = ((14/4,000 P-Y) * 5 Years) = 0.01750.
Step 2	Add the two MRΔts together: (0.06667 + 0.0170) = 0.08367.
Step 3	Take the negative of the result in step 2: $-(0.08367) = -0.08367$.
Step 4	Raise e (≈ 2.72) to the power resulting from your result in step 3: $e^{-0.08367} = 0.919$.
Step 5	Subtract the result from step 4 from 1: $1 - 0.919 = 0.081$ (8.1%).

In this example, there are only two segments of Δt. The formula, however, is appropriate for any number of segments of Δt and IRs.

Suppose, in this example, the 15y-CI had been calculated ignoring the age-specific MRs. How, if at all, would the numerical result have been different? The calculation of the 15y-CI, ignoring the age-specific MRs, would be based on the crude MR (24/5,500 P-Y) and an unsegmented Δt equal to 15 years, as follows: $15y\text{-}CI = 1 - e^{-((24/5,500\ P\text{-}Y) * 15\ \text{years})} = 0.063$, or 6.3%. This calculation for the 15y-CI does not result in the correct answer of 0.081 (= 8.1%). Is the difference between 6.3% and 8.1% large enough to be meaningful epidemiologically? Probably it is, because 8.1% is almost 29% higher than 6.3% ((8.1%/6.3%) = 1.286).

Box 6.3 describes two other proportions used in epidemiology: case fatality or case fatality rate; and proportionate mortality. Although neither of those proportions is a measure of disease frequency, each proportion is useful in different circumstances to convey information of interest to epidemiologists.

BOX 6.3

OTHER USEFUL PROPORTIONS

There are two other proportions that often are used in the epidemiologic literature. These proportions are "case fatality" and "proportionate mortality."

Case Fatality

Case fatality, or case fatality rate (these phrases often are used interchangeably), is defined as the number of people who die from a particular disease or injury divided by the number of people who have that particular disease or injury. Case fatality is not a measure of disease occurrence in the same sense in which IR, P, and CI (or attack rate) are measures of disease or injury occurrence. For example, case fatality is not a rate (recall that a rate is a change in one variable relative to a change in another variable of which it is a function); it is a *proportion*. In addition, case fatality, unlike P and CI, is not a mathematical function of the IR of disease or injury. Instead, the case fatality associated with a certain disease or injury is the proportion of people who have that disease or injury who will die from it (that is, who will not recover or die from some other disease or injury).

As an example, the overall case fatality associated with breast cancer among women in the United States is approximately 30–35 percent. Notice that the denominator for case fatality in this example is the number of women who have been diagnosed with breast cancer. There is no reference to the size of the population of women from whom these cases of breast cancer were diagnosed, nor is there reference to some number of woman-years. Thus, case fatality does not convey information about how rapidly or slowly a disease or an injury is occurring in a population. Case fatality, however, may convey information about how rapidly or slowly a person with a particular disease or injury will die from that disease or injury. This information is conveyed, for example, by referring to a disease's or injury's "one-year case fatality" or "five-year case fatality," in other words, what *proportion* of cases die within the first or fifth year following diagnosis.

Proportionate Mortality

Proportionate mortality is the proportion of people who die from a particular cause among all people who die (that is, from all causes of death combined) in a certain population. Like case fatality, proportionate mortality is not a measure of disease or injury frequency in the same sense in which IR, P, and CI are measures of disease and injury occurrence. Also, like case fatality, proportionate mortality is not a mathematical function of the IR, nor does it convey information about the magnitude of IRs or MRs in a population.

Proportionate mortality is used often in occupational epidemiologic studies in which data are available on the number of workers who have died and their causes of death but little information is available on the numbers of person-years that gave rise to those deaths; thus, MRs cannot be calculated. As just stated, it is important to appreciate that the size of the proportionate mortality associated with a particular cause of death

Box 6.3 continued

in a particular population does not provide information about the magnitude of the MR from that cause in the population. For example, if 20 percent of all people who died in an occupational group died from lung cancer (a large percentage of all deaths), it cannot be inferred that the MR from lung cancer in that occupational group is unduly high compared, for example, with the lung cancer mortality rate for adults in the United States. To the contrary, it may be that both the overall (all causes) MR and the lung cancer MR are relatively low, as illustrated in the following hypothetical example.

In this example, the number of person-years in each population is known. In the type of epidemiological study in which proportionate mortality typically is calculated, the numbers of person-years would be unknown; thus, neither the overall nor the lung cancer–specific MRs would be available to compare with the MRs for some other population.

Population	A	B
Total deaths	100	100
Lung cancer deaths	20	5
Person-years	10,000	1,000
Overall MR	100/10,000P-Y = 10/(1,000 P-Y)	100/(1,000 P-Y)
Lung cancer MR	20/10,000 P-Y = 2/(1,000 P-Y)	5/(1,000 P-Y)
Proportionate mortality from lung cancer	20% (20 of 100 deaths)	5% (5 of 100 deaths)

The proportionate mortality for lung cancer in Population B (5%) is less than the proportionate mortality for lung cancer in Population A (20%), although the lung cancer MR in Population B (5/(1,000 P-Y) is higher than the lung cancer MR in Population A (2/(1,000 P-Y). This example demonstrates that the relative sizes of the proportionate mortality for lung cancer in these two populations does not convey information about the relative size of the lung cancer MR for each population.

OVERVIEW OF MEASURES OF DISEASE/INJURY FREQUENCY

The table on page 141 summarizes and compares the three primary measures of disease frequency discussed in Chapters 4 through 6.

REVIEW QUESTIONS

1. Define "cumulative incidence" (CI).
2. What is the range of possible values for CI?
3. CI can be estimated using two approaches. How is CI estimated in each of these two approaches?
4. Define and give examples of "cohorts."
5. List four assumptions that underlie the calculation of CI.
6. Define "competing causes of lost to follow-up" as this term pertains to CI.

Summary of the Three Primary Measures of Disease/Injury Frequency Used in Epidemiology

Measure of Disease Frequency	Formulae	Interpretation
Incidence rate (IR)	IR = # *new* cases/*person-time*	An instantaneous quantity; the *rate* at which people either develop a disease or injury or die from a disease or injury
Mortality rate (MR)	MR = # deaths/*person-time*	
	IRs and MRs sometimes are expressed as • # cases/# people/year; or • Annual rate = # cases/# people	
Prevalence (P) or prevalence rate	P = # *existing* cases/size of the *population*	The *proportion* of a population who have an *existing* disease or injury at a specific point in time
	P = IR * D/(1 + (IR * D)), where D is the average duration of disease or injury	
	P sometimes estimated as P = (IR * D)	
Cumulative incidence (CI), also known as "risk" or, for a short period of follow-up (= short Δt), "attack rate"	CI = # *new* cases/size of the *population* followed for a specific period of time $CI = 1 - e^{-\Sigma(IR\Delta t)}$	The *proportion* of people who *develop* a disease or injury *over a specified period of time*

REVIEW EXERCISES

1. a. Using these hypothetical data, calculate the age-specific cumulative incidence (CI) of injury for each age interval. Then, calculate the crude 65y (= 0–64 years) CI of injury and the 65y-CI taking the age-specific IRs into account. Use as your "Δt" the width of each age interval. For example, Δt for the first age interval, 0–2 years, is 3 years, and the Δt for the second age interval, 3–9 years, is 7 years.

Age Category (years)	Injury IR	Δt (years)	CI ?
0–2	273/(2,490 P-Y)	3	
3–9	201/(10,973 P-Y)	7	
10–14	84/(9,714 P-Y)	5	
15–19	151/(11,450 P-Y)	5	
20–24	65/(11,206 P-Y)	5	
25–64	307/(57,924 P-Y)	40	
65 and older	172/(1,469 P-Y)	Unknown	
All ages	1,253/(105,226 P-Y)	Unknown	

    b. Can the CIs for age categories "65 and older" and "all ages" be calculated? Why, or why not?

    c. One of the assumptions of the CI calculation is that people can experience the outcome of interest at most one time. How realistic is that assumption with respect to the incidence rates for injuries?

    d. What assumption must be made to calculate the CI of injuries for people aged 65 years and older?

2. Calculate the 5y-CI of disease in the following (hypothetical) cohorts. Each cohort was followed for 5 years.

Cohort	# People in the Cohort	# Cases of Disease Over 5 Years	5y-CI ?
A	752	87	
B	1,189	52	
C	3,009	177	
D	2,667	344	

3. A population of size 5,046 was followed for 8 years. Over this 8-year period, 833 cases of disease occurred with an average duration of 3 months. Using these data, calculate the 8y-CI of disease using two different approaches.

See selected answers for exercises 1–3 on page A–5.

## CHAPTER 7

Design Strategies: Descriptive Studies

"Design strategies" are the types of studies epidemiologists use to assess the distribution and determinants of disease and injury in human populations. Design strategies can be divided into two major categories: descriptive studies and analytic studies. Within each of those two major categories are several study-design options (Figure 7.1). In addition, there are a number of "hybrid" study designs that sometimes are used. The primary study-design options within the category of descriptive studies are the correlational study (also known as an ecological study), the cross-sectional study, and the case report or case series. Within the category of analytic studies are intervention (experimental) studies and two types of observational studies, the case/control study and cohort studies. Intervention studies consist of community trials and clinical trials, and cohort studies consist of prospective cohort studies and retrospective cohort studies. This chapter discusses the descriptive study designs. Chapter 9 discusses the analytic study designs.

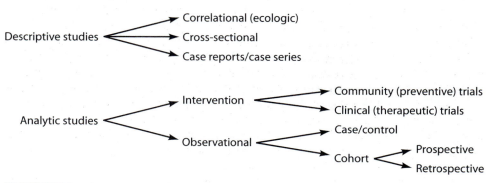

FIGURE 7.1
Options in study design.

OBJECTIVES OF DESCRIPTIVE STUDIES

In general, the objectives of descriptive studies are to provide data for better understanding the distribution of disease and injury in a population, to provide data for planning health services needs and prevention programs, and to provide data for developing epidemiologic hypotheses that then are evaluated in analytic studies. Descriptive studies are not hypothesis-evaluating; that is, descriptive studies cannot be used to evaluate epidemiologic hypotheses but only to suggest the existence of associations between exposures and outcomes. Thus, descriptive studies measure the distribution or variability of exposure, disease and injury occurrence, and utilization patterns of health-care services in human populations. Analytic studies, on the other hand, seek to identify the determinants (causes) of human disease and injury.

Descriptive studies ask questions such as, In which geographic areas do disease and injury occur with high or low frequency? In which age, gender, or occupational populations are certain diseases or injuries more or less common? By which characteristics of people or of their physical, social, economic, or political environments do disease and injury incidence rates vary?

Descriptive studies often are based on previously collected data such as routinely collected vital statistics, census data, data from mandatory disease reporting and disease and injury registries, mandated environmental sampling data, national health survey information, and administration data. Because of their reliance on previously collected data, descriptive studies typically are low in cost (time and money) and are used as a "first look" at the plausibility of an association between a particular exposure and a health outcome.

PRIMARY USES OF DESCRIPTIVE STUDIES

Quantifying Variation in Exposures and Health Statuses

Descriptive studies are useful for at least two reasons. First, descriptive studies provide the requisite information about variation in exposure status, and in disease and injury frequency, with which to predict health services needs or to target preventive programs. For example, overall in the United States, approximately 20–30 percent of women seen in medical care facilities may be victims of physical abuse. Similarly, a woman's lifetime risk of being battered in the United States is estimated to be between 20 and 30 percent (www.ama-assn.org, accessed on April 2000). Those descriptive statistics help health-care professionals estimate the need for medical and emotional support services for abused women, and aid prevention specialists in estimating the extent and type of programming efforts needed to control this major public health problem.

Examples of Descriptive Studies

Other examples of descriptive studies are the series of studies conducted following the meltdown of a reactor at the Chernobyl nuclear power plant in the Ukraine on April 26, 1986. The reactor caught fire, spewing large quantities of radioactive materials into the environment. Public health professionals from many countries responded to the disaster, providing medical assistance to injured workers, measuring radiation exposure levels, and monitoring health effects in the general and the occupationally exposed populations. Radioactive contamination from the damaged reactor circulated worldwide, affecting even remote communities. For example, in Labrador, reindeer (a primary source of nutrition for the local inhabitants) were rendered inedible because of the high levels of radioactive substances in their natural plant foods.

Descriptive studies of the population exposed to radiation, especially among people who resided close to the Chernobyl plant, yielded alarmingly high levels of exposure. Based on those descriptive data, estimates were made of the numbers of new cases of cancers, birth defects, and other health ailments expected to occur, and to require medical treatment, as a result of the exposure to radiation. Later data, released by the Ukraine government in 2000, validated the earlier estimates. Approximately 4,000 deaths occurred among workers who participated in the clean-up effort, and 70,000 people were disabled as a result of environmental exposure to radioactive substances. Overall, an estimated 3.4 million of the Ukraine's 50 million inhabitants, including 1.26 million children, were expected to suffer now or at some point in the future from some form of ill health because of the meltdown (Sysoyeva 2000).

Box 7.1 provides an example of a descriptive study whose primary objective was to provide information concerning the current health status of a population pursuant to the planning and implementation of clinical and preventive programs. The population studied lives in the Kono District of northeast Sierra Leone, a region decimated by war and now being repopulated. The descriptive data show that the prevalences of malnutrition (wasting) and of severe, acute malnutrition are high and compounded by other health-related challenges in the region such as fevers and the possibility of a measles epidemic. Those data are being used to help identify and prioritize unmet health needs in the Kono District with the hope of better targeting public health programs.

BOX 7.1

PRACTICAL EPIDEMIOLOGY IN A PUBLIC HEALTH SETTING: NUTRITIONAL ANTHROPOMETRICS SURVEY, KONO DISTRICT, SIERRA LEONE

EXECUTIVE SUMMARY, SEPTEMBER 2001

HEINKE BONNLANDER, R.N., M.S., PH.D.

HEALTH MANAGER, WORLD VISION INTERNATIONAL, SIERRA LEONE

Kono district is situated in the northeast of Sierra Leone and was one of the most populated among the 12 districts in Sierra Leone. It is known for its diamonds. During civil war that started in 1991, major settlements were destroyed, homes, health centres and grain stores looted and in excess of 80% of the population displaced to Guinea and Liberia. Health care has been virtually unavailable in the region for the last 10 years. In October

Box 7.1 continued

2000, World Vision International (WVI) once again moved into Kono South where it traditionally has operated, providing commodities, agricultural aids, and health services.

After disarmament of the Revolutionary United Front between August and September 2001, WVI expanded its Primary Health Care (PHC) program to ten chiefdoms now supporting 20 clinics. Refugees and the internally displaced population (IDP) are returning daily to their respective villages, resulting in a rapidly changing village population, though many appear to remain near the Guinean border cautious to move inland (eyewitness report).

Study Objectives

The study objectives were:

- To assess the nutritional status among children aged 6 to 59 months or between 65 and 110 cm in length;
- To estimate the measles immunization coverage rate;
- To assess the mortality rate and suspected causes of deaths for the last four months (beginning of the rainy season) among the aged <5 years and 5 years or older population.

Methodology

The survey was conducted from September 8th to 13th of 2001. The survey was carried out in Kono's three southern chiefdoms of Gorama, Nimiyama and Nimikoro. The two-stage anthropometrics survey used cluster sampling (24 clusters with at least 30 children per cluster) sampling a total of 750 children aged 6 to 59 months. Standard UNHCR/WFP/MSF methodology was followed. The results for weight and height index values were based on the Reference Population Table of the NCHS/CDC/WHO 1982.

Results

Nutritional

Total/Global acute malnutrition (wasting) of both sexes among the 6–59 months population was:

−2 Z-score and/or oedema:	17.1%	(95% CI: 11.5%–22.7%)
<80% median and/or oedema:	14.7%	(95% CI: 9.9%–19.5%)

Severe acute malnutrition was:

−3 Z-score and/or oedema:	4.7%	(95% CI: 3.3%–6.3%)
<70% median and/or oedema:	3.7%	(95% CI: 2.3%–5.4%)

Note: A Z-score comes from a normal distribution having a mean value of 0 and a variance, or measure of the dispersion of the scores, equal to 1.0. A Z-score equal to minus 2 (−2) or minus 3 (−3) means that the children surveyed were well below the average values for healthy children. (A.R.)

Box 7.1 continued

Measles Vaccination Coverage

The documented measles immunization coverage rate was 16.4% among the <5 year old population.

Mortality Rate

The mortality rate among children <5 years was 6.1/10,000 persons/day for the last four months. The mortality rate of the 5 years or older population was 1.4/10,000 person/day for the last four months. Among the children <5 years of age, 42% reported fever as the most common cause of mortality compared to 23% of the 5 years or older population.

Conclusions

- The total and severe malnutrition rate among the <5 year old population was significant in Kono's chiefdoms of Gorama, Nimiyama and Nimikoro and indicates a nutritional emergency situation.
- The measles immunization coverage rate was minimal, posing a high mortality risk should an epidemic occur.
- The mortality rate among the <5 year old population was alarmingly high; fever was reported as the most common cause of death.

Recommendations

- Provide supplementary feeding programs in the district, targeting children identified as high risk as soon as possible until stability returns to the region;
- Explore the opening of a therapeutic feeding center (TFC) for severely malnourished children;
- Conduct periodic nutritional surveys until the movement of refugees and IDP's has decreased or stabilized;
- Conduct mass immunization campaigns to reduce all preventable diseases as soon as feasible among the <5 year old population;
- Add, maintain and improve medical facilities to increase PHC accessibility including the establishment of clinics for children <5 year old;
- Introduce a nutritional surveillance system in all health facilities as soon as possible;
- Increase mobile clinic activities targeting populations without health care access;
- Train all clinic Maternal Child Health aides and In-charges on nutritional topics including growth monitoring;
- Establish a community-based nutritional education system addressing the prevention of malnutrition, including the importance of breast-feeding and the demonstration of cooking with local foods;

Box 7.1 continued

- Introduce malaria prevention programs among the most vulnerable populations, providing bed nets and stressing early treatment of fevers;
- Continue rehabilitation of wells and gravity systems to increase access to clean water.

Source: The survey was made possible with funding from CIDA and OFDA. Special thanks go to the supervisors and the team members for their hard work under difficult conditions during the survey as well as to those who provided direct support. During this study, Dr. Bonnlander was Health Manager, World Vision International.

Figure 7.2 presents a web of causation showing the causes of low birth weight in Yemen, a problem whose underlying causes are similar to the health problems among newborns in Sierra Leone. As stated in *The World Factbook* (www.cia.gov/cia/publications/factbook/, accessed July 2004):

> North Yemen became independent of the Ottoman Empire in 1918. The British, who had set up a protectorate area around the southern port of Aden in the 19th century, withdrew in 1967 from what became South Yemen. Three years later, the southern government adopted a Marxist orientation. The massive exodus of hundreds of thousands of Yemenis from the south to the north contributed to two decades of hostility between the states. The two countries were formally unified as the Republic of Yemen in 1990. A southern secessionist movement in 1994 was quickly subdued. In 2000, Saudi Arabia and Yemen agreed to a delimitation of their border.

Current environmental challenges in Yemen include limited natural fresh water supplies and potable water, overgrazing, soil erosion, and consequently **desertification** (usable land becoming arid or desertlike because of land mismanagement and/or climate change). The median age for both females and males is 16.5 years, with approximately 45 percent of the population between the ages of 0 and 14 years. The per capita gross domestic product is US $800; unemployment is at 35 percent (www.cia.gov/cia/publications/factbook/, accessed July 2004).

Box 7.2 provides another use of data from a descriptive study to assess the need for health services. The study focuses on the mental health needs of children living in Benton County, Oregon.

Forming Hypotheses

A second primary use of descriptive studies is to provide data on which to formulate **epidemiologic hypotheses** about the causes of human disease and injury. An epidemiologic hypothesis is a statement, tentatively held to be true, that relates a specific dose of exposure with a specific amount of a health outcome in a certain population over a specified period of time. The definition of an epidemiologic hypothesis includes the phrase "ten-

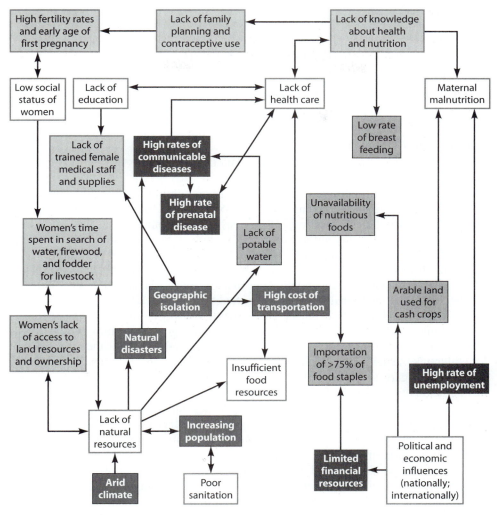

FIGURE 7.2
Causes of low birth weight in Yemen.
Source: Lisa Kirk, M.P.H.

tatively held to be true." This phrase means that an epidemiologic hypothesis, like other scientific hypotheses, conveys a working idea about how the laws of nature—in this case, the laws of exposures and health outcomes in human populations—operate. An epidemiologic hypothesis, like hypotheses in other fields of science, is subject to modification as new information becomes available. Ideally, an epidemiologic hypothesis has at least five components: an exposure, a health outcome, a **dose-response** (how much of the exposure results in how much of the outcome), a **time-response** (how

BOX 7.2

PRACTICAL EPIDEMIOLOGY IN A PUBLIC HEALTH SETTING: EPIDEMIOLOGY ON THE FRONT LINES— ASSESSING THE MENTAL HEALTH NEEDS OF BENTON COUNTY, OREGON, CHILDREN

DOROTHY TIBBETTS, M.P.H.

EPIDEMIOLOGIST, BENTON COUNTY, OREGON HEALTH DEPARTMENT

Mental health is indispensable to personal well-being, family and interpersonal relationships, and contribution to community and society. The cost to society of mental illness is high and includes direct costs of services for the mentally ill, as well as indirect costs from lost productivity at the workplace, school, and home resulting from mental health disability. Lifelong mental disorders may start in childhood or in adolescence. It has been estimated that at least one in five children and adolescents between ages 9 and 17 years has a diagnosable mental disorder in a given year (Healthy People 2010).

Federal, state, and local initiatives in recent years have called for improved child mental health programs. A U.S. Surgeon General's report issued in 2000 established several goals in the area of child mental health, including goals to (a) improve the assessment and recognition of mental health needs in children, (b) improve the infrastructure for children's mental health services, (c) increase access to and coordination of quality mental-health-care services, and (d) monitor access to and coordination of quality mental-health-care services (U.S. Department of Health and Human Services 2000).

The Oregon Mental Health Alignment Workgroup assembled during 2000 to explore issues associated with Oregon mental health services. The workgroup found that more services are needed for children and adolescents. Because schools often have the first indication of need, the workgroup recommended that screening for children who show early signs of mental health disorders take place in schools.

At the local level, the Benton County Public Health Planning and Advisory Committee focused on childhood mental health services in Benton County during the year 1999–2000 and recommended that the county conduct a comprehensive needs assessment of childhood mental health services.

The Benton County Health Department responded to those recommendations by implementing the Benton County Child Mental Health Needs Assessment study to determine the mental health needs of Benton County children. A project steering committee, consisting of school staff, parents, and other local stakeholders, was created to help guide the planning and implementation of the assessment. A preexisting survey instrument, the Strengths and Difficulties Questionnaire,* was used to measure mental health symptoms among fifth graders attending Benton County public schools (see http://www.sdqinfo.com).

---

*The Strengths and Difficulties Questionnaire (SDQ) was developed in Great Britain by Dr. Robert Goodman. It has been adapted for use in other countries, including the United States.

Box 7.2 continued

A letter was sent to the parents of Benton County public school fifth graders describing the purpose and importance of the project and requesting their participation. Accompanying the letter was information about child mental health promotion and about child mental health services that are available in the community. A second mailing included the survey instrument and an envelope in which the anonymously completed survey could be sealed for the child to return to the school. A third mailing served as a thank-you to those parents who completed the survey and a reminder to those who had not yet completed the survey. The completed survey forms were collected from the schools, entered into a statistical software program, and analyzed.

The survey generated information about how children rated on five difficulty scales, a prosocial scale that measured positive mental health behaviors, and an impact scale that measured the impact that reported difficulties had on the child's home life, friendships, classroom learning, and leisure activities. For each of the scales, children's scores could be classified as normal, borderline, or abnormal.

The results of the survey suggested that the Benton County community is "average" with respect to child mental health symptoms; that is, the results were consistent with the estimate that at least one in five children and adolescents between ages 9 and 17 years has a diagnosable mental disorder in a given year.

It may seem that those results are unremarkable. On the contrary, the Benton County Child Mental Health Needs Assessment Project provided essential information to help Benton County Health Department staff to

- Demonstrate the need for child mental health services in the community
- Conduct an analysis of services currently available in the community to determine whether they are adequate to meet the need demonstrated by the assessment
- Gather support for the development of school-based mental health promotion programs
- Establish baseline data for future monitoring and program evaluation activities

In addition, because the mailings to parents included education and outreach materials about child mental health promotion and services, the project helped to promote public awareness of children's mental health issues and reduce the stigma associated with mental illness.

Finally, the Benton County Child Mental Health Needs Assessment project was a success because it provided a foundation for effective partnerships among health department staff, school staff, parents, and other community members concerned about the mental health of Benton County children. Such partnerships are essential to the work of successful local county health programs.

REFERENCES

Healthy People 2010. *Healthy People in Healthy Communities.* http://www.health.gov/healthypeople/About/.

U.S. Department of Health and Human Services. Office of the Surgeon General. 2000. *A Report of the Surgeon General's Conference on Children's Mental Health: A National Action Agenda.* http://www.surgeongeneral.gov/cmh/childreport.html.

long after the exposure the health outcome occurs), and the population to whom the hypothesis applies. There are a number of different types of dose responses, three of which are depicted pictorially in Figure 7.3.

The magnitude of a health response does not always increase monotonically with the dose of exposure and/or length after exposure. For example, cancer rates may decrease following a large dose of a carcinogen compared with lower doses because of cell-killing: Dead body cells do not divide and hence do not produce cancers.

An example of using the results of a descriptive study to formulate an epidemiologic hypothesis is the following study, conducted in Marseille, France. In an effort to reduce HIV transmission, investigators in Marseille conducted a descriptive study of the use of syringe vending machines among injection drug users. The study found that 21.3 percent of the respondents used syringe vending machines as their primary source for clean syringes. In addition, primary users of syringe vending machines tended to be younger than thirty years old, to report no prior involvement with drug maintenance treatment, and to report no sharing of needles or other injection equipment. The authors concluded that "syringe vending machines can be a useful adjunct to existing needle exchange programs and pharmacy sales of sterile syringes without prescription" in Marseille and suggested that such programs may have merit in other settings, such as in the United States (Obadia et al. 1999). Thus, the authors developed a hypothesis about the use of syringe vending machines and reduced transmission of HIV among a certain population of injection drug users, a hypothesis that later could be evaluated in analytic epidemiologic studies in other cities in France and in other countries.

Another example of the use of data from descriptive epidemiologic studies to develop a hypothesis about disease causation comes from the study of hepatitis C and **parenteral** antischistosomal therapy (PAT) in Egypt. Parenteral, in this context, means from a needle injection. Specifically, potassium antimony tartrate was injected into people twelve to sixteen times in an attempt to kill schistosomal flukes in the blood. **Schistosomiasis** is a serious disease caused by infestation by the parasitic fluke *Bilharzia*. The fluke lives in human blood vessels and often damages the liver and the spleen. A characteristic symptom of the disease is blood in the urine.

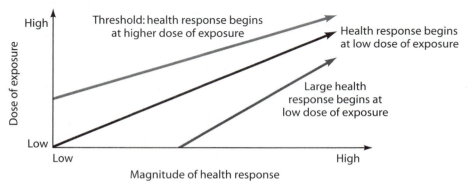

FIGURE 7.3
Pictorial representations of dose-responses.

Hepatitis C is a viral infection that can cause chronic liver disease, cirrhosis, and hepatocellular carcinoma. It was observed, from descriptive studies, that approximately 20 percent of Egyptians test positive for hepatitis C, a prevalence that is considerably higher than the prevalence of hepatitis C infection in neighboring countries and elsewhere having comparable socioeconomic conditions. In addition, children have a lower prevalence of hepatitis C than do adults, and the prevalence of infection increases markedly with age (Abdel-Wahab et al. 1994; Darwish et al. 1996). Within Egypt, people living in the desert regions have the lowest prevalence of infection, and people living in the urban areas, especially in the Nile Delta region (Lower Egypt), have the highest prevalence (El-Sayed et al. 1996). Coupled with those descriptive observations were data concerning the use of PAT in mass-treatment programs of the Egyptian population. PAT was initiated in Egypt in the 1920s to prevent and cure schistosomiasis. After extensive use, PAT was discontinued in the 1980s.

Based on those descriptive observations, a hypothesis was developed that hepatitis C transmission was occurring because of the reuse of contaminated needles in the PAT program. A subsequent analytic study provided strong evidence in support of that hypothesis, finding a 31 percent increase in the seroprevalence of hepatitis C antibodies among persons scoring high on an index of exposure to the PAT programs. This finding suggests that Egypt's mass PAT programs may be the world's largest **iatrogenic** (inadvertently caused by a clinician or by medical treatment) transmission of a blood-borne pathogen (Frank et al. 2000).

TYPES OF DESCRIPTIVE STUDIES

Case Reports and Case Series

The first type of descriptive study is the **case report** or **case series.** In a case report or case series, an investigator studies one or more people (that is, one or more cases) who ostensibly have an unusual disease or injury and sometimes an unusual exposure that may or may not have caused the disease or injury. These studies comprise only cases; no person who lacks the disease or injury of interest is included in the study. Case reports and case series typically are published in medical journals rather than in epidemiology or public health journals. (See Box 7.3 for a discussion of a case series used in a social, rather than medical, context.)

The major difficulty in interpreting case reports and case series is the omission of a group of people who lack the disease or injury of interest. Without a **comparison group** who lack the disease or injury of interest, it is not possible to evaluate whether the exposure experiences of the case group really are "unusual." For example, if 25 percent of cases in a series (people with the disease **"of interest"**) work at the same industrial plant (a large percentage), it is tempting to conclude that some exposure at the plant is causing ill health. That conclusion is unwarranted. It may be, for instance, that although 25 percent of the cases work at the plant, 30 percent of a comparison group (people without the disease **"of interest"**), if such a group had been assembled, would be found to work at the plant. These large percentages might be found, for example, if the plant were the major employer in the region. Thus, the exposure of "working at the

BOX 7.3

ETHICS MATTERS: US AND THEM—PUBLIC HEALTH ETHICS IN AN AGE OF "OTHERNESS"

ANNETTE M. ROSSIGNOL, SC.D., AND PHILIPPE A. ROSSIGNOL, PH.D.

"Modern" public health in the United States had its genesis in the latter decades of the 19th century. The disease that catapulted sanitary reform, the hallmark of modern public health, was not tuberculosis, the foremost but slow killer at the time, but cholera. Cholera was a mysterious disease that struck both the rich and the poor alike, and killed with terrifying speed. The rich could hide from many of the diseases and injuries that afflicted the poor, but they could not hide from cholera. The advent of piped public water supplies in the major United States cities at the end of the 19th century assured that both rich and poor would reap the benefits of having piped water but also suffer the diseases, such as cholera, that water carries.

The epidemics of cholera began to form the distinct culture of public health in the United States. This culture centered on perceived "class status," with diseases and injuries that affected "undesirable" classes (them) allowed to exist unabated, whereas diseases and injuries that affected those in power (us) were targeted for control. What was undesirable changed from time to time as new waves of immigrants came to the United States but often focused on characteristics such as skin color, gender, economic status, or ethnicity.

The divisive class culture of public health is visible in the history of other diseases and injuries in the United States. For example, there was little public concern for preventing or controlling HIV/AIDS as long as these diseases affected primarily homosexual men, Haitians living in the United States, and intravenous drug users (them). As another example, there were few funds for teenage suicide prevention programs until this tragedy moved from the primarily Black, low income intercity areas (them) to the more affluent, primarily Caucasian suburbs (us).

Public health focuses on bringing "us" and "them" together to achieve a high level of population health for all. More specifically, the ethical underpinnings of public health challenge society to regard health status as a basic human right that dissolves the classist distinction of "us" and "them." Public health holds society as a whole responsible for quality health for all without class distinctions about who deserves to have good health and who deserves none. It challenges the convictions of some individuals that people in poor health are to be blamed for their unenviable health statuses or even held morally accountable for their poor health because of actions, whether real or imagined, they may have taken to precipitate their poor health.

Progress in public health is slow. Part of this slowness is economic: The United States spends between 1 and 1.5 cents per health dollar on public health with the remainder (98.5–99 cents) spent on clinical care, most of which, unlike public health, is used for the treatment of ill individuals rather than for the prevention of disease or injury. Part of the slowness in the progress of public health is sociopolitical: Public health

Box 7.3 continued

asks people to consider in what kind of society they wish to live. The choices are: a society in which power is shared, including the power to live, work, and learn in safe environments and to have access to preventive health services and health care, or a society in which power is hoarded.

The events of September 11, 2001, and their aftermath have challenged public health programs, public health education in general, and the teaching of ethics in public health in particular in a way not encountered for many decades. The perceived distinctions between "us" and "them" have been blurred into an "otherness" that regards people in the "other" category (often Muslims or people of Middle Eastern heritage) as inhuman and thus undeserving of rights as specified in the United States Bill of Rights and federal laws. These rights include the right to travel freely, the right not to be imprisoned without legal representation, freedom from personal assault and mockery, freedom from intrusions into personal conversations and affairs, equal access to education and health services, freedom from fear, and the right to pursue happiness. Ethics education in public health must emphasize the salience of these rights as precursors to a just society in which disease and injury are not imposed willingly on certain classes of people.

Thus, the challenge for public health educators today is to hold steadfastly to their defining ethical principles as the culture of public health in the United States once again swings toward a bitter divide between people who are deemed desirable and those whose hopes and dreams are to be crushed.

Source: A. M. Rossignol and P. A. Rossignol, "Us and Them: Public Health Ethics in an Age of 'Otherness'"; *Reflections* 10, no. 1 (March 2003): 8. Reprinted with permission from the Program for Ethics, Science, and the Environment, Department of Philosophy, Oregon State University.

plant" actually is underrepresented in the case series and therefore may not be a cause of the cases' ill health.

A comparison group provides the investigator with a baseline, or representative accounting of the typical exposures and experiences for people who are similar to the cases but who lack the disease or injury of interest. Investigators sometimes misinterpret case reports and case series as demonstrating a relationship between the disease or injury of interest and some prior exposure, conveying the idea that the exposure is the cause of the disease or injury. Inclusion of a comparison group in the study usually avoids that kind of error. Case reports and case series, like other descriptive studies, are used to generate hypotheses about disease and injury etiology but should not be interpreted as hypothesis-evaluating.

A classic example of a medical treatment that initially was based on a case series is gastric freezing as a treatment for ulcers. In 1962, a new treatment for duodenal ulcers was initiated. The treatment involved placing a tube down a person's throat into the stomach and circulating a cold liquid through the tube, thereby freezing the person's stomach (Wangensteen et al. 1962). The procedure was intended to ease the symptoms caused by the ulcer. Patients who had their stomachs frozen generally reported a lessening of symptoms. The procedure was not evaluated using a comparison group until 1969 (Ruffin et al. 1969). In this evaluation, people who had their stomachs frozen reported the same severity and prevalence of symptoms related to their ulcers as did a comparison group of patients with ulcers who had not had their stomachs frozen. Thus, the initial conclusion about the efficacy of gastric freezing, based solely on the case series, was incorrect.

What comparison treatment should be used in evaluating whether gastric freezing is an effective treatment for duodenal ulcers? Clearly, a person would know whether a tube was placed down his or her throat and cold liquid circulated. Such knowledge might **bias** (be systematically in error) study subjects to report a lessening of symptoms associated with stomach freezing if the subjects believed that they would benefit from the procedure. For this reason, the study investigators placed tubes down every subject's throat and circulated a cold liquid down each tube. For the comparison subjects, however, the cold liquid traveled only as far as the esophagus and did not enter the stomach; thus the stomachs of the comparison subjects were not frozen, although they, and all subjects in the study, believed that their stomachs had been frozen.

Why did the patients whose stomachs were not frozen report a lessening of symptoms when, apparently, no benefits accrued as a result of the treatment? It is not unusual for subjects, in a variety of different settings and having different health conditions, to report short-term improvements in symptoms in response to treatment regimens that are ineffective. These alleged improvements are an example of **placebo effects.** Such effects can be quite large, at least over the short term.

Placebo effects occur as a response to increased attention given to people who are ill; that is, the mere fact of being in a study or being given a treatment (regardless of its physiologic helpfulness) can result in people's reporting reduced prevalence and severity of symptoms. Such effects tend to be especially large for health conditions whose symptoms are vague, etiologies are unclear, and treatment options are limited. Examples of such health conditions are "sick building syndrome," premenstrual syndrome, chronic fatigue syndrome, and post-traumatic stress disorder. People having these health conditions may have been told by their clinicians that the reason for their ill health is "psychological," with the implication that the condition is not "real." Clinical validation that a health condition is "real" may have a strong although often time-limited placebo effect, reducing the perceived number and severity of symptoms.

Errors in medical treatment have been made because treatment options have been based on case reports and on case series. Those errors include performing unnecessary mastectomies for breast cancer and unnecessary coronary bypass surgery for people with coronary heart disease. In the latter example, when clinical trials eventually were conducted in the 1980s to evaluate the efficacy of coronary bypass surgery in comparison with the most practical drug treatment available at the time for people having coronary heart disease, it was found that some patients in the surgery group suffered more short-term morbidity than did the drug treatment group, paid higher medical costs, and showed no improvement in long-term prognosis such as in age-specific mortality. In the breast cancer example, studies indicated that for some women, the benefits of lumpectomies plus radiation or chemotherapy were equal to the results achieved through performing mastectomies.

Cross-Sectional Studies

The second type of descriptive study is the **cross-sectional study.** The strict definition of a cross-sectional study is a study in which information about exposure and about disease or injury refers to the same point in time. For that reason, it can be unclear whether the exposure preceded or was modified by the health outcome of interest. The strict definition of a cross-sectional study probably is too narrow. The characteristic that renders a study "cross-sectional" is lack of clarity about whether the exposure under study preceded the health outcome under study *far enough in time* to possibly be a cause of the health outcome. "Far enough in time" means at least as long as the minimum latency period between the exposure and the health outcome. *An epidemiologic study that neglects to include an accurate time-response may inadvertently be cross-sectional even if the exposure and the health outcome under study refer to different points in time* (Figure 7.4). In Figure 7.4, any exposure occurring within the ten-year latency period for the health outcome of interest cannot be a cause of the health outcome. A study relating exposures within the ten-year latency period to the health outcome is not valid in the sense of having a **latency period bias.**

An example of a cross-sectional study is the study of smoking habits and health outcomes conducted among 8,040 students aged 13–18 years in Nord-Trondelag County, Norway. In this study, 13.3 percent of the 372 boys who currently smoke tobacco daily reported nervousness or restlessness "often" last month, and 18.5 percent reported "sleep problems in the last month." The corresponding percentages for the 1,789 nonsmoking boys were 4.2 percent and 7.9 percent (Holmen et al. 2000). Note that in these data, both the exposure (current daily smoking) and the outcomes (nervousness/restlessness and sleep problems in the last month) refer to essentially the same point in time. For that reason, it is unclear whether daily smoking caused some or all of the increase in nervousness/restlessness or difficulty sleeping among the boys who smoked. As the authors correctly pointed out, it may be, to the contrary, that because the boys were nervous or restless, or had trouble sleeping, they began to smoke daily. This difficulty in ascertaining the true time sequence between the exposure and the health outcome is the hallmark challenge in interpreting a cross-sectional study.

Another example of a cross-sectional study is a report of consumption of caffeine-containing beverages and the prevalence and severity of premenstrual syndrome (PMS) (Rossignol and Bonnlander 1990). The investigators queried 841 resident undergraduate students at a public university in Oregon. The study questionnaire solicited information about the presence and severity of menstrual and premenstrual symptoms, demographic characteristics, use of over-the-counter drugs containing caffeine, and typical daily consumption of beverages, including caffeine- containing beverages. Analysis of the data revealed a strong **dose-response relationship** between usual, daily consumption of

FIGURE 7.4
Depiction of a cross-sectional study for a disease having a ten-year latency period.

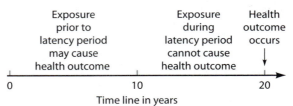

caffeine-containing beverages and premenstrual symptoms that was not explained by differences in daily total fluid consumption. As noted previously, a dose-response relationship is an association between an exposure and an outcome in which an increase or a decrease in the dose results in a systematic increase or a decrease in the health response. Specifically, in the caffeine-and-PMS example, as the level of exposure to caffeine-containing beverages (the "dose") increased from zero cups per day to eight to ten cups per day, the prevalence of premenstrual symptoms increased 6.5-fold.

Interpreting the results of this study is problematic. Does caffeine cause PMS, or do women who experience PMS drink caffeine-containing beverages to overcome the tiredness or other symptoms caused by premenstrual syndrome? There is some evidence to suggest that both of those interpretations may be true. Caffeine may cause PMS, and, in addition, women with PMS may self-medicate with caffeine in response to their symptoms, thereby exacerbating the severity of their PMS (Rossignol et al. 1991).

PMS is an interesting example of a health condition that probably is initiated anew during each menstrual cycle or, at least, over a relatively few number of cycles. Thus, whether or not PMS is caused or exacerbated by caffeine probably could be evaluated straightforwardly by having women refrain from consuming caffeine-containing beverages and cease using medications that contain caffeine. An investigator could then observe the effects, if any, on the presence and severity of the women's premenstrual symptoms. For other exposure-health status associations identified in cross-sectional studies, evaluating whether the association is causal is considerably more difficult. That difficulty could be especially challenging if the time between exposure and outcome is long. Did the exposure occur *long enough* before the health outcome to be a cause of the health outcome? That challenging question arises in studies of many of the chronic diseases such as the heart diseases, cancers, and cerebrovascular diseases. In contrast, the difficulty in determining whether an exposure preceded or was modified by a health outcome does not occur in cross-sectional studies in which the exposure of interest is a long-standing characteristic that does not vary over time. Such characteristics include blood type and gender.

As a further example of the challenges in interpreting exposure-heath associations in cross-sectional studies, few people would disagree that tobacco smoking causes lung cancer. It is not the cigarette a person smoked yesterday, however, that resulted in his or her lung cancer that was diagnosed today (one day later). There is a physiologically-determined interval in time between the exposure and the development of disease (i.e., the latency period). Could the cigarettes a person smoked five years ago have caused a lung cancer diagnosed today? If not, then those cigarettes should not be counted as contributing to the development of the lung cancer. Perhaps only cigarettes smoked at least ten years earlier can be causal. Or, perhaps only cigarettes smoked twenty or more years earlier can result in a lung cancer diagnosed today. The length of the latency period for a particular exposure-health association must be quantified in order to determine whether a study is cross-sectional (even though the exposure and health condition refer to the same point in time). In addition, ideally, exposures, if any, that affect the length of a latency period for a particular exposure-health association should be identified and quantified; any changes in the lengths of a minimum latency period must be taken into account when determining whether a study is cross-sectional.

A related issue is how to measure the dose of exposure when exposure occurs over a long period of time and at different doses over time. Again, cigarette smoking provides an excellent example. How should the latency period be determined? Should a person's first smoked cigarette be the start of the latency period, even though one cigarette in all likelihood will not result in a lung cancer? If not, after how many cigarettes and in what pattern of smoking should the latency period start?

Another related difficulty is the question of whether early symptoms of the health outcome could have altered exposure, such as may occur, for example, when early symptoms of heart disease cause a person to alter his or her diet, exercise, or tobacco use habits. This change in habits may occur either in an attempt to reduce the severity of the symptoms or because the symptoms make certain habits, such as strenuous exercise, difficult. Finally, it is important to appreciate that latency periods, like random variables, often follow probability or other distributions (see Chapter 11 for a discussion of distributions). For this reason, the length of a latency period may differ from one person to another, for the same exposure-health condition association.

Correlational Studies

The third type of descriptive study is the **correlational study,** also often referred to as an **ecological study.** In a correlational study, data about disease or injury, and about exposure, are collected for *groups of people (and not for individual people),* and then those data are correlated with one another. "**Correlate,**" in this sense, means that the data points for each exposure and outcome pair are plotted on a grid, and then the *linear association* between the exposure and the outcome is calculated. A grid, in general, takes the following form (Figure 7.5). Note that a grid may be drawn with the exposure either on the *y*-axis as in Figure 7.3 or on the *x*-axis as in Figure 7.5.

As an example of correlational studies, Figures 7.6 and 7.7 summarize part of the findings from a correlational study of coronary heart disease mortality among men aged 55–64 years in forty countries in relation to an index for cholesterol and saturated fat and in relation to milk intake (Artaud-Wild et al. 1993).

In each figure, the number of coronary deaths per 100,000 person-years for men aged 55–64 years is given on the vertical (or *y*) axis, and either the average per capita cholesterol and saturated-fat index (Figure 7.6) or the average per capita milk intake (Figure 7.7) is given on the horizontal (or *x*) axis. In the study, the cholesterol–saturated-fat index, or CSI, was calculated as CSI = (1.01 × grams saturated fat) + (0.05 mg cholesterol).

In the original figures, the authors showed the location on the grid for each of the forty countries included in the study. Figures 7.6 and 7.7 show only the locations of the data for Finland and for France and the regression line summarizing the association between the coronary heart disease mortality rate and either the CSI or the average milk intake for all forty countries. Notice that the "dots" (small triangles) for Finland and for France represent the coronary heart disease mortality rate and the average exposure status for the entire population in each country and *not* for individual people.

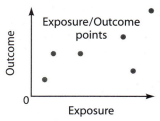

FIGURE 7.5
Grid of exposure versus health outcome.

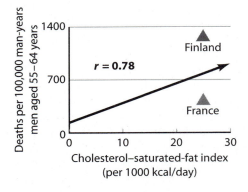

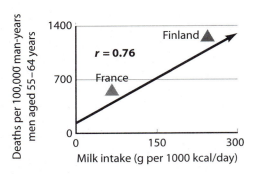

FIGURE 7.6
Coronary heart disease mortality in relation to cholesterol–saturated-fat index.

FIGURE 7.7
Coronary heart disease mortality in relation to milk intake.

Source: Figures 7.6 and 7.7 suggested by data from Artaud-Wild et al. 1993.

Both Figure 7.6 and Figure 7.7 show strong linear associations between exposure status and coronary heart disease mortality. (This association is more easily appreciated by looking at the regression lines that are based on the authors' original figures.) In other words, as the value for the average CSI or milk intake increases, coronary heart disease mortality tends to increase linearly, and vice versa. France and Finland are highlighted in these figures because of their unusual positions in Figure 7.6 but not in Figure 7.7. This finding suggests that perhaps people in Finland have a diet high in foods other than those containing cholesterol and/or saturated fat that cause coronary heart disease. Figure 7.6 suggests that perhaps people in France have a diet high in foods that, on balance, prevent coronary heart disease regardless of the population's overall diet that is high in cholesterol and/or saturated fat.

Thus, the CSI may be an **indicator,** or **marker,** for the presence or absence of another exposure or other exposures, related to coronary heart disease mortality, that differ between Finland and France. An indicator, or marker, is a **variable** (a factor that can have more than one value) that is **associated** with another variable; this other variable is the true cause of the health outcome under study. "Associated" means that the presence or the severity of a variable is more prevalent among people who have a certain exposure than among people lacking this exposure. As an example, unrelated to Figures 7.6 and 7.7, carrying matches or a lighter is a risk indicator for lung cancer because most people who carry matches or a lighter on a regular basis do so to light their cigarettes, and smoking cigarettes is a true cause of lung cancer. This association can be depicted pictorially as:

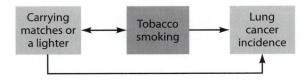

The challenge posed by disease and injury indicators is common in many correlational studies. In other words, one of the difficult aspects of interpreting the results of correlational studies is determining whether the exposure under study is in itself related to the disease or injury under study or whether it is an indicator for some other exposure of etiologic importance. As another example, correlational studies fairly consistently have shown a **positive** linear relationship between per capita meat consumption and countries' mortality rates from colon cancer. ("Positive," as used here, means that as a country's per capita meat consumption increases, the country's colon cancer mortality rate tends to increase. A **negative** or **inverse** association would mean that as a country's per capita meat consumption increases, the country's colon cancer mortality rate tends to decrease.) Determining whether this association is causal is complicated by the fact that many factors vary with per capita meat consumption, such as average income; fruit, vegetable, and grain consumption (a negative association); and population density.

Often, the results from a correlational study, as in Figures 7.6 and 7.7, are summarized using the statistic **r.** This statistic, called the **correlation coefficient,** measures the degree of *linear association* between two **normally distributed** variables. (The phrase "normally distributed" is discussed in the next paragraph.) The possible values for r range from -1 to $+1$, with both -1 and $+1$ indicating a perfect linear association between the two variables (-1, a perfect negative association, and $+1$, a perfect positive association) and 0 indicating no linear association between the two variables. "Perfect," as used here, means that all the observations lie exactly on the correlation line. In the study of coronary heart disease mortality just discussed, r was equal to 0.78 for the association with CSI and 0.76 for the association with milk intake.

A variable that is normally distributed belongs to a family of variables that have distinct "bell-shaped" curves, as depicted below. In the depiction, the y-axis shows the *percentage* of values for the variable that are contained *within a certain range of values* for that variable. The x-axis shows the actual values for the variable. For variables that are normally distributed, the sum of all the percentages for values of the variable (the shaded area "under the curve") equals one (1.0) μ is the **mean** (average value) of the variable.

Although a full discussion of probability distributions is beyond the scope of this text, it is important to appreciate that the analysis of epidemiologic data, especially data used to evaluate an epidemiologic hypothesis, depends on identifying the underlying probability distribution for the data. Each type of probability distribution has its own set of characteristics that distinguish it from other probability distributions. In the case of a variable that has a normal distribution, the distribution

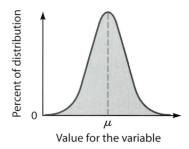

Depiction of a variable that is normally distributed.

- Has a single peak value in its center that is equal to the mean for the distribution
- Is symmetrical around the mean value
- Has values along the x-axis from negative infinity to positive infinity
- Has an area under the probability curve equal to 1.0

The defining characteristic of a correlational study, and the defining limitation, is the fact that the data used in the study refer to groups of people as a whole, and not to individual people. Thus, neither the exposure nor the health status is known for any individual person in the study, nor is it known whether the people in the study who have the disease or injury of interest are the same people who have the exposure of interest. This difficulty means that correlational studies, like other descriptive studies, cannot be used to evaluate epidemiologic hypotheses but can be used only to suggest associations between exposures and outcomes—that is, to help develop epidemiologic hypotheses. It is a serious error to interpret the results of a descriptive study, such as a correlational study, as implying a causal association between the exposure and the outcome under study. Further epidemiologic research using analytic study designs is necessary to evaluate whether the suggested associations are causal.

When the results of a correlational study are misinterpreted as implying causation, the resulting error often is called an **ecologic fallacy.** "Ecologic fallacy" refers to the error of drawing conclusions about disease or injury causation in individuals based on data from groups. For example, group data may be available on average nutritional level and average number of traffic injuries, suggesting a linear association between the two variables. An ecologic error would occur if those data were interpreted to mean that having a low nutritional level increases a person's risk of sustaining a traffic-related injury.

There is one additional feature of the correlational study design that is problematic. Because data are collected for groups of people, and not for individuals, it is not possible to control for the **confounding effects of variables** during the data analysis phase of the study. For instance, in the example of poor nutritional status and traffic injuries, it may be that having a poorer nutritional status is related to an increased use of alcoholic beverages, and it is the use of those beverages and not the poorer nutritional status that increases the risk of sustaining a traffic-related injury. Recall that confounding variables are factors that are associated with the exposure under study and that are independent causes of the health outcome of interest. Quite often in epidemiologic studies, the presence or magnitude of an association between an exposure and a health outcome results not because there is a causal association between the two variables (or a causal association that is smaller or larger than the "true" causal association). The association occurs because some other variable (a confounding factor) associated with the exposure is the true cause of the disease or injury under study. Figure 7.8 shows a pictorial depiction of confounding.

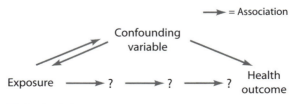

FIGURE 7.8
Pictorial representation of confounding.

Confounding variables obscure the true size of association between an exposure and a health outcome of interest because they exert an effect on the association that is "mixed in," to an often unknown extent, with the true effect. Prevention and control of confounding is the primary challenge in epidemiologic study design and data analysis confounding will be discussed in detail in Chapter 12.

SUMMARY

In summary, each of the three major types of descriptive studies has strengths, which lie in providing basic epidemiologic data on which to plan for health services and other programmatic needs and for generating epidemiologic hypotheses that later are evaluated in analytic epidemiologic studies. Each type of study also has major weaknesses, as summarized in Table 7.1.

As you think about the different types of descriptive studies, think about what descriptive data would be most useful to you in your professional field, and how and where you might conduct a descriptive study to obtain those data. For example, if you are interested in health promotion and health behaviors, what data might you need to focus an educational intervention on populations at high risk for teenage pregnancy? Where might you obtain those data inexpensively? Does a community, state, or federal survey routinely collect such data, and, if so, are the data readily available to the public at little or no monetary cost? When using routinely collected data that were collected with a different objective in mind (that is, without your study in mind), what limitations might the data have with respect to the definitions of variables used, the time frame surveyed, the people specifically included in or excluded from the study, or to questions not asked? Is a codebook available that clearly defines each variable? Were the questions asked unambiguous? Was the response rate (the proportion of people targeted for inclusion in the survey who actually participated) high enough to have prevented substantial bias in the data from this source? Although many descriptive studies rely on previously collected data and hence may serve as a good first look at a health problem, it nevertheless is worthwhile to adopt a critical view of the data. "Critical" means asking the types of questions just mentioned to assess how useful the data will be in meeting

TABLE 7.1

Major Limitations of Each Type of Epidemiologic Descriptive Study

Type of Study	Definition	Major Limitation
Correlational	Data for populations and not for individuals	No data on exposure or health outcome for individuals; lack of control for confounding
Cross-sectional	Data on exposure and outcome either refer to the same point in time or refer to points in time closer than minimum latent period for a disease	Lack of clarity regarding whether the exposure preceded the outcome and so may be a cause of the outcome, or was modified by the outcome
Case reports; case series	Data for cases but no data for a comparison group	No comparison group

your particular professional needs. As will become clearer in the discussions of the analytic epidemiologic studies (Chapters 9 and 10), obtaining accurate data about exposures, confounders, and health outcomes in human populations is a challenging endeavor. All epidemiologic data contain at least some errors. The challenge is to be able to discern which data are useful and the extent to which they are useful and which data lack the accuracy and rigor necessary to serve as a basis for epidemiologic inquiry.

REVIEW QUESTIONS

1. List the major types of study designs.
2. List the primary objectives of descriptive studies.
3. Define "epidemiologic hypothesis." Then list at least five components of an epidemiologic hypothesis.
4. List and define the three main types of descriptive studies. What is the primary limitation(s) of each type of study?
5. Define an "indicator" or "marker" for an exposure or a disease. Then provide three examples of exposure indicators and three examples of disease indicators that might be useful to measure and include in the data collected for an epidemiologic study. What does each of the indicators you provided measure?
6. Define "correlation coefficient." In which type of descriptive study is a correlation coefficient used?
7. Define "ecologic fallacy." In which type of descriptive study is an ecologic fallacy most likely to occur?
8. Define "confounding effect." Why do you think that prevention and control of confounding is a major challenge in epidemiology?
9. Cross-sectional studies usually are defined as studies in which the exposure and the outcome of interest refer to the same point in time. What modification to this definition is useful when the health outcome of interest is a disease with a long latent period?
10. Define "comparison group" as this phrase is used in the context of case reports or case series.
11. Define "placebo effect." What do you think causes placebo effects?

REVIEW EXERCISES

1. What descriptive epidemiologic data might you wish to assemble before initiating an analytic study evaluating whether meat consumption is a cause of colon cancer? Where might you find these descriptive data; that is, what sources of data (for example, routinely conducted surveys, governmental sources, Web sites, product sales data) might you review? What possible confounding variables might concern you as you review and interpret the descriptive data you assemble?
2. Find examples of descriptive studies in epidemiology journals. Review each article with respect to the type and objective(s) of descriptive study, plan for data collection, plan for data analysis, possible sources of error, results, and interpretation of study findings.

## CHAPTER 8

Causation

CAUSATION

Before discussing the analytic epidemiological studies, it is helpful to understand the epidemiologic concept of **causation** and how epidemiologists determine whether or not an association between an exposure and an outcome is causal. Ideally, analytic studies evaluate whether an exposure is causally related to (and not just "associated with") a certain health outcome. For that reason, it again is helpful to understand the process by which associations come to be viewed as "causal relationships."

Most people have an intuitive understanding of what causation means. The crowing of a rooster does not cause the sun to rise, but dropping a glass of milk does cause the milk to spill. In the first example, most people rely on their knowledge of physics to conclude that the rooster has no control over the sun. In the second example, repetition (every time I drop the glass, the milk spills) and physical, scientific plausibility help guide the decision about causality.

Conclusions regarding causality are considerably more difficult to determine in epidemiology. At times, a **strong association** between an exposure and a health outcome is observed that eventually is found not to be causal. A strong association means that the frequency of disease is more or less common among exposed people than it is among people who are not exposed. An example of a strong association that eventually was determined not to be causal is following: Many well-conducted case/control studies documented a strong, consistent association between beta-carotene (after ingestion, beta-carotene can be converted in the body to Vitamin A) and a reduced frequency of certain cancers (Peto et al. 1981). More-definitive studies (intervention trials, as discussed in Chapter 9) found that the association was not causal (Hennekens, Buring, and Manson 1996).

A second example is the repeatedly observed and assumed causal association between hormone replacement therapy (HRT) for menopausal symptoms and a reduced risk of heart disease. A more definitive study (again an intervention trial) of

HRT and heart disease demonstrated that the reduced risk of heart disease was not causally related to HRT. Instead, women who had greater access to health services and who generally enjoyed lower risk factors for heart disease were the women receiving HRT. When these other causes of heart disease were taken into account in the HRT trial, no reduction in heart disease associated with HRT was observed (Grady et al. 2002).

How can epidemiologists establish causation between an exposure and a health outcome, such as a chronic disease, when the biophysical connection between the exposure and the outcome usually is not directly observable and may be separated by long distances in time? Although a number of different strategies can be employed to determine causation in epidemiology, most epidemiologists try to determine whether an exposure causes a certain health outcome by asking (and answering) a prescribed set of questions about the observed association. Some of the most commonly asked questions or criteria used to evaluate causation, based on the pioneering work of A. Bradford Hill, are the subjects of the following sections.

CRITERIA FOR EVALUATING CAUSATION

1. How Strong Is the Association between Exposure and Outcome?

All else being equal, a stronger association is more likely to be causal than is a weaker association. For example, a lifetime habit of smoking a pack of cigarettes each day is associated with an approximately 40 percent increase in the incidence rate of cardiovascular disease (see Box 8.1) and a 900 percent increase in the incidence rate of lung cancer. Based solely on that information, this criterion for establishing causation suggests that the association between smoking and lung cancer is more likely to be causal than is the association between smoking and coronary heart disease. This conclusion reflects the substantially larger increase in the IR and MR of lung cancer associated with smoking than the increase in cardiovascular disease. (In reality, both associations are causal.)

2. Is the Association Biologically Credible?

For instance, does the exposure come into contact with the organ or anatomic site of the health outcome, or is the exposure metabolized or excreted by the target site or organ? It is biologically credible that smoking causes lung cancer because tobacco smoke comes into contact with the lung. In addition, because some of the mutagenic constituents and metabolites of tobacco smoke are excreted in urine, it makes sense biologically that smoking may be a cause of bladder cancer.

3. Are the Results of Epidemiologic Studies Generally Consistent with Respect to the Presence and Size of an Association between Exposure and Outcome?

If there is consistency in the size of the association between the exposure and the health outcome in different studies, then the association is more likely to be causal than is an association that is not consistent among studies. Almost always, many epidemiologic studies evaluating whether there is an association between a certain exposure and a certain disease outcome are conducted in different populations before a possible interpretation of causality is warranted. That repetition of studies is necessary because the vast majority of epidemiologic studies are **observational** (not experimental); thus, **bias** (systematic error) is a possible explanation for study results. As an example, approximately fifty studies of the relationship between tobacco smoking and lung cancer had been conducted before the Surgeon General of the United States indicated that smoking *may* be a cause of lung cancer.

In an observational study it is important to appreciate that a particular exposure-health outcome association may *not* be causal even if the magnitude of the association is consistent among studies. A study investigator does not assign study participants to an exposure(s), as occurs in an experimental study. It may be that, as in the HRT and coronary heart disease studies, all the results of the studies were consistent because all the studies incorporated the same biases into their study designs. In other words, sometimes the process by which people come to have certain exposures results in a fundamental noncomparability among participants with respect to their risks of disease and injury. For example, a person who smokes cigarettes may be more likely to drink alcoholic beverages and/or to exercise sparsely than is a person who does not smoke cigarettes. For that reason, smokers and nonsmokers may have different risks of developing certain diseases and injuries over and above the differences that result from their tobacco habits or lack thereof. That "residual noncomparability" manifests in epidemiologic studies as bias, usually confounding bias.

4. Is the Time-Response between the Exposure and the Health Outcome Appropriate?

In other words, did the exposure occur at a time far enough before the outcome to have been a cause of the outcome? As mentioned previously, sometimes, in the study of a chronic disease, an exposure precedes the disease in time but does not precede the disease far enough in time to be a cause, taking the disease's latent period into account. For example, bladder cancer has a **latency period** (the time between the occurrence or the accumulation of a sufficient amount of the causal agent(s) and the occurrence of the disease) of at least twenty-five years and sometimes as long as forty years. Thus, it is unlikely that an exposure occurring ten or fifteen years before the onset of a bladder cancer is a cause of the cancer. There may be exceptions to a typical time-response pattern for a certain disease, however. For example, BCME (Bis-Chloromethyl Ether), an occupational carcinogen, can cause lung cancer, even in young (40–49-year-old) people, after a latency period of only five years rather than a more typical latent period for other causes of lung cancer (twenty years or longer) (http:www.epa.govirissubst0375.htm).

5. Is There a Dose-Response Relationship between the Exposure and the Health Outcome?

When there is a dose-response relation between an exposure and a health outcome, the incidence rate of the health outcome increases or decreases as a mathematical function of the amount and/or duration of the exposure. All else being equal, the presence of a dose-response relationship supports an interpretation of causation. For example, as the amount and/or duration of tobacco smoking increases, the incidence rate of bronchogenic carcinoma (one type of lung cancer) increases. Similarly, as the level of physical fitness increases, the incidence rate of coronary heart disease decreases.

The absence of a dose-response relationship does not necessarily mean that the association is not causal. It may be that there is a threshold amount of the exposure that, once accumulated, increases or decreases the risk of disease to a certain extent regardless of any additional amount of the exposure. Such a model seems to apply to the association between DES (diethylstilbestrol) and adenocarcinoma, a cancer of the vagina that is rare in young women who were not exposed in utero to DES (Herbst et al. 1971). DES was prescribed for pregnant women from 1938 through 1971 to help prevent miscarriages.

Similarly, the presence of a dose-response relationship does *not* guarantee that the association is causal. A dose-response relationship might be observed if the amount of a confounding factor mirrors any changes in the amount of exposure. In that situation, a dose-response relation would be observed only because of the increased magnitude of confounding associated with increases in exposure.

6. Are the Henle-Koch Postulates Satisfied?

The Henle-Koch postulates are the historical reference point for establishing causation for the acute onset infectious diseases. The postulates state that to be a cause of a particular disease, the infectious agent must be able to be isolated from *all* cases of the disease, grown in culture in a laboratory, and, when injected into a susceptible host, cause the disease. In addition, the infectious agent must be able to be isolated from these new cases and grown in culture (Rivers 1937).

These postulates in their strict meaning, though still sometimes used in microbiology, often are no longer helpful in establishing causation for certain diseases, especially diseases that do not have an infectious etiology. In addition, there are obvious ethical constraints associated with injecting an alleged causal agent into a susceptible host to evaluate causality. Interestingly, however, the postulates have been modified to apply to noninfectious diseases and to chronic diseases with an infectious etiology (Evans 1978). Thus, using a modified version of the postulates, it might be posited that tobacco use is a cause of lung cancer because it is a habit of many people who develop lung cancer (and is a more common habit in people who develop lung cancer than in people who do not develop lung cancer); more cigarettes can be manufactured; and when those cigarettes are used by populations of previous nonsmokers, lung cancer begins to occur after an approximately twenty-year latency period.

As more of the criteria (questions 1–6) are satisfied, generally the possibility that an exposure–health association is causal increases (Table 8.1). There are, however, no definitive criteria or standards that can guarantee that an association between a certain exposure and health outcome is causal.

TABLE 8.1
Summary of Criteria for Evaluating Causation

Criterion	Criterion for Evaluating Causation
1	How strong is the association between exposure and outcome?
2	Is the association between exposure and outcome biologically credible?
3	Is the presence and size of the association consistent among epidemiologic studies?
4	Is the time-response relation between the exposure and the outcome appropriate?
5	Is there a dose-response relation between the exposure and the outcome?
6	Are the Henle-Koch postulates satisfied?

7. Prelude to Intervention Studies

In evaluating epidemiologic hypotheses, the gold standard of studies is the **intervention study,** discussed in detail in Chapter 9. In an intervention study, the investigator **randomly assigns** the study participants to different treatment/exposure groups. Random assignment means that every participant in the study has the same probability of being in any of the treatment/exposure groups as does every other participant. Because of random assignment, concerns about whether the study results are in error because of bias (and, in particular, because of confounding bias) are minimal as long as the assignment of treatment/exposure is random and a large enough number of participants is included in the study. The results of intervention studies are easier to interpret and lend themselves more readily to interpretations of causality than do the observational studies, because observational studies lack the random assignment of treatment/exposure.

A MODEL FOR DISEASE/INJURY CAUSATION

One other aspect of causation warrants discussion. Most, if not all, chronic diseases are caused by more than one exposure, even in an individual person. Consequently, various models of causation in disease and injury have been developed in an attempt to provide useful, conceptual frameworks for understanding the multidimensional aspects of causality (Rothman 1976). At least one aspect of those models can be particularly useful both theoretically and practically. That aspect is the distinction among necessary component causes of a health outcome, component causes, and sufficient causes. A **necessary component cause** is a component cause that must be present in *every* case of a particular disease or injury. Necessary component causes are exposures whose presence does not guarantee that a certain health outcome will occur but whose absence guarantees that the outcome will not occur. Examples of necessary component causes are infection with *Mycobacterium tuberculosis* for tuberculosis and exposure to silica for silicosis.

A **component cause** is an exposure that contributes to a certain health outcome but whose presence, by itself (that is, without other component causes), will not result in the health or injury outcome. A **sufficient cause** is a constellation of component causes

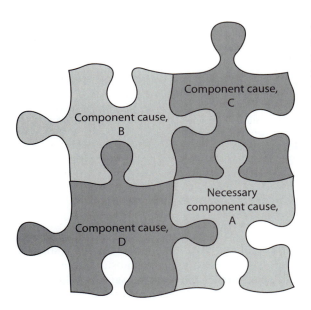

The interaction of A + B + C + D = a sufficient
cause for a hypothetical disease

FIGURE 8.1

Depiction 1 of necessary component causes, component
causes, and sufficient causes.*

*Following Rothman 1976.

or of a necessary component cause in addition to component causes that, acting together, will result in a certain disease or injury unless some intervening event, such as death or administration of an antidote for the sufficient cause, occurs. Figures 8.1 and 8.2 depict the differences among necessary component causes, component causes, and sufficient causes. In Figure 8.1, there is only one sufficient cause for a hypothetical disease, whereas in Figure 8.2, there are three sufficient causes for a different hypothetical disease.

In Figure 8.2, exposure A is a necessary sufficient cause. Removal of A from this population would not allow *any* of the sufficient causes to form, because each sufficient cause requires A as one of its component causes. One hundred percent of the disease or injury would be prevented by removal of component cause S would prevent all disease or injury caused by either the first or the third sufficient cause because each of these two sufficient causes requires component cause S. Eighty-five percent of the disease or injury (50% from SC1 + 35% from SC3) would be prevented. Elimination of component causes L, W and/or X would result in a 15 percent reduction in disease or injury in this population. Removal of component cause C would result in a 35 percent decrease. If feasible, an effective prevention program would target the necessary component cause A because its elimination would result in a 100 percent decrease in the incidence. This preventative approach, however, may not be feasible. For example, if A is an unalterable exposure, such as a certain genotype, A is "too expensive" to remove, or if its removal would result in non-preventable harm to people and/or their environments, then removal of A may/will be problematic. The diagrams presented in Figure 8.2 may apply only to populations in which the component causes are similarly prevalent. For example, in a population lacking exposure C, and having no other significant causes than sufficient causes 1 and 2, all of the disease or injury would be cause by sufficient causes 1 (77% [50%/65%]) and 2 (23% [15%/65%]). (The percent of disease or injury caused by SC1 and SC2 is obtained by dividing the percent of disease or injury when all three sufficient causes are present by the percent of disease or injury attributable to SC1 and SC2 (50% to 15% = 65%).

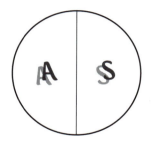 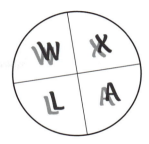 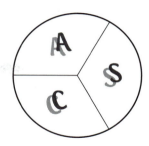

SC1[†] causes 50% of disease in this population	SC2[†] causes 15% of disease in this population	SC3[†] causes 35% of disease in this population
CC[‡] = A, S	CC[‡] = A, L, W, X	CC[‡] = A, C, S

FIGURE 8.2

Depiction 2 of necessary component causes, component causes, and sufficient causes for a disease having three sufficient causes.*

*Following Rothman 1976.

[†]Sufficient cause.

[‡]Component cause.

As an example of a component cause, cigarette smoking causes heart disease in the presence of other component causes. When these other component causes are missing, cigarette smoking does not result in heart disease. Usually (perhaps always), these other component causes are not known; their existence can be inferred, however, from the fact that not all people who smoke cigarettes develop heart disease, even if they live longer than the "usual" maximum latency period for smoking and heart disease.

Whenever a component cause is absent, disease or injury will not result from any sufficient cause of which that particular component cause is a part. In other words, without each component cause present, the sufficient cause is incomplete.

The practical importance of realizing that the absence of a component cause renders its corresponding sufficient cause(s) incomplete lies in the area of disease and injury prevention. To prevent disease or injury from a particular sufficient cause, it is necessary to prevent only one of the component causes (perhaps the easiest and most cost-effective component cause to prevent). It is not necessary to know each of the component causes of a particular disease or injury to prevent its occurrence. For instance, people who are exposed to both asbestos and tobacco smoke have an approximately ninetyfold increase in the incidence rate of lung cancer compared with people who are not exposed to either tobacco smoke or asbestos. Prevention of tobacco smoke exposure (active and environmental) among asbestos-exposed people will prevent most of the lung cancers in this group of people. Their incidence rate of lung cancer, all other exposures being comparable, will be about twice (instead of ninety times) the incidence rate for people who are not exposed to tobacco smoke or asbestos. If the alternative preventive strategy is undertaken, prevention of asbestos exposure, the incidence rate of lung cancer in this group of people will be about ten times the incidence rate among people who have neither exposure. Notice, in this example, that there must be at least three sufficient causes of lung cancer: One sufficient cause has both tobacco and asbestos exposures as component causes; a second sufficient cause has tobacco exposure but not asbestos exposure as a component cause; and a third sufficient cause has asbestos exposure but not tobacco exposure as a component cause.

SUMMARY

Boxes 8.1 through 8.4 present case studies of several aspects of causality in epidemiology. The boxes address, respectively

1. What Causes Cardiovascular Disease?
2. Why Do Some Consumer Products Kill?
3. Genetic versus Environmental Causes of Disease. (Also see the special case study on biocolonialism that follows Chapter 8.)
4. The Epidemiologist as Forensic Scientist.

As you read through these boxes, think how the authors applied the six criteria for establishing causation presented in this chapter. Which criteria were used most often, which were modified to apply to a specific situation, and which were inapplicable to the question at hand? Were other criteria to establish causation used and, if so, how were those criteria used?

Epidemiology is a dynamic science, presently undergoing rapid changes in its scopes of inquiry and modes of application. Although it is still directed toward solving new or long-standing health challenges such as preventing the leading causes of death and injury in the United States and/or elsewhere. While this is true, the webs of disease and injury causation, and thus prevention, within which epidemiologic inquiry proceeds often have become more complicated. For example, the emergence or resurgence of epidemic diseases such as tuberculosis, West Nile virus, certain food- or water-borne diseases, and HIV/AIDS in countries previously largely unaffected or, at least, not known to be affected, occurs in increasingly complicated global social and environmental systems. (HIV/AIDS in India is a case in point, with current estimates projecting an epidemic of the disease in massive proportions over the next decade.) In addition, epidemiologists are participating in new areas of concern such as surveillance and control of the potential effects of bioterrorism and the effects of "natural disasters" such as the tsunami that struck South Asia in 2004 and the extensive environmental and social health challenges caused by the 2005 flooding in New Orleans, Louisiana.

As you read through the case studies, as an epidemiologist or some other public health professional, think which public health problems you would like to help solve and how you might proceed to do so. What kind of personal and professional networking might you need in helping to solve the heath problems you deem important and also of personal interest? The networking necessary to solve public health problems begins now, with your soon-to-be professional colleagues and current mentors.

BOX 8.1

WHAT CAUSES CARDIOVASCULAR DISEASE?

California was the first state in the United States to begin experiencing a decrease in mortality from cardiovascular disease. The year was 1963, and by the late 1960s, many other states were experiencing a similar decrease. Data from epidemiologic studies initiated in the 1950s (for example, the Framingham Heart Study in Framingham, Massachusetts, and the Tecumseh Heart Study in Tecumseh, Michigan) and thereafter firmly established high blood pressure, tobacco use, inactivity, obesity, and serum cholesterol as major risk factors for cardiovascular disease. The association between serum cholesterol and cardiovascular disease later was refined to differentiate among high-density lipoproteins (HDLs), low-density lipoproteins (LDLs), and triglycerides, with the HDLs being beneficial for cardiovascular health and the LDLs and triglycerides detrimental to cardiovascular health.

What was puzzling about the associations between these known risk factors and cardiovascular disease was that none of them, alone or in combination, fully explained the dramatic increase and then decrease in cardiovascular disease mortality in the United States. Clearly, there were other, as yet unidentified, causes of cardiovascular disease.

Recent epidemiologic studies have begun to solve this puzzle. For example, it has been discovered that the level of C-reactive protein is a strong predictor of adverse cardiovascular events and, in fact, may be a stronger predictor than is a person's level of LDLs (Ridker et al. 2002). C-reactive protein increases in response to inflammation. Such inflammation appears to increase the development and increase of plaque within the artery walls, leading to atherosclerosis and cardiovascular disease. This discovery may explain why taking a small amount of aspirin either daily or every other day prevents not only a second myocardial infarction (MI) but also a first myocardial infarction. In addition, early treatment with aspirin following a cardiovascular event substantially lowers mortality from the event.

A second recent discovery, that elevated levels of homocysteine (an amino acid produced in the human body) probably contribute to elevated cardiovascular risk, furthers understanding of the risk factors for this disease. Homocysteine may act by irritating blood vessels, leading to atherosclerosis. In addition, in one study, treatment with folic acid (1 mg/day), vitamin B_{12}, and vitamin B_6, which together lower homocysteine levels, reduced the occurrence of major cardiovascular disease (Schnyder et al. 2002).

Cardiovascular events in the United States now are occurring less often to older individuals than in the past few decades and case fatality rates have dropped. These changes are attributable to the advent of improved therapies for cardiovascular events in addition to better adherence to preventive behaviors and medical interventions such as control of high blood pressure and reduction of LDLs. Increasingly, cardiovascular disease, rather than being a rapidly fatal occurrence, is becoming a chronic disease with death, often from congestive heart failure, occurring many years after the initial event. Some people have questioned whether this reduction in early mortality is contributing to an improvement in public health. For instance, a cardiovascular event that is survived

Box 8.1 continued

by an 85-year-old person may result in more years of life, but those years may be marked by extreme frailty, dementia, and/or limited independence.

REFERENCES
Ridker, Paul M., Nader Rifai, Lynda Rose, Julie E. Buring, and Nancy R. Cook. 2002. Comparison of C-reactive protein and low-density lipoprotein cholesterol levels in the prediction of first cardiovascular events. *New England Journal of Medicine* 347 (20): 1557–1565.
Schnyder Guido, Marco Roffi, Yvonne Flammer, Riccardo Pin, and Otto Martin Hess. 2002. Effect of homocysteine-lowering therapy with folic acid, Vitamin B12, and Vitamin B6 on clinical outcome after percutaneous intervention. The Swiss Heart Study: A randomized clinical trial. Journal of the American Medical Association 288:973–79.

BOX 8.2

ETHICS MATTERS: WHY DO SOME CONSUMER PRODUCTS KILL?

Injury epidemiologists know only too well the toll that certain consumer products have taken on peoples' lives: infamous products such as the Ford Pinto with its gas tank precariously close to a screw that impaled the gas tank and set off a fiery explosion after even a minor rear-end collision; an airplane, the DC-10, whose rear door fell off in flight just as it had during the end stage of testing in an on-ground vacuum encasement but which was allowed to fly without modification; torch sweaters, whose fluffy cotton material burned from waist to neck in a matter of seconds if brought close to an ignition source.

The public health literature is replete with examples of consumer products that kill. Why were those products allowed to reach the marketplace? The story of cyanide-laced Tylenol is instructive. In 1982, a person entered a grocery store and laced several bottles of Tylenol with cyanide. Seven people died after ingesting the tainted Tylenol. Because of those deaths and the fear that followed, pharmaceutical companies developed tamper-resistant containers for their products within several days. The irony of the story is that many consumers, and especially consumers with young children, had asked both companies and federal regulatory agencies for tamper-resistant drug containers to protect their children from inadvertent overdoses of the drugs. The pharmaceutical industry responded that it was "too difficult" to manufacture a tamper-resistant container. When concern over market share arose, however, tamper-resistant containers were made available. As a final irony, the initial tamper-resistant containers, while preventing young children from opening the container, were difficult for some people, particular elderly individuals and people with arthritis, to open the containers to obtain their needed medications.

As another illustrative example of a poorly designed consumer product is the household stove. Controls on many stoves can turn directly from Off to High, without having to go through the Low and Moderate temperature settings. Curious young children find crawling on stoves an adventure, particularly if colorful spice or other bottles are placed on the back edge of the stove or if items such as cookies are kept in cabinets above the stove. Many children crawling atop a stove have knocked a control knob to

Box 8.2 continued

High, with the result that the burner's temperature soars high enough to ignite the child's clothes and cause extensive burns (personal observation, Shriners Burns Institute, Boston). When stove manufacturers were asked why the control knobs were not made with a two-way process (for example, push down and then turn to Low, then Medium, then High), they responded that such a control was too difficult to manufacture. One such conversation with a stove manufacturer occurred during the year that the first American walked on the moon. How could making a safe stove control be more difficult than sending a person to the moon?

How do consumer-product manufacturers evaluate the safety of the products they design and produce? The education processes are rather secretive and certainly vary from manufacturer to manufacturer, but in one approach, the product is designed to function well and, after tooling for the product is compete or nearly complete, is reviewed and approved by a "product safety committee"—too late to modify the design of the product.

The typical product (or other) engineer receives little education in health and safety evaluation during his or her undergraduate experiences. Although the Accreditation Board for Engineering and Technology (ABET), the national board that accredits undergraduate engineering programs, requires education in health and safety for accreditation, to my knowledge, no engineering educational program has been denied accreditation because of failure to meet the health and safety requirement.

The list of consumer products that have killed includes a wide variety of products: certain types of cribs with slats too far apart, allowing an infant's body, but not the head, to slip through two slats, resulting in strangulation; certain Firestone tires, whose outer layer comes off, resulting in tire failure and crashes; automobiles that flip over when making a turn even at relatively low speeds; children's plastic toy cars with metal axles that puncture children's skulls when fallen upon. Those and other consumer products are monitored and regulated by United States Consumer Product Safety Commission (CPSC), the federal agency charged with safeguarding the public from dangerous consumer products.

Among the worst consumer products, in terms of health and safety, is the cigarette, even though, unfortunately, cigarettes explicitly were exempted from regulation by the CPSC. Cigarettes not only cause numerous diseases but also are responsible for most deaths by burning in the United States, especially as the ignition source for house fires. There have been a number of patents issued for cigarettes that self-extinguish when not "puffed on" for a few minutes. Requiring all cigarettes sold to be self-extinguishing, as has the state of New York (in 2004), would prevent many cigarette-related burn deaths in this country. Why did the tobacco companies state until recently that developing a self-extinguishing cigarette was too difficult a task?

Note: In June 2004, several tobacco companies reported that they had pilot-tested or shortly will pilot-test self-extinguishing cigarettes in several cities within the United States. Preliminary results indicated overall satisfaction with the cigarettes except for complaints from some consumers that the cigarettes self-extinguished before the consumer had finished smoking the cigarette.

BOX 8.3

GENETIC VERSUS ENVIRONMENTAL CAUSES OF DISEASE

Many diseases cluster within families; that is, some families and/or extended families experience higher frequencies of certain diseases than do others. Why does such clustering occur? The two primary possibilities are (1) similarity of genetic makeup within family members with certain genes predisposing people to particular diseases and (2) similarity in exposure to environmental and/or lifestyle factors that cause particular diseases. Separating genetic from environmental/lifestyle causes of disease can be a challenging endeavor. The difficulty lies in the fact that most children in a nuclear family share similarities in both genetic makeup and/or in environmental/lifestyle exposures. Monozygotic twins (twins arising from fertilization of one ovum) have exactly the same genetic makeup, and other siblings, given the same mother and father, have approximately 50 percent of their genetic makeup in common. Siblings within a nuclear family also share many of the same environmental and lifestyle exposures, including housing, food choices, physical-activity levels, air quality, psychosocial variables, and factors associated with the family's income level. Thus, the difficulty in separating genetic from environmental/lifestyle causes of disease lies in part on the fact that the closeness or remoteness of similar genetic and environmental/lifestyle causes of disease tends to co-vary. This concept can be depicted graphically as follows:

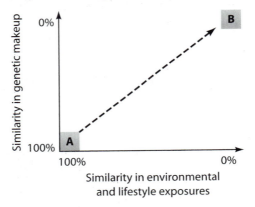

A = monozygotic twins living in the same household and "doing everything together."
B = unrelated people having polar opposite environmental and lifestyle exposures.

Given the tendency for genetic makeup and environmental/lifestyle exposures to vary together, how can these two potential causes of disease be studied separately? Some study designs provide a means for keeping the genetic makeup of study participants constant but varying their environmental and lifestyle exposures, or keeping study participants' environmental and/or lifestyle exposures constant and varying genetic

Box 8.3 continued

makeup. This concept is analogous to moving either vertically or horizontally on the preceding figure. Examples of study designs that can separate genetic from environmental/lifestyle exposures are depicted graphically as follows:

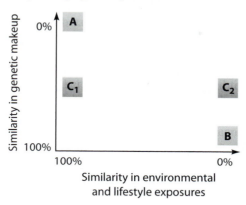

A = children adopted by the same family at birth who have different and unrelated, biologic mothers and fathers and who "do everything together."

B = monozygotic twins adopted by different families at birth and whose environmental and lifestyle exposures are polar opposites.

C = C_1 siblings (who therefore share approximately 50 percent of the same genetic makeup) living in the same family household who "do everything together" compared with C_2 siblings separated at birth and whose environmental and lifestyle exposures are polar opposites.

Another approach for separating genetic from environmental/lifestyle causes of disease includes studying migrant populations and their offspring. In these studies, migrant populations "bring their genes with them" but may move into an environment that differs substantially from the environment in which they formerly lived. The children of migrant populations tend to more quickly adopt the lifestyles prevalent in the new environment than do their parents, thus providing an opportunity to compare the effects of the new environment while keeping genetic similarity constant. The health of migrant populations also can be compared with the health of people from the same home area who did not migrate, although, in those comparisons, it is necessary to take into account the reasons why some people migrated and other people from the same area did not migrate. Understanding those reasons is important because the reasons may be associated with risk factors for disease. Epidemiologic studies of the kind depicted in the figure above and investigations of migrant populations offer intriguing opportunities for epidemiologists to better understand the causes of human disease. Indeed a new field of epidemiology inquiry, "genetic epidemiology," makes use of new methods for rapidly sequencing DNA explicitly for the purpose of discovering the genetic basis for human disease.

BOX 8.4

THE EPIDEMIOLOGIST AS FORENSIC SCIENTIST

MICHAEL D. FREEMAN, PH.D., D.C., M.P.H.

FORENSIC TRAUMA EPIDEMIOLOGIST, DEPARTMENT OF PUBLIC HEALTH AND

PREVENTIVE MEDICINE, OREGON HEALTH SCIENCES UNIVERSITY SCHOOL OF MEDICINE

On March 15, 44 B.C., Julius Caesar was the victim of a homicide, stabbed to death by a number of Roman senators. The killers believed that if they all participated in the murder, they could obscure the culpability of any single individual. The physician Antistius claimed to be able to determine the individual blow that pierced the emperor's heart and who delivered it, and threatened to expose the killer in front of the Senate in the Forum. Whether or not that would have been possible, the term "forensic" is said to originate from those events, referring to the presentation of Antistius's evidence in front of the "Forum." In present times, the term **forensic** is used to refer to any **expert testimony** (testimony that does not consist of knowledge regarded as commonly known to a layperson) that is suitable for presentation in court. There are forensic pathologists, forensic anthropologists, forensic accountants, forensic computer scientists, forensic entomologists, and numerous other forensic specialists.

Judges and juries in the civil and criminal legal system may rely on epidemiologic testimony in arriving at their conclusions and, ultimately, their verdicts. Such testimony has become a regular fixture in trials in which a fact finder (either judge or jury) is expected to determine whether an exposure and a disease/injury are related—for example, a pesticide and a birth defect, a car crash and a herniated disc in the spine, or a repetitively performed task and carpal tunnel syndrome. The epidemiologist is uniquely qualified to opine on such issues, because determinations of causation require solid educational backgrounds and experiences in study design and extrapolability, as well as the ability to recognize the presence of confounding and other biases. In practice, one of the most important tasks for the forensic epidemiologist is to weigh the likelihoods of outcomes other than those observed in a particular case. An example is testimony given when an injury has occurred in a motor vehicle crash in which an occupant was unrestrained; expert testimony frequently is sought as to whether the injuries would have been mitigated had a seat belt been in use.

Epidemiologists also are consulted in **toxic tort** cases, in which an injury or a disease is claimed to result from exposure to an environmental toxin. The epidemiologist may be required to study the problem *de novo,* with no established literature base from which to perform a **meta-analysis** (a statistical process that results in an overall or "composite" estimate of the effect of an exposure on a health outcome) or even evaluate the relevant variables of the problem. In such cases, the experience of clinical experts and other scientists may be helpful in designing a systematic approach to the problem. In other instances, the epidemiologist must evaluate the literature carefully to make a determination of the strength of the link between an exposure and an outcome

Box 8.4 continued

that may require in-depth knowledge of the physiological and/or pathological nature of a particular disease or injury.

The standard for testimony in a civil trial is that it be rendered as a **reasonable probability,** meaning that the expert is more than 50 percent certain that his or her opinion is accurate. This standard does not correlate with any numerical values that can be derived from scientific study; it is merely an expression of the certainty of the expert that the testimony is true and correct. For example, a condition that can result from an exposure to a toxin only 1 in 10,000 times cannot be ruled out in a particular instance because of the remote probability of the relationship, anymore than a lottery winner is denied a prize because of the low probability of winning the lottery.

It is important to understand that, from a scientific perspective, it is much easier to find a potential link between an exposure and an outcome than to rule it out. There are a multitude of reasons why that is true; however, foremost is the fact that a 0 percent probability of an association between an exposure and an outcome is virtually impossible to verify because of the effects of confounding, limited sample sizes and variance, and the limited extrapolability of the results of experimental studies to what occurs in the real world.

The phrase "forensic epidemiologist" is appropriate to use when referring to scientists who are educated and experienced in epidemiologic methodology and are able to apply this methodology to contested issues of fact, and to the presentation and interpretation of testimony relating to relevant findings with respect to exposures and health outcomes. In addition, subspecialties such as forensic trauma epidemiologist are used to describe individual scientists in specific fields of expertise.

REVIEW QUESTIONS

1. List and summarize six criteria used to evaluate whether an association between an exposure and a health outcome is causal. Then, provide examples from the epidemiologic literature for each criterion. Which criteria seem to be most compelling to you? What other criteria might be useful in establishing causation?

2. Why are observational epidemiologic studies (unlike experimental or intervention studies) almost always repeated many times in different populations before a causal interpretation of an association between an exposure and a health outcome is warranted?

3. Why are intervention studies often regarded as the "gold standard" for evaluating whether exposure-outcome associations are causal?

4. Define, differentiate between, and provide examples of "component causes," "necessary component causes," and "sufficient causes." In what way(s) are concepts of causation useful in planning programs to prevent disease and injury?

REVIEW EXERCISES

1. About fifty studies of ill effects associated with tobacco smoking had been published before the U.S. Surgeon General published the first Report on Smoking and Health in 1964. The report, nonetheless, concluded only that smoking *may* (not *does*) cause adverse health effects. Suggest several reasons why the report was so conservative in its interpretation of the epidemiologic studies of smoking and ill health.

2. There exists a dose-response relationship between coffee consumption and the incidence rate of myocardial infarction (MI). The association between coffee consumption and the incidence rate of MI, however, probably is not causal. If it is true that the association is not causal, what factors might account for the observed dose-response relationship between coffee and MIs? How might you evaluate whether your suggested explanation for the observed dose-response relationship is correct?

3. How were the Henle-Koch postulates (as originally stated or modified) used in determining sufficient component cause of AIDS?

4. List several examples in which it would be unreasonable and/or unethical to target a particular sufficient component cause in designing a disease and/or injury prevention program. As an example, it may be that a certain genetic component is a sufficient component cause for a particular disease. Even so, it would be unethical to attempt to reduce the incidence of this disease by removing people with this genetic makeup or passing legislation forbidding people with this genetic component from having children.

5. With a review of the epidemiologic literature as a basis, construct sufficient causes for a particular disease, such as one of the cancers. Clearly, you will not be able to identify all sufficient causes, and all component causes of each sufficient cause, for the disease or injury you select. Work with this exercise, though, long enough to gain a good sense for how the results of epidemiologic studies are used to construct models of causation for a particular disease or injury.

6. How do the ideas about causation presented in this chapter complement the ideas of "webs of causation" and "signed digraphs" presented in Chapter 1?

■ SPECIAL CASE STUDY:
Insights into Biocolonialism
Kathy Blaustein, M.P.H.

Concern for man and his fate must always form the chief interest of all technical endeavors. Never forget this, in the midst of your diagrams and equations.

ALBERT EINSTEIN

Biocolonialism Defined

Exploration and conquest of the natural world are activities as old as the human race, driven by a natural curiosity about new lands and the desire to obtain new sources of food, natural resources, and labor. The conquests of Africa, Latin America, the Caribbean, the Middle East, and parts of Asia by the British, French, Portuguese, and Spanish during the last five hundred years are generally referred to as colonialism, originally a neutral term that meant the establishment of a settlement by emigrants. Today it carries the derogatory connotation of the exploitation of a weaker country by a stronger one that uses the weaker country's resources to strengthen and enrich itself. As the fields of molecular biology and biotechnology have expanded, new techniques have allowed scientists in Western countries to explore and harness the biological resources of developing nations. This ability is called biocolonialism, defined as "the taking of knowledge and biological resources from an indigenous people without compensation. A term synonymous with biocolonialism is biopiracy" (Buzzwatch.com 2003). The development and commercialization of biological resources of developing nations and their indigenous peoples have bioethicists concerned about biosafety and medical ethics, especially regarding culturally appropriate informed consent (Roughan 2002) and the treatment of DNA as a marketable commodity (Senituli and Boyes 2002). This paper will discuss two cases of biocolonialism: attempts to purchase human gene pools and xenotransplantation experiments.

Case Study 1: Purchasing Human Gene Pools

In October 1999, Autogen Ltd., an Australian biotech company, announced an agreement to form an alliance with Merck Lipha, the German manufacturer of metformin, the world's top-selling drug for treating Type 2 diabetes. Under this agreement, Merck Lipha would control 15 percent of Autogen's shares and fund Autogen's Human Genetics Project, dedicated to the discovery of the human genes involved in weight imbalance, Type 2 diabetes, and insulin resistance, and to the development of drug treatments and diagnostic tests (Senituli and Boyes 2002). In November 2000, Autogen announced that it had struck a deal with the government of Tonga, a nation archipelago in the South Pacific (population 108,000), to gain exclusive rights to the genetic makeup of native Tongans. Genealogical studies indicate that Tongans are probably descended from a single Polynesian family. That fact combined with Tonga's geographical isolation has produced a genetically homogeneous population (Weber 2000). Obesity and diabetes are two major health problems in Tonga. By purchasing the rights to the Tongan gene pool, Autogen hoped to be able to isolate genes involved in diabetes, patent them, and use them for commercial gain. In return, Autogen promised to provide annual research funding to Tonga's Ministry of Health, pay royalties on revenues generated by any successful commercialization of Tongan gene research, and provide new therapies developed from the research free of charge to the population.

Tongan activists reacted immediately by attempting to find out which government officials were responsible for striking the deal. Tonga is a constitutional monarchy with the day-to-day running of the government conducted by a prime minister and Cabinet of Ministers handpicked by the king. The prime minister and the king denied making an agreement. The minister of health admitted to having discussions with Autogen but denied reaching any agreement. Many activists suspected that the premature announcement was intended to coerce the Tongan government into acting quickly before local opposition had a chance to respond. Opposition was, however, well organized and extremely vocal, led by the Tonga Human Rights and Democracy Movement (THRDM).

Initially, the opposition objected to the proposed sale on the basis of a lack of public discussion on the issue. Autogen's plan could lead to the commercialization and patenting of the DNA of the indigenous people of Tonga disguised as a public health program funded by the Australian government (Harry 2002). Criticism was also leveled at Autogen's statement on ethics emphasizing informed consent by individual volunteers. Individual consent ignores the unique processes for group decision making in traditional Tongan society, in which the extended family has a major voice in the granting of consent. In addition, genetic material is reflective of the extended family's genetic makeup, not just the individual's. The proposed research is in fact group research, but Autogen's ethics policy does not address group rights. Even if genetic material is collected from a limited number of individuals, the homogeneity of the Tongan population makes the research plan an issue for the total population (Burton 2002).

In response to the lack of monitoring systems to protect participants, the Tongan government approved the establishment of the National Health Ethics and Research Committee. The committee will scrutinize future proposals for legal, scientific, cultural, and ethical requirements before any consideration or negotiation is conducted (Anonymous 2002a). In August 2001, Autogen withdrew its interest in studying the Tongan human gene pool (Senituli and Boyes 2002).

The search for a genetically homogeneous population took the U.S.-based biotech company deCODE Genetics to Iceland. The 270,000 present-day inhabitants originated from a single group that settled the island about one thousand years ago (Nicholson 2000), and genealogies dating back centuries are readily available (Senituli and Boyes 2002). In 1998, Iceland's parliament passed a law allowing deCODE to use existing health, genetic, and genealogy data to establish a national health database to study the genetic basis of inherited diseases. The law assumed citizen participation, requiring Icelanders unwilling to participate to formally file notice to "opt out" within six months of the law's passage (Lewis 1999). A parliamentary act claimed informed consent on behalf of the entire Icelandic population. An intense debate involving the medical, scientific, and legal communities ensued. Informed consent and privacy protection were major concerns. The association of Icelanders for ethics in science and medicine, Mannvernd, claimed the law was an infringement of human rights (Lewis 1999). Ethicists questioned how well the public really understood the scientific issues raised. Although deCODE claimed the support of 88 percent of Iceland's population, a 1998 Gallup poll showed only 13 percent of a representative sample of citizens understood the law (Lewis 1999).

In contrast to the furor in Iceland, the Baltic nation of Estonia is proceeding with plans for a national databank that enjoys large popular support. The program will be administered by a not-for-profit government-controlled foundation that will geno-type any Estonian willing to participate. In contrast to Tonga and Iceland, Estonia is an ethnic mix from the Russian, Swedish, German, and Danish invaders who left their genetic heritage. Genetically it is as diverse as any European nation or the United States and would be a representative population for almost any White popu-lation. Once a precise gene is identified with a disease, a diverse population con-taining a large number of genetic variants, such as the Estonian population, would be useful to test drug therapies. No payment or incentives will be offered in exchange for participation. Patient information will be decoded and anonymous. It is hoped that the database will encourage the development of the biotech and phar-maceutical industries in Estonia as well as provide information to the international community (Kangilaski 2001). Despite widespread support, the plan has some detractors concerned about privacy issues, unauthorized release of data, and corrup-tion from the lucrative market for population-based genetic information.

The cases presented describe three different responses to the dilemma of genetic research using human genomic databases. Analysis reveals some issues common to all three countries and some issues that are unique to a particular culture. All three nations are small and trying to find a place in the global economy. Their economies rely heavily on natural resources. Iceland and Estonia historically have been ruled by a variety of larger foreign nations. Although Tonga has never been colonized, it has been heavily influenced by European culture brought by Christian missionaries. The polarizing debates that occurred in Tonga and Iceland are due primarily to the lack of citizen involvement in the decision-making process. In both cases, the gov-ernment negotiated with for-profit companies with little or no communication with their citizens. In both Tonga and Iceland, the issue of informed consent was para-mount to the opposition. Autogen and the Kingdom of Tonga neglected to address the culturally sensitive issue of group decision making in the consent process. The Icelandic Parliament assumed that consent was implied and required citizens who did not wish to participate to formally opt out of the program. The Estonian program avoided contentious debates by involving the citizenry in the discussion from the beginning. Open public debate is essential when deciding on issues that directly affect the medical and genetic heritage of every citizen. The Estonian plan also dif-fers in that the project will be administered by a government-controlled foundation rather than giving a for-profit company access to peoples' records. In addition, no incentives will be offered, allowing people to decide whether to participate without feeling pressured to do so. One issue common to all but the most high-income countries is the lack of existing infrastructure to monitor medical research and protect participants. That issue must be addressed before any research programs begin and must be culturally sensitive to the population involved.

Case Study 2: Xenotransplantation (XTP) Studies

Organ transplantation is one of modern medicine's most remarkable success stories. For many diseases, transplantation is the treatment of choice and may be the only way to save the patient's life (Bach, Ivinson, and Weeramanty 2001). It has become so common that there is a human organ shortage in most Western countries. In 2001, there were 62,000 Americans waiting for a liver, kidney, or pancreas transplant. It is estimated that only 25 percent of potential donors give their consent. This shortage has fueled research into the procedure of XTP, in which cells, tissues, or organs from nonhuman animals are transplanted into humans. The domestic pig has become the donor of choice because of similarities in size and anatomy with humans, abundance, familiarity, and historical acceptance. The use of nonhuman donors carries two significant risks: (1) the more acute and severe host-versus-implant reaction resulting from the different immunologies of the two species and (2) transmission of viral and prion diseases from the organ to the human host.

The first risk is being addressed in several ways. New immunosuppressive drugs are being developed to prevent the host from rejecting the donated organ. Genetic engineers are breeding cloned pigs, called "knock out" pigs, that lack the gene that causes rejection (Dobson 2002). Transplanting cells and tissues instead of whole organs may produce a milder immune response in the host (Melo et al. 2001).

The transmission of diseases is even more controversial. The genetic coding of pig viruses lies in the DNA of all the pigs' cells. The viruses of most concern are the porcine endogenous retroviruses, PERV, belonging to the same family of retroviruses that causes AIDS. Laboratory experiments have demonstrated that PERV can infect human cells in vitro (Paradis et al. 1999). This does not imply that PERV could produce an infection in one person that could be transmitted to others, resulting in an epidemic. It simply shows that PERV are capable of being passed from donor to host under some conditions. There may be other viruses or prions present that we are unaware of at this time. Since the danger is unknown, the scientific community is debating whether clinical XTP trials should be conducted. Proponents argue that as long as patients are educated and give informed consent, then trials should proceed. Opponents argue that until the disease risk is thoroughly understood, no clinical trials should be conducted. With so many unknowns, the true risks of XTP cannot be explained to patients, so their consent is not truly informed. They believe that XTP is a public health issue because the possibility exists that an infected recipient could start an epidemic. Because people other than the recipient are at risk, informed consent by the public, not just the individual, should be required. Another important consideration that will not be discussed in this paper is the issue of animal rights and the ethics of harvesting animal organs for human use.

In 2001, the New Zealand biotech company Diatranz and Rafael Valdes, a Mexican physician, reported the results of a Phase 1 clinical trial conducted on twelve Mexican children with Type 1 diabetes, aged 10–15 years. Patients received two transplants, six months apart, of pig pancreatic islet cells and Sertoli cells. The Sertoli cells provide immune protection for germ cells developing in the testes and were used in place of immunosuppressive drugs to improve the chances of a successful transplant. The donor cells were harvested from pathogen-free pigs bred by Diatranz. The entire procedure was new and had never been tested in primates or other large animal models. Valdes reported that four of twelve patients showed a decrease in daily insulin requirements of at least 40 percent. At the end of a year, two of those patients continued to show reduced insulin requirements. In addition, one patient showed evidence of microchimerism in the blood, meaning donor cells were found circulating in the blood (Valdes et al. 2001). Valdes believed that those data indicated some promise for the procedure and reported plans for further studies involving twenty-four new patients.

Reaction to the report was swift. Although the work was acknowledged as potentially groundbreaking, many scientists were skeptical. There was a lack of hard data, the trial was conducted in Mexico outside internationally recognized regulatory conditions, and no controlled testing in nonhuman model systems had been conducted (Anonymous 2002b; Birmingham 2002). Because the patients were children, the exact extent of informed consent remains uncertain (Archer and McLellan 2002).

In 2001, Diatranz sought permission to conduct similar experiments in New Zealand on patients with Type 2 diabetes. The application was refused mainly because of concerns about PERV. Diatranz then took its proposal to the Cook Islands, a small island state in the South Pacific with a high rate of diabetes (Archer and McLelland 2002). Many opponents believed Diatranz was trying to avoid the stringent regulatory controls on XTP research by going to a small country lacking effective biosafety and ethics monitoring systems. Diatranz offered to share profits with the Cook Islands if the treatment became marketable. In early 2002, the Cook Islands government announced that they would likely approve the Diatranz application. That announcement unleashed an international debate about the safety and ethics (or lack there of) of the Diatranz proposal. Some questioned why such a clinical trial should take place on patients with Type 2 diabetes, which is more appropriately treated with diet and lifestyle changes. Maori leaders worked hard to successfully defeat the Diatranz proposal, and the government withdrew its support (Permanent Forum on Indigenous Issues 2003).

In 2000, the Canadian Public Health Association (CPHA) formed a public advisory group to educate the public about XTP and determine the extent of public support for the procedure. Understanding of and support for the procedure were determined using mail, phone, and Web surveys (Wright 2002). A series of six regional citizen fora were conducted in which panelists representing different regions of the country met with experts in transplantation, infectious disease, ethics, law, and animal welfare. A transplant recipient also sat on each panel. Experts gave presentations for the lay panel and answered questions. Lay panelists discussed their findings and voted on whether they would support proceeding with XTP research. At first, many panelists supported continued research, but after learning about the risks, the majority (53 percent) voted against proceeding (Wharry 2002). Although some scientists were critical about certain aspects of the consultation process (Wright 2002), it was valuable for two reasons: It provided an opportunity to educate the public about a highly technical and controversial scientific process, and it provided stakeholders the opportunity to understand the public's concerns so that they can be addressed when making public policy. In effect, it was an exercise in gathering informed consent on a very large scale (Ivinson and Bach 2002). The Canadian model is an outstanding example of involving the public early in the discussion of public health issues.

Conclusion

These case studies illustrate the difficulty of conducting biomedical research on humans. The issue becomes more complex when the research is being conducted by a more powerful nation or a multinational corporation on a less powerful nation or on a group of indigenous peoples. Any human research must be driven by compassion, ethical concern for patients, and sensitivity to cultural and ethnic variables. Although the political system must be engaged in the process, it should not be used to circumvent citizen involvement as happened in Iceland. Biosafety and bioethics must be held to the highest standards. If research is being conducted in a country lacking a regulatory infrastructure, the standards required in the country conducting the research or international standards must prevail. Before any research begins, an independent agency must be in place to monitor issues of informed consent, safety, adherence to protocol, adverse reactions, and patient welfare. The world is a global village in which various people and cultures have increasing contact with one another. However, this global village should not lead to Westernization on a massive scale. Globalization allows dialogue with different people around the globe. Every effective dialogue must include the willingness not just to talk but also to listen.

REFERENCES

Anonymous. 2002a. The gene hunters. *New Internationalist.* 349:13–15.

———. 2002b. Diabetes trial stirs debate on safety of xenotransplants. *Nature* 419:5.

Archer, K., and F. McLellan. 2002. Controversy surrounds proposed xenotransplant trial. *Lancet* 359:949.

Bach, F., A. Ivinson, and H. Weeramantry. 2001. Ethical and legal issues in technology: Xenotransplantation. *American Journal of Law and Medicine* 27 (2001): 283–300.

Birmingham, K. 2002. Skepticism surrounds diabetes xenograft experiment. *Nature Medicine* 8 (10): 1047.

Burton, B. 2002. Proposed genetic database on Tongans opposed. *British Medical Journal* 324:443.

Buzzwatch.com Web site. http://www.buzzwhack.com/buzzcomp/indac.htm (accessed July 2003).

Dobson, R. 2002. Scientists produce genetically engineered cloned pigs for xenotransplantation. *British Medical Journal* 324:67.

Harry, D. 2002. FACTSHEET: Human genetic research and indigenous people. Paper presented at the South-South Biopiracy Summit, "Biopiracy—Ten Years Post Post-Rio." http://www.biowatch.org.za/dharry.htm (accessed July 2003).

Ivinson, A., and F. Bach. 2002. The xenotransplantation question: Public consultation is an important part of the answer. *Canadian Medical Association Journal* 167 (1): 42–43.

Kangilaski, J. 2001. The devil in the details. *Scientist* 15 (4): 6.

Lewis, R. 1999. Iceland's public supports database, but scientists object. *Scientist* 13 (15): 1.

Melo, H., C. Brandao, G. Rego, and R. Nunes. 2001. Ethical and legal issues in xenotransplantation. *Bioethics* 15 (56): 427–442.

Nicholson, D. 2000. Banking on genes. *The Scientist Daily News,* December 4, 2000. http://www.biomedcentral.comnews20001204/03/ (accessed July 2003).

Paradis, K., G. Langford, Z. Long, W. Heneine, P. Sandstrom, W. Switzer, L. Chapman, C. Lockey, D. Onions, and E. Otto. 1999. Search for cross-species transmission of porcine endogenous retrovirus in patients treated with living pig tissue. *Science* 285 (5431): 1236–41.

Permanent Forum on Indigenous Issues. 2003. Risks posed by substance abuse, environmental pollutants and lack of health services. Press release. http://www.un.org/News/Press/docs/2003/ hr4668.doc.htm (accessed July 2003).

Roughan, P. D. 2002. The diversity resource? Genetic research in Pacific Island futures. 2002 Pacific Research Development Symposium. http://www.fdc.org.au/events/pdrsecdev.htm/ (accessed July 2003).

Senituli, L., and M. Boyes. 2002. Whose DNA? Tonga and Iceland, biotech, ownership and consent. Paper presented at the Australasian Bioethics Association Annual Conference, Adelaide, February 14.

Valdes, R., R. Elliott, L. Dorantes, N. Garibay, O. Garkavenko, E. Bracho, C. Masias, M. Silva, and P. Valencia. 2001. Safety and preliminary efficacy of porcine islets and Sertoli cells implanted into an autologous collagen generating device in Type 1 diabetic humans. Abstract no. 9. *Xenotransplantation* 8. Suppl. no.1, August. abstract number 9.

Weber, W. 2000. Tonga sells genetic heritage to Australian firm. *Lancet* 356:1910.

Wharry, S. 2002. Canadians not ready for animal-to-human transplants. *Canadian Medical Association Journal* 166 (4): 493.

Wright, J. 2002. Alternative interpretations of the same data: Flaws in the process of consulting the Canadian public about xenotransplantation issues. *Canadian Medical Association Journal* 167 (1): 40–41.

## CHAPTER 9

Design Strategies: Analytic Studies Part 1—Intervention Studies

Now that we have thought about what is meant by causation and how to establish causation in epidemiologic studies (Chapter 8), this is an opportune time to discuss **analytic epidemiologic studies.** Unlike descriptive epidemiologic studies (discussed in Chapter 7), which often are hypothesis-generating, analytic studies are hypothesis-evaluating. In other words, an analytic study is designed to evaluate a specific epidemiologic hypothesis. Probably every person learned in grade school that a hypothesis is an "educated guess" about how some aspect of the world works; the hypothesis tentatively is held to be true until data are generated that show it to be false or in need of modification. To be useful, a hypothesis must be exceedingly specific. "Useful" in this context means "able to be tested" or "able to be refuted." "Specific" means that each of the components of an epidemiologic hypothesis must be delineated in as much detail as current knowledge and measurement tools permit.

In epidemiology, the hypothesis of interest states a relationship between certain exposures and health outcomes. Some of the more commonly used components of an epidemiologic hypothesis include the following:

1. Exposure(s) of interest.
2. Health outcome(s) of interest.
3. Population(s) to whom the hypothesis applies. For example, does the hypothesis apply only to men? only to women? only to people over the age of 40 years?
4. Dose-response. What amount of the exposure(s) results in what frequency of the health outcome(s) of interest?
5. Time-response. How long is the time interval between exposure and the occurrence of the health outcome; that is, how long after exposure does the outcome occur?

Other commonly used components include delineations of the relationships between the exposure-outcome association and different aspects of specific people, places, and time variables.

As noted in Figure 7.1 (page 143), there are two broad types of analytic studies in epidemiology:

- **Intervention studies,** which include the community (or preventive) trial and the clinical (or therapeutic) trial. (**Trial** is a synonym for experiment.)
- **Observational studies,** which include the case/control study and the prospective and retrospective cohort studies.

The more frequently conducted types of analytic studies are the observational studies. The defining distinction between intervention studies and observational studies is how the study participants become exposed or not exposed, as discussed later in this chapter.

Regardless of which type of analytic study is contemplated, the basic study design, developed before the implementation of the study, focuses on several plans. These plans include, but are not limited to

- The plan for the type of analytic study (which type of study will be conducted).
- The plan for the selection of subjects (how subjects will be identified and enrolled in the study).
- The plan for randomly assigning exposure, if an intervention study (what methods will be used to randomly allocate subjects to an exposure/treatment category).
- The plan for data collection (which types of data will be collected; what sources of data will be utilized).
- The plan for data analysis (how the data will be analyzed).
- An assessment of how many participants must be included in the study to achieve a reasonable expectation of precisely evaluating the hypothesis under study and for avoiding a Type II error. (See Chapter 12 for a discussion of Type II errors.) Type II errors occur when the hypothesis of interest is false but the study data fail to disclose that falseness.

In addition to those plans, a plan is developed for preventing and/or controlling confounding bias, usually as part of one or more of the other plans. **Preventing confounding bias** means designing a study in such a way that confounding bias does not enter into the study, whereas **controlling confounding bias** refers to removing confounding bias during the data analysis phase of the study. Methods to prevent or control confounding are discussed in Chapter 12.

INTERVENTION STUDIES VERSUS OBSERVATIONAL STUDIES

In an **intervention study,** also known as an **intervention trial,** the study investigator **randomly assigns** exposure to or withholds exposure from the study subjects. Although study subjects may **withdraw from a trial prematurely** (withdraw before the end of the trial), theoretically the assigned exposure for each study subject is under the control of the investigator. **Random assignment** means that each subject in the trial has the same predetermined probability of being in any of the exposure groups. The study investigators decide the predetermined probabilities of subjects' being in a particular exposure group. The predetermined probabilities of being in a certain exposure group need not be the same. For example, it may be that in a clinical trial, an exposure group of "usual care" is twice as large as the exposure group composed of subjects receiving "the new medical treatment"; thus the predetermined probabilities would be 0.67 and 0.33, or 67 percent and 33 percent, respectively. It is *essential* conceptually to understand that every participant in an intervention study is offered some treatment or exposure, even if the treatment or exposure offered is a participant's "usual exposure or usual treatment."

The distinction between intervention studies and observational studies does not lie in the presence or the absence of a control group. Both intervention and observational studies have at least one control group made up of subjects having a level of an exposure different from the level in the exposed/treatment group. In both types of studies, subjects in the different exposure groups are compared with one another with respect to their frequencies of the health outcome(s) of interest. In addition, in both types of studies, one exposure level group is the "control" or comparison group for the exposed group(s).

In intervention studies, the importance of random assignment arises from the unpredictability (randomness) and equality with which particular subjects are assigned to each exposure group. Almost always these two characteristics (unpredictability and equality) prevent confounding bias from occurring in an intervention study as long as the number of subjects in the study is large. Randomly assigning exposure also prevents confounding bias by both *known* and *unknown* potential confounding variables. Random assignment guarantees, at least for well-conducted intervention trials that include a large number of subjects, that the study groups are comparable with one another with respect to their baseline (preintervention) risk of the health outcome(s) under evaluation in the trial. This baseline comparability among the exposure/treatment groups means that any differences among the groups in their postintervention frequencies of disease are *not* attributable to confounding bias. Random allocation prevents confounding bias by blocking the association between the exposure and a potential confounding factor, as shown pictorially in Figures 9.1 and 9.2.

Observational studies do not have a guarantee that confounding bias will be prevented in the study design, because the investigator does not randomly allocate the exposure/treatment to the study participants. The implications of that distinction are profound. The possible explanations for the findings from an intervention study are either **chance** (**random error**—the unsystematic, unpredictable error inherent in a study, in contrast to **bias** or systematic error)—or cause (the exposure caused the outcome). In contrast, the possible interpretations for the findings of an observational

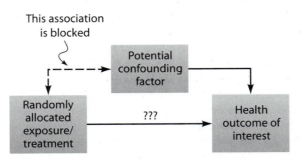

FIGURE 9.1
Strategy for preventing confounding bias.

study include not only chance and cause but also **bias,** and especially confounding bias. Other types of bias are discussed in Chapter 12.

If intervention studies tend to have less bias than observational studies, why are most analytic epidemiologic studies observational rather than intervention studies? The answer to that question resides in the many **ethical constraints** associated with intervention studies.

First, intervention studies

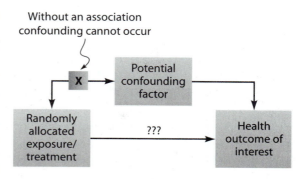

FIGURE 9.2
Pictorial representation of prevented confounding bias.

can be conducted only when there are good reasons to believe that the exposure or treatment of interest is a preventive or cure of disease or injury. In other words, it is unethical to randomly allocate study subjects into exposure groups when the exposure is a suspected or known cause of disease or injury or in the absence of compelling evidence to the contrary.

Second, it may be unethical to randomly allocate subjects into an exposure group when the exposure is suspected to be less efficacious (although helpful) than is some other exposure. The U.S. Food and Drug Administration's guidelines for establishing the therapeutic value of new drugs provides an example of standards that some epidemiologists have questioned as being unethical (see, for example, www.fda.gov; click on "Drugs," under "Products FDA Regulates") (Rothman and Michels 1994). The ethical challenge centers in part on the fact that the efficacy of a potential new drug is determined by comparing the drug's effectiveness with "no treatment" rather than with the most effective currently available drug or other therapeutic modality.

INTERVENTION STUDIES

As mentioned previously, there are two main types of intervention studies: the community (or preventive) trial and the clinical (or therapeutic) trial. Both types of trials seek to evaluate the relative benefit of a new preventive or cure of ill health either relative to a currently used preventive or cure or relative to a placebo.

Like other types of scientific experiments, intervention trials seek to alter only one factor (the treatment or exposure under evaluation) at a time. By changing only one factor, researchers can attribute any differences between the health outcomes of the compared groups to the one factor whose presence, absence, or dose was varied.

The primary difference between community and clinical trials pertains to the preintervention health of the study subjects. In a **community (preventive) trial,** study subjects are free of the health outcome of interest, and the intervention under evaluation seeks to keep the subjects free of that outcome. In other words, the intervention under evaluation is an assumed preventive of the health outcome. The unit of study in

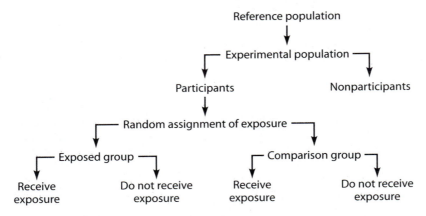

FIGURE 9.3
Basic design for an intervention study.

a community trial can be either individual people or some larger unit. Examples of larger units are "all children in certain school classes," "all people residing in a particular town or city," and "all members of a managed care organization."

In a **clinical (therapeutic) trial,** on the other hand, the subjects have a certain health condition, and the intervention seeks to reduce adverse health consequences related to that condition. The intervention of interest, therefore, is a medical, a lifestyle, or some other form of curative or palliative therapy. Clinical trials almost always are conducted with individuals as the unit of study. The basic design for an intervention study, either a community trial or a clinical trial, is shown in Figure 9.3. See Box 9.1 for further discussion.

BOX 9.1

PRACTICAL EPIDEMIOLOGY IN A CLINICAL SETTING: DIABETES MELLITUS—OVERVIEW OF CLINICAL AND PUBLIC HEALTH IMPLICATIONS

MARTHA BELL-HART, B.A., R.N., C.D.E., AND CARLA SHAW BEYER, M.P.H.

Diabetes mellitus is a chronic disease caused by a failure of the body to properly metabolize food components, especially carbohydrates, for energy. This faulty metabolism is caused by insufficient amounts of the hormone insulin, or by ineffective insulin action.

Box 9.1 continued

Those defects result in abnormally high blood-glucose levels, because without insulin, glucose cannot be transported through cell walls. Cells thus are deprived of necessary energy.

Diabetes is a common disease worldwide and affects 6.2 percent of the United States population (Centers for Disease Control and Prevention 2002). Approximately one-third of those with diabetes are not yet diagnosed. Certain age and ethnic groups are disproportionately affected. Americans age 65 years and older have a prevalence of 20.1 percent, whereas those less than 20 years of age have a prevalence of 0.19 percent. American Blacks, Hispanics, Pacific Islanders, and American Indians have higher rates of disease, with the highest rate (25.7 percent) observed in Southwest Indians.

Two main types of diabetes are recognized, Type 1 and Type 2 diabetes. Type 1 diabetes, accounting for 10 percent of all diabetes, usually is diagnosed in children or young adults. In Type 1 diabetes, there is an absolute lack of insulin caused by auto-immune destruction of insulin-secreting islet cells of the pancreas. Persons with Type 1 diabetes require daily administration of insulin, usually by injection, with the goal of normalizing blood-glucose levels as much as possible. Hypoglycemia (low blood glucose) can at times be a troublesome iatrogenic acute complication caused by insulin therapy. On the other hand, if adequate amounts of insulin are not administered, a life-threatening emergency known as diabetic ketoacidosis can develop.

In Type 2 diabetes, which accounts for 90 percent of all diabetes, there is a relative lack of insulin that is due either to decreased insulin secretion or to insulin resistance at the cellular wall. Type 2 diabetes usually is diagnosed in adults. For many persons, nutrition and exercise therapy lower blood-glucose levels sufficiently. When that is not the case, various oral medications or insulin injections may be prescribed. Persons with Type 2 are likely to have hypertension, hyperlipidemia, and obesity as comorbidities. Although there usually is a genetic predisposition to both Type 1 and Type 2 diabetes, lifestyle issues are responsible for a dramatic increase in the incidence of Type 2 diabetes in the United States. Sedentary lifestyle and poor eating habits resulting in obesity increase the risk of developing diabetes. Unfortunately, as obesity is on the rise among America's youth, the incidence of Type 2 diabetes appears to be increasing in that age group (American Diabetes Association 2000; Rocchini 2002). Research into the prevention of Type 2 diabetes has shown that weight loss and routine physical exercise can reduce the incidence of diabetes in persons with slight elevations in blood-glucose levels (often a precursor of Type 2 diabetes) (Diabetes Prevention Program Research Group 2002).

Normalization of blood-glucose levels is crucial because hyperglycemia seems to damage tissues, especially blood vessels and nerves. Long-term hyperglycemia increases the risk of chronic complications affecting especially the heart, retina, kidneys, and nerves (Diabetes Control and Complications Trial Research Group 1993; U.K. Prospective Diabetes Study Group 1998). Large-blood-vessel disease can lead to heart attack and stroke, and heart disease is the leading cause of death among persons with diabetes, with death rates two to four times greater than for nondiabetic adults. Diabetes is the leading cause of new blindness in adults aged 20 to 74 years. It is the leading cause of end-stage kidney disease, with almost 115,000 people receiving dialysis

Box 9.1 continued

or kidney transplantation in 1999. Neuropathy occurs in 60 to 70 percent of all persons with diabetes, with peripheral neuropathy in the feet being most common. This neuropathy can lead to lack of sensation in the feet, which is a significant risk factor for lower-extremity amputation, as is peripheral vascular disease. Diabetes is responsible for the majority of nontraumatic amputations in the United States (Centers for Disease Control and Prevention 2002).

For diabetic women who are pregnant, significant hyperglycemia in the first several weeks of pregnancy is associated with high rates of major birth defects. Women of childbearing age who have diabetes require prepregnancy counseling and care so that blood-glucose control is meticulous at conception and throughout the pregnancy (Kitzmiller et al. 1996). In a small percentage of nondiabetic women, a temporary form of insulin resistance occurs in the last trimester of pregnancy, resulting in hyperglycemia. Women with gestational diabetes have an increased risk of developing Type 2 diabetes later in life (American Diabetes Association 2003).

Optimal management of diabetes requires not only treatment from the medical team but also great involvement of the diabetic person, whose daily self-management ideally includes monitoring of finger-stick blood glucose, careful measurement and distribution of carbohydrate foods, medication administration if needed, exercise, and foot care. Understandably, for some the daily pressures to maintain control of blood glucose can seem overwhelming at times, and depression occurs more commonly in persons with diabetes. Long-term clinical and self-care can be quite burdensome, not only in terms of psychological and lifestyle impact, but also in financial terms: The total cost per year in the United States is 98 billion dollars, based on 1997 estimates (Centers for Disease Control and Prevention 2002), with direct medical costs accounting for 44 billion dollars of that figure. Efforts at optimal clinical and self-care are worthwhile, however, because a large clinical trial published in the 1990s shows that standardized intensive efforts to control blood-glucose levels and prevent or promptly treat complications greatly reduce the negative impact on health, finances, and quality of life (Diabetes Control and Complications Trial Research Group 1996).

REFERENCES

American Diabetes Association. 2002. Type 2 diabetes in children and adolescents (Consensus Statement). *Diabetes Care* 23:381–89.

———. 2003. Gestational diabetes mellitus (Position Statement). *Diabetes Care.* 26. Suppl. no. 1: S103–S105.

Centers for Disease Control and Prevention. 2002. National diabetes fact sheet: General information and national estimates on diabetes in the United States, 2000. Atlanta, GA: U.S. Department of Health and Human Services, Centers for Disease Control and Prevention.

Diabetes Control and Complications Trial Research Group. 1993. The effect of intensive treatment of diabetes on the development and progression of long-term complications in insulin-dependent diabetes mellitus. *New England Journal of Medicine* 329:977–86.

———. 1996. Lifetime benefits and costs of intensive therapy as practiced in the diabetes control and complications trial. *Journal of the American Medical Association* 276:1409–15.

Diabetes Prevention Program Research Group. 2002. Reduction in the incidence of type 2 diabetes with lifestyle intervention or metformin. *New England Journal of Medicine* 346:393–403.

Box 9.1 continued

Kitzmiller, C., John L. Andrew, Thomas A. Buchanan, Siri Kjos, C. A. Combs, Robert E. Ratner. 1996. Preconception care of diabetes, congenital malformations, and spontaneous abortions. *Diabetes Care* 19 (5): 514–41.

Rocchini, Alpert P. 2002. Childhood obesity and a diabetes epidemic. *New England Journal of Medicine* 346 (11): 854–55.

The **reference population** (Figure 9.3) is the group of people to whom the results of the intervention study apply, and the **experimental population** is the group of people from whom study subjects are selected. All **study participants** must give their **voluntary, informed consent** to be subjects in a study. Intervention studies can be conducted ethically only among people who volunteer to be subjects in a study and who understand the potential adverse risks, benefits, and expectations of participation. There probably is no intervention study that lacks some potential adverse risks, even if those risks are remote and/or of minor consequence (for example, anxiety caused by participating in the trial).

Sometimes the characteristics of the reference population, experimental population, and participants differ. For example, trials of therapeutic drugs have been conducted among White adult males with the expectation that the study results would apply to non-White males, to adult females, and to children of either gender and of any ethnic identification. Those expectations are not always valid (other trials of the therapeutic drug later were conducted in populations not comprising White adult males and had different results), or their validity is not known (trials in other populations have not been conducted).

In response to a general lack of information on women's health, the National Health, Lung, and Blood Institute (NHLBI) within the National Institutes of Health (NIH) established the Women's Health Initiative (WHI) in 1991. The WHI is a series of studies that address the most common causes of death, disability, and impaired quality of life—including cardiovascular disease, cancer, and osteoporosis—among postmenopausal women. The fifteen-year multi-million-dollar initiative is one of the largest series of related prevention studies ever conducted in the United States. The three primary elements of the WHI are "a randomized controlled clinical trial of promising but unproven approaches to prevention; an observational study to identify predictors of disease; and a study of community approaches to developing healthful behaviors" (http://www.nhlbi.nih.gov/whi/).

EXTERNAL VALIDITY

The example of the evaluation of therapeutic drugs only in White males raises a critical idea in epidemiology, namely the concept of "**external validity,**" also known as "**generalizability.**" External validity refers to the extent to which the findings of a study are applicable to (can be generalized to) people who were not included in the study. External validity indicates lack of bias in the application of study results to a wider group of people than the group in whom the study was conducted. An epidemiologic study is meaningful, from a scientific perspective, mainly to the extent to which its findings help to improve the health of people who were not included in the study. Otherwise, any health benefits identified by the study would help, at most, only the limited number of actual study participants. The process of generalizing the results of an epidemiologic study to nonparticipants differs materially from the process used in some other scientific fields, such as classical statistics.

The topic of external validity is discussed in greater detail in Chapter 12. The essential point to appreciate at this time is the need to consider, during the design phase of an analytic study (trial or observational study), what types of people make up the intended reference population. The characteristics of the study participants should permit generalization to that population.

ADHERENCE TO THE INTERVENTION PROTOCOL

Once participating individuals (or some larger study units) are identified and enrolled in the trial, the participants or units are randomly assigned to an exposure category. Recall that randomly assigning exposure prevents confounding bias, thereby ensuring (except for "bad luck" or large random error) that the groups formed by randomization are comparable with respect to their preintervention risks of the outcome(s) of interest. That concept and its consequences are crucial to understand. For instance, one consequence of randomization concerns study participants who become nonparticipants. If participants decide to leave the trial or are lost-to-follow-up after randomization has occurred, the remaining groups in the study may no longer be comparable with one another with regard to their preintervention risks of the health outcome(s) of interest. Thus, the primary benefit of randomization (prevention of confounding bias) may be lost.

Sometimes investigators analyze data from an intervention study assuming that **subsets** of the groups formed by randomization also are comparable to one another (MRFIT Research Group 1982; Stallones 1983). A subset, as the term is used here, refers to a proportion of all subjects randomly allocated to a certain exposure/treatment group. An error of this type can be serious and may undermine the entire value and interpretability of a study's findings.

Again, once the exposure groups are formed by randomization (Figure 9.3), each group is offered its assigned treatment or exposure. Although the goal is for all subjects to receive the full treatment or exposure offered, some study participants may change their minds and no longer wish to participate in the intervention or may wish to participate only on an intermittent or partial basis. The scientific merit of a trial depends upon having most subjects or units receive the full treatment or exposure assigned. Nevertheless, trials can be conducted only among volunteers; thus, allowing subjects to change their minds about participating must be permitted.

Because the groups that are comparable to one another are the groups formed by randomization, to maintain comparability, even subjects who do not complete the assigned treatment or exposure protocol must be included in the data analysis as though the protocol were followed in its entirety. For that reason, the results of intervention studies reflect not only the differences, if any, between the assigned treatment or exposure and the health outcome of interest but also the palatability of the interventions themselves.

Sometimes, **differential levels of adherence to the treatment or exposure protocol** occur between the groups in the trial. For example, one group may be assigned a onetime surgical intervention while the other group is assigned a six-month rigorous exercise program. Differential adherence to the assigned intervention might easily occur in such a trial because the surgery group has been asked to agree once, for a one-time procedure, whereas the other group must renew a commitment to exercise every day for six months. Differential adherence to a treatment or exposure protocol can be a serious threat to the validity of a trial, because the study results compare outcomes for groups that have dissimilar opportunities for the assigned treatment to demonstrate an effect. Contributing to that difficulty is the fact that people who do not complete assigned treatment protocols tend to differ from people who complete such protocols in ways that affect disease and injury risk. For example, people who do not comply tend to use tobacco and alcohol more often than do people who comply.

LOST-TO-FOLLOW-UP

Among subjects who either do or do not receive the assigned treatment or exposure, the health outcome(s) of interest in the trial either are or are not known. For example, some subjects may complete the treatment protocol but then leave the study area without notifying the investigator of their health outcome(s). Those subjects are referred to as **lost-to-follow-up** and can present an investigator with a difficult challenge: Subjects whose outcomes are not known cannot be included in the data analysis and trial results. The groups formed by randomization (and who, therefore, are comparable) may become less comparable to the extent that subjects are lost-to-follow-up. As with people who change their minds about fully participating in an intervention study, people who are lost-to-follow-up typically differ from people who are not lost-to-follow-up in ways that are related to health. People who are lost-to-follow-up are self-selected individuals whose absence may introduce bias into the trial. For example, people may even leave the trial because they have developed the health outcome under study.

The best way to assure that lost-to-follow-up is not introducing confounding bias into a trial is to have few subjects whose outcomes are unknown. There is no "magic" number or percent of the study participants that equates to "few." To help avoid bias from lost-to-follow-up, the study protocol should include vigorous procedures for follow-up. Sometimes the choice of the population in whom the trial is conducted enhances follow-up. For example, groups of United States military veterans typically are easier to follow than are some other groups because the benefits veterans receive encourage contact with the U.S. Veterans Administration; hence, the veterans' contact information is available. As the benefits offered to veterans decrease, as currently is occurring, this group of individuals may become harder to follow. As an alternative to enrolling subjects that inherently are easier to follow, an investigator might initiate an extensive follow-up of a subset of subjects who were lost-to-follow-up. Data from those subjects might provide useful information concerning how subjects who were lost may differ from the subjects who remained in the trial.

Several additional points about participants who are lost-to-follow-up warrant mention. First, there can come a point in a trial when the proportion of study subjects who are lost-to-follow-up becomes "too large"; in other words, too many participants are lost for the study to proceed or for results to be reported. That situation is more likely to occur if the length of follow-up is long or with difficult-to-follow treatment protocols. There have been trials reported in the scientific literature in which lost-to-follow-up has exceeded 50 percent or even 80 percent. Such studies exceed the threshold of acceptable lost-to-follow-up because of the potential, indeed the likelihood, of having considerable bias introduced into the trial by the large proportion of subjects who were lost-to-follow-up.

Second, sometimes investigators think it is "unfair" to include, in the trial results, outcomes for subjects who failed to adhere to the assigned treatment protocol. At times, it seems that an investigator is "sure" that a beneficial outcome from a new intervention would have been observed "if only adherence to the treatment protocol had been better." There are at least two conceptually important responses to that concern. The first response pertains to the validity of the trial. Removing subjects who fail to complete the treatment protocol from the trial undermines the comparability among treatment groups established by the process of randomly allocating the treatment. Probably no other aspect of a trial except ethical considerations is more central than maintaining the benefits of randomization. The second response pertains to the potential benefits, if any, from the new treatment. In real-life situations, the effectiveness of a treatment depends only in part on the treatment's intrinsic benefits, if any. Effectiveness also depends on the ease and cost of treatment delivery and on the acceptability and perceived benefits of the treatment. A treatment that is unacceptable to the target population or whose delivery is difficult will not result in the intended medical or public health benefits, regardless of the treatment's intrinsic worth. Additional research may find improved methods for delivering the treatment or rendering the treatment more acceptable to the target population. For any given trial, however, interpretation of the study results encompasses the actual, measured benefits of the new treatment (all subjects whose outcome are known included) plus the acceptability of the treatment to the target population.

As a final, related point, almost always the proportion of subjects who comply fully with a treatment protocol, and therefore who potentially will benefit from a new treatment, is higher during the intervention trial than in subsequent use of the new treatment. This higher compliance occurs because the investigative team will work extremely hard to keep study participants in the trial and adhering to the treatment protocol to allow for the most accurate evaluation of the benefits, if any, of the new treatment.

EXAMPLES OF PREVENTIVE TRIALS

1954 POLIOMYELITIS VACCINE TRIAL

The community vaccine trials for certain infectious diseases conducted during the 1930s–1950s were marvels of methodological ingenuity. The strategies for successfully conducting large-scale community trials were developed and implemented during those trials. A stellar example of that newfound ingenuity is the 1954 poliomyelitis trials of the Salk vaccine conducted among children in the school grades 1–3 (Francis et al. 1955). "Observed control" sites (127 sites) in 33 states with a combined first through third school-grade population of 1,080,680 and 84 "placebo control" sites in 11 states with a combined first through third school-grade population of 749,236 participated in the trial. In the "observed control" sites, children in the second grade were offered the vaccine, whereas children in the first and third grades served as unvaccinated ("observed") controls. In the "placebo control" sites, half of the children in grades 1–3 received the polio vaccine whereas the other half received a placebo injection. The large number of children recruited to participate in the trials was required to ensure that an adequate number of incident polio cases occurred among the study children to yield statistically meaningful results. The trial results found that the vaccine was 60–70 percent effective against paralytic polio caused by Type I polio virus and 90 percent or more effective against paralytic polio caused by Types II and III polio viruses.

It is interesting to view the polio trials in their secular context. From incidence rates of approximately 20–40/100,000 person-years in the United States before availability of the vaccine, and higher incidence rates elsewhere, polio in the year 2004 is nearing eradication worldwide.

NEWBURGH-KINGSTON DENTAL CARIES TRIAL

The Newburgh-Kingston Dental Caries Trial was an ingenious trial to evaluate the efficacy of reducing the prevalence of decayed, missing, and filled (DMF) teeth by enriching public drinking-water supplies with fluoride (Ast, Finn, and McCaffrey 1950). Previous investigators had observed that residents of communities whose public drinking water naturally was high in fluoride had a reduced prevalence of dental caries. Too much naturally occurring fluoride, however, caused teeth to become mottled (darkened), and very high levels could cause skeletal fluorosis, a serious condition causing the bones to become either hard and brittle, or soft. At a concentration of 1ppm fluoride in drinking water, most of the benefits of fluoride in reducing dental caries and few of the risks of mottled teeth were observed.

On the basis of the observed benefits and risks of naturally occurring fluoride in drinking water, the community of Newburgh was randomly allocated to have its public water supplies enriched to 1ppm. The other trial community, Kingston, at first did not have its drinking water enriched. (Before the trial, neither Newburgh nor Kingston had substantial naturally occurring fluoride in its public water supplies.) Both before and after fluoridation, the DMF experiences of the resident children in the two trial communities were monitored and compared over time.

The trial results found an estimated 70 percent reduction in the prevalence of DMF teeth among children residing in Newburgh compared with their prefluoridation DMF prevalence and compared with the DMF prevalence among the children residing in Kingston. Later fluoridation of the drinking-water supplies in Kingston produced a similar reduction in the prevalence of DMF teeth.

In this trial, the unit of randomization was the community. One of the two participating communities was randomly allocated to receive fluoridation while the other community served as the control community. The trial can be viewed as having only two "subjects": one that received enrichment with fluoride and one that did not. For that reason, it was important for the investigators to evaluate the similarity between the pretrial dental experiences between the two communities. The investigators needed to be certain that any postfluoridation differences in the dental experiences in the two communities were attributable to differences in the fluoride concentration of their drinking waters and not to differences in their pretrial prevalences of DMF teeth.

Three interesting ramifications of the fluoride trial warrant mention. First, enriching drinking water with fluoride changed the epidemiology of dental health in some populations in the United States. In those populations, DMF teeth no longer were prevalent dental health problems. Instead, orthodontics became a larger area of emphasis. (In other populations, dental problems including DMF teeth, abscessed teeth, and gingivitis continued to be major public health problems.)

Second, adding fluoride to public water supplies became a political issue during the 1970s and thereafter in the United States. There was concern, later demonstrated to be unfounded, that fluoride might cause cancers or birth defects. Communities repeatedly voted against referenda proposing to enrich public drinking water with fluoride.

And third, adding fluoride to public water supplies resulted in widespread environmental contamination with fluoride. Increased mottling of teeth begins at about 2ppm of fluoride, and plants such as tea bioaccumulate fluoride. Communities that decided not to fluoridate their drinking water began to experience the same 70 percent reduction in the prevalence of DMF teeth as did communities that chose to fluoridate. That reduction occurred because little of the fluoride added to water supplies is taken up by water drunk by residents in fluoridated communities; the rest is recycled to water supplies and plant foods consumed by residents of other communities. In addition, concerns surfaced about possible adverse effects of fluoride on the bone health of adults, individuals whose dental health was not affected by fluoridating water. Fluoridation of public water supplies is an excellent example of a highly effective, inexpensive public health measure whose potential limitations and adverse environmental consequences may not have been adequately contemplated before implementation.

PHYSICIANS' HEALTH STUDY

The Physicians' Health study was a randomized trial of aspirin as a preventive of cardiovascular mortality and beta-carotene as a preventive of cancer incidence that was conducted among approximately 22,000 physicians, residing in the United States, who were between the ages of 40 and 84 years at the beginning of the study in 1982. Previous epidemiologic data had suggested that aspirin was effective in preventing secondary cardiovascular events. Whether aspirin could prevent first events had not been evaluated. Thus, one of the two primary objectives of the trial was to evaluate whether aspirin intake every other day could prevent primary cardiovascular events.

Similarly, previous epidemiologic data had demonstrated that people who consume large quantities of vegetables containing beta-carotene, a precursor of Vitamin A, had a reduced incidence of certain cancers, such as lung cancer. What was unknown was whether people who consume large quantities of foods containing beta-carotene differ from people who do not consume those foods in ways that might reduce their risks of cancer. Thus, the second primary objective of the trial was to evaluate whether a beta-carotene supplement, taken every other day, would reduce cancer incidence.

The participating physicians were randomly allocated to receive one of four treatments: both aspirin and beta-carotene, aspirin plus a beta-carotene placebo, beta-carotene plus an aspirin placebo, or both placebos. The trial results were intriguing.

The aspirin component of the trial was ended early, before its planned termination date, because of a large reduction (47 percent) in total cardiovascular events (fatal plus nonfatal) in the aspirin group (Steering Committee of the Physicians' Health Study Research Group 1988). That large reduction meant that continuation of the aspirin component of the trial would be unethical, because it would be unethical to withhold aspirin, given its beneficial health effects, from the aspirin placebo group. (A recent trial, however, failed to find an aspirin effect in women.)

Results of the beta-carotene component of the trial were equally intriguing. There was essentially no difference in cancer incidence between the beta-carotene group and the beta-carotene placebo group (Hennekens, Buring, and Manson 1996). Contrary to the multitude of well-designed observational epidemiologic studies showing an association between consumption of foods containing carotene and a reduced incidence of cancer, the trial results failed to find a benefit. A previous prevention trial conducted among male smokers also found no benefit. In that study, the incidence of lung cancer among the beta-carotene group was higher than the incidence among the beta-carotene placebo group (Alpha-Tocopherol Beta Carotene Cancer Prevention Study Group 1994).

Knowledge of the beneficial effects of aspirin on cardiovascular health has transformed the treatment and outcomes for some cardiovascular patients and for people at increased risk of cardiovascular disease. For example, in one large study conducted in Minneapolis and St. Paul, treatment with aspirin of patients having coronary heart disease increased from 13 to 81 percent between 1985 and 1990. That change, together with increases in thrombolytic therapy (treatment designed to dissolve a blood clot) (from 13 to 30 percent), in patients receiving coronary angioplasty (5 to 21 percent), and in the administration of heparin (53 to 75 percent), resulted in a 41 percent decrease in in-hospital mortality from coronary heart disease and a 17 percent decline in out-of-hospital mortality (McGovern et al. 1996).

EXAMPLE OF A CLINICAL TRIAL

POLYP PREVENTION TRIAL

The Polyp Prevention Trial Study evaluated the hypothesis that a diet low in fat (20 percent of total calories) and high in fiber (18 grams of dietary fiber per 1,000 kcal) and fruits and vegetables (3.5 servings per day) would reduce the development of recurrent colorectal adenomas (Schatzkin et al. 2000). Adenomas are precursors of most cancers of the large bowel. Numerous prior epidemiologic and laboratory data had supported an association between certain dietary factors and the incidence of colorectal cancer, one of the most common cancers in the United States. For that reason, evaluation of the benefits, if any, of a low-fat, high-fiber diet on the recurrence of colorectal adenomas had potentially significant public health consequences.

Over two thousand men aged 35 years or older who had had one or more histologically confirmed colorectal adenomas removed within the past six months were randomly assigned to either the special-diet group or a comparison group. Participants of the comparison group received an informational brochure and advice to follow their usual diets.

After an approximately four-year follow-up, the proportion of subjects in each group who had at least one recurrent adenoma was nearly identical (39.7 percent in the special-diet group and 39.5 percent in the comparison group), suggesting that the low-fat, high-fiber diet did not alter the risk of subsequent adenomas. The benefits of this diet, if any, on other health outcomes, such as cardiovascular health, were not evaluated. A similar trial evaluating the effects of a high-fiber (wheat bran) diet on the incidence of recurrent colorectal adenomas reached the same conclusion of no benefit (Alberts, 2000).

VACCINES AND SOCIAL CHANGE

Previously in this chapter, it was stated that the community vaccine trials for certain infectious diseases conducted during the 1930s–1950s were marvels of methodological ingenuity. An assumption underlying the development of the vaccines evaluated in those trials was that having vaccines to prevent diseases is "good" even if changes in environmental and/or social conditions might produce the same reduction in the incidence of disease. (See, for example, the successful environmental changes used to reduce the incidence rate of paralytic polio in the United States before the discovery of polio vaccines.) Is that assumption true for all diseases for which a vaccine might be possible? Box 9.2 provides an example in which the development of a vaccine for African trypanosomiasis raises several ethical challenges that place environmental priorities, and political and economic realities, in opposition to potential but perhaps short-term human health benefits. If the decision to proceed with vaccine development and distribution were your decision to make, what would you do?

BOX 9.2

ETHICS MATTERS: A RIFT IN THE RIFT VALLEY

PHILIPPE A. ROSSIGNOL, PH.D., AND ANNETTE M. ROSSIGNOL, SC.D.

Scientific advances in tropical medicine can provide protection against lethal parasitic diseases. Such protection, however, may allow populations to reside in areas that previously were hostile. Their presence would then put them in direct competition with native animals and plants.

African trypanosomiasis, or sleeping sickness, is caused by a microorganism transmitted by tsetse flies. The disease occurs only in equatorial Africa. Many wild animal species, particularly ungulates (gazelles, wildebeests, and warthogs), have a high prevalence of the parasite but generally suffer little if at all from the disease. People, however, generally are very susceptible, and the disease is almost always lethal. Cattle also are vulnerable. For this reason, people have not settled in vast areas of the Rift Valley. These savannas remain the last areas on earth where vast migratory herds of large mammals, such as gazelles, wildebeests, and zebras, in addition to elephants, rhinoceros, giraffes, and hippopotami, may be found. The governments of countries in parts of the Rift Valley derive substantial revenues from eco-tourism.

The rise of modern biology, particularly molecular biotechnology, has brought about intense interest in the parasite of trypanosomiasis because the microorganism has so-called "jumping genes" that readily are expressed. Tremendous contributions to basic biology already have arisen from studies of these genes. It is widely believed that an effective human and cattle vaccine or some other "cure" for trypanosomiasis will arise from further work in this area. Current drug therapy is dangerous and expensive,

Box 9.2 continued

and attempts to control the tsetse fly have not been effective. A novel vaccine or cure would allow people rapidly to settle on the savannas in the Rift Valley where they would compete for space and other resources with wild animals. From studies of surrounding areas, scientists believe that long-term coexistence of people and large herds of mammals is unlikely. The last remaining migratory herds of large mammals on earth would become extinct.

The people in the areas surrounding the Rift Valley currently live in subsistence conditions with overcrowding and malnutrition, often with famine rampant. Many of the people are pastoralists whose livelihoods depend on the quality and quantity of grazing land. Under current conditions, areas safe for cattle and their owners are restricted and consequently overgrazed. Nearby urban areas are economically sterile, overcrowded, and unhealthy. None of the countries with lands in the Rift Valley have funds to support research that could lead to a vaccine or cure for trypanosomiasis.

Almost all funds for research in tropical disease come from North American or European nations, some of which (Belgium, Great Britain, France, Germany, and Portugal) colonized parts of the Rift Valley at one time or another. By denying or approving funding to study trypanosomiasis, these countries in effect would still be creating policy regarding the fate of the people living near the Rift Valley. Many of these people, as did their ancestors, recall the fact of being colonized with substantial bitterness.

Given this scenario, it is instructive to ask whether a vaccine or cure for trypanosomiasis vigorously should be pursued and, if so, which countries or organizations should fund the required research and later distribution of the remedy.

Source: Reprinted from P. A. Rossignol and A. M. Rossignol, "A Rift in the Rift Valley," *Reflections* 5, no. 2 (1998): 2. Reprinted with permission from the Program for Ethics, Science, and the Environment, Department of Philosophy, Oregon State University.

SUMMARY

Intervention studies serve as the gold standard for evaluating the presence of a causal association between an exposure/treatment and a health outcome. Nevertheless, because of ethical concerns, intervention studies are limited in the types of associations that they can evaluate, namely to possible preventives and cures of disease or injury. Random allocation of exposure/treatment, the defining characteristic of all intervention studies, ensures an accurate (precise and unbiased) assessment of the magnitude of association between an exposure/treatment and a health outcome as long as the study size (number of participants) is large and subject participation and follow-up are high.

Observational studies, discussed in the next chapter, also are analytic (hypothesis-testing) studies but do not include the random allocation of exposure/treatment as part of their study designs. For that reason, the possible explanations for the findings from observational studies include not only random error and cause, as in the case of intervention studies, but also bias, such as confounding bias. That difference notwithstanding, intervention studies should serve as the design "goal" for the observational studies in the sense that the design of an observational study should try to mirror the rigor of the intervention studies to the extent that ethics and natural circumstances permit. Recall from Chapter 2 the historical importance of John Snow's "natural experiment" in determining which sources of piped water held the highest risk for cholera. Snow's natural experiment was an observational study that cleverly mirrored the random allocation (in this case, of water source) found in true experiments.

As you read through the next chapter, try to keep the paradigm of the intervention studies in mind. What plans for the selection of participants in an observational study most reflect the rigor of an intervention study? Which plans for data collection and for data analysis best reflect that rigor? What design strategies might you employ to prevent or control for confounding bias given that the random allocation of exposure/treatment is not available as a design option for preventing that bias?

REVIEW QUESTIONS

1. Define "analytic study." In what ways do analytic epidemiologic studies differ from intervention studies?
2. Define "hypothesis." Why must a hypothesis be specific to be useful?
3. List and define at least five components of an epidemiologic hypothesis.
4. List and define the two main types of analytic studies. Then, list and define the "plans" that compose the study designs for the analytic studies.
5. What is the difference between "preventing confounding bias" and "controlling confounding bias"?
6. Define "random assignment." Why is random assignment central to the design and interpretation of intervention studies? How do the possible interpretations of intervention studies differ from the possible interpretations of observational epidemiologic studies?
7. List several of the most important ethical considerations associated with conducting intervention studies.
8. Define "control or comparison group." Which types of analytic studies have comparison groups?
9. Define "placebo." What is the purpose of having a placebo in an intervention study?
10. List, define, and provide examples of the two main types of intervention studies.
11. List and define the main components in the design of intervention studies.
12. What is meant by "external validity"?
13. Why does random assignment prevent confounding bias?
14. Why must the subjects in an intervention study who later "drop out" of the study still be included in the data analysis if information concerning their health outcomes is known?

15. What are the consequences, if any, of "differential levels of adherence to the treatment protocols"?

16. Define "lost-to-follow-up." Why is lost-to-follow-up a potentially large source of error in an intervention study?

REVIEW EXERCISES

1. Suggest five reasons why the results of the Polyp Prevention Trial Study may have differed from the previous epidemiologic and laboratory data.

2. Go to the World Wide Web and read about ongoing clinical and preventive trials. What are the typical proportions of participants who are lost-to-follow-up? What are the demographic characteristics of participants in the trials? Which diseases or injuries most often are the targets of trials? If you were setting national priorities for funding trials, which exposures/treatments and/or diseases and injuries would you fund first? Why?

## CHAPTER 10

Design Strategies: Analytic Studies
Part 2—Observational Studies

The majority of analytic epidemiologic studies are observational rather than intervention studies. In an observational study, the subjects' exposure statuses are not randomly allocated by the study investigator, as occurs in an intervention study. Instead, the study participants acquire certain exposures in ways that are outside the control of the study investigator. Those exposures may be acquired in a workplace setting, by nutritional preferences, from environmental sources such as air or water quality, or by a myriad of other personal, social, or economic situations.

Observational studies tend to contain more bias, and especially more confounding bias, than do intervention studies. Nevertheless, because of ethical restraints, observational studies are the mainstay of epidemiologic research when hypothesized causes of disease and injury are being investigated. Hypothesized causes of disease or injury cannot ethically be randomly allocated to study participants.

There are two main types of observational epidemiologic studies: the **cohort study** and the **case/control study.** The primary difference between a cohort and a case/control study pertains to the criterion by which subjects are enrolled into each study.

The basis for enrollment in a cohort study is whether subjects have the exposure under investigation (are "**exposed**") or do not have the exposure under investigation (are "**unexposed**"); then the subjects' subsequent frequencies of disease and/or injury are compared. In contrast, the basis for enrollment in a case/control study is whether subjects have the disease or injury of interest (are "**cases**") or do not have the disease or injury of interest (are comparison subjects or "**controls**"); during the study, information about the subjects' exposure histories is collected and then compared. The difference in the criteria by which subjects are enrolled into each type of observational study determines a study's options for the selection of subjects, data collection, and data analysis.

COHORT STUDIES

In a strict sense, the term "cohort," means a fixed group of people that is followed over time. "Fixed" means that once the cohort is established, no person may enter or leave the cohort. An example of a cohort that truly is fixed is a birth cohort comprising all people born in the same calendar year. Once the year has ended, no one else may enter the cohort because no one else can be born in that year. Other cohorts, in a less strict sense of the term, are "dynamic," meaning that membership in the cohort may change over time. An example of a dynamic cohort is the resident population of a town, where some people become new residents and some current residents move elsewhere.

The cohorts that are established in a cohort study are groups of exposed and unexposed subjects. People having different exposure levels (different doses and/or durations of exposure) are assembled into cohorts whose subsequent disease and/or injury frequencies are measured and then compared. For instance, the frequencies of disease in a cohort of tobacco smokers may be compared with the frequencies of disease in a cohort of never-smokers.

The hypothesis under investigation in a cohort study usually is that the exposure under study may be a cause of the health outcomes of interest if the observed frequency of the health outcomes is higher in the exposed cohort than in the unexposed cohort. Conversely, the hypothesis sometimes is that the exposure under study may be a preventive of the health outcomes of interest if the observed frequency of the health outcomes is lower in the exposed cohort than in the unexposed cohort. The important epidemiologic information is contained in the comparison of the disease and/or injury frequencies between the cohorts. In other words, it is the *relative* magnitude of disease or injury frequencies in the cohorts that conveys valuable information rather than the *absolute* frequencies.

Cohort studies can be either prospective or retrospective, although sometimes of a combination of designs is implemented. The timing of the exposure(s) and the health outcome(s) of interest with respect to the implementation of the study determines whether the cohort study is prospective or retrospective.

In a **prospective cohort study,** subjects are enrolled in the study on the basis of their current exposures, and then the cohorts are followed forward in time to measure their frequencies of disease and/or injury. Thus, the investigators age along with the study subjects. The issue of aging investigators usually is not an obstacle to the successful completion of a cohort study when the period of follow-up is short. For long periods of follow-up, however, not only is the aging of the investigators an issue, but also other challenges emerge, such as maintaining contact with the study participants over the long time frame of the study. As an example, the original members of the cohort in the Framingham Heart Study, an ongoing, prospective cohort study originally designed to identify causes of heart disease, were enrolled in 1950. Thus, some members of the study were followed for decades. (For more information about the Framingham Heart Study, see http://framingham.com/heart/ and http://www.nhlbi.nih.gov/about/framingham/.)

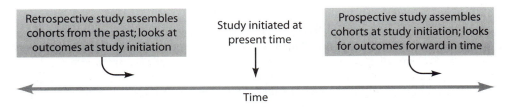

FIGURE 10.1
Prospective versus retrospective cohort studies.

In a **retrospective cohort study,** the subjects are enrolled in the study on the basis of their exposure statuses at some point or points in the past. These groups then are compared with respect to their frequencies of disease or injury up to the present time (that is, up to the time when the study is initiated). A long-term prospective cohort study requires more time and money to complete than does a comparably sized retrospective cohort study, although there are other trade-offs when deciding between the two study designs. A prospective design provides opportunities to collect detailed information about the subjects and their exposures that may not be available in a retrospective design. These opportunities arise because current exposures may be measured at different points in time as the cohorts are followed forward in time. In contrast, in a retrospective study, information about airborne occupational exposures or prescription drug use, for example, may not be available from written records or from participants' recall. Prospective designs also provide opportunities for the investigator to establish mechanisms to enhance the completeness of follow-up. Figure 10.1 summarizes the overall design of prospective and retrospective cohort studies.

Table 10.1 summarizes several of the important questions to consider when designing a cohort study. In addition to the questions listed in Table 10.1, plans for the collection of data, following up on study participants, and data analysis are part of the overall study design strategy.

TABLE 10.1
Pertinent Questions to Consider When Designing a Cohort Study

Question	Choices/Objectives
Who is exposed?	How much (dose and duration) of an exposure counts as "exposed"?
What is the source of the exposed subjects?	Which exposed people should be enrolled in the study? For a common exposure, should subjects be placed into exposure categories after enrollment in the study? For uncommon exposures, how can exposed individuals be identified and enrolled into the study?
Who is unexposed?	How much (dose and duration) of an exposure counts as "unexposed"?
What is the source of the unexposed subjects?	Which unexposed individuals are comparable to the exposed cohort? Comparability between the exposed and the unexposed cohorts is the primary goal. Choices for the unexposed cohort members include internal comparisons (for common exposures), the general population, and a cohort that is a subset of the general population but external to the exposed cohort.

IMPORTANT QUESTIONS TO CONSIDER WHEN DESIGNING COHORT STUDIES

Who Is Exposed?

It often is difficult to measure whether or not a person is exposed and, if it is determined that exposure has occurred, to estimate accurately the dose and the duration of exposure. Difficulties in measurement can arise even for easily observed exposures such as tobacco smoking. Is a person who smokes one cigarette each month considered a "smoker" or a "nonsmoker"? How can lifetime tobacco smoking be summarized taking into account changing patterns of use over time? Other exposures can be even more daunting to estimate. For example, what methods work best in determining the long-term nutrient content of a person's diet? How can lifelong exposure to pesticides be assessed? How can an accurate measure of illegal drug use be determined? The objective in measuring exposure is to identify cohorts of people whose varying levels of exposure have different pathophysiologic consequences. What are the biologically important levels of exposure that increase or decrease the frequency of disease or injury, and how can those levels be measured accurately?

Data concerning exposure (or lack of exposure) status can be gleaned from a variety of sources, including personal interviews with potential study participants, review of existing medical, occupational, or other records, and analyses of biologic samples such as blood, hair (for example, for metals), saliva, or urine. In addition, environmental samples can be taken to measure constituents in air, drinking water, foods, or soil. Three-day, seven-day, or other durations of dietary intake may be recorded by potential study participants if some dietary nutrient is the exposure of interest.

Sources of the Exposed Cohort

Two general approaches for establishing an exposed cohort are used. The first approach entails specifically identifying exposed individuals and then enrolling them into the study. For instance, an investigator might establish a cohort of asbestos-exposed people by identifying all people who worked in certain underground asbestos mines over a specified period of time. The investigator also might attempt to establish levels of exposure to asbestos by categorizing each worker by job type/task and duration of work experience. Using this approach, the investigator specifically enrolls asbestos-exposed people into the cohort study. This first approach for establishing an exposed cohort almost always needs to be used whenever the exposure of interest is rare, making exposed subjects in the general population difficult to identify.

The second approach for establishing an exposed cohort is used when the exposure of interest is common among the targeted general population for the study. In this approach, individuals are enrolled in a study without regard for their exposure statuses and then are categorized by exposure level after enrollment. As an example, in the Framingham Heart Study that began in 1950, two-thirds of the eligible residents of Framingham, Massachusetts, were enrolled in the study without regard for their levels of the exposures of interest. Those exposures included tobacco use, serum cholesterol levels, exercise habits, and weight for height, among others. Because each of the levels for those exposures was common among the target population residing in Framingham, enrolling subjects in the study without regard for exposure status and then later categorizing them into exposure categories was a satisfactory and relatively efficient plan for the selection of both the exposed and the unexposed cohorts.

Who Is Unexposed?

Primary considerations in establishing an unexposed cohort are lack of exposure and **comparability** with the exposed cohort. The idea of comparability means that the frequencies of disease and/or injury in the unexposed cohort are used to estimate what those frequencies would have been in the exposed cohort if the cohort had not been exposed. In other words, the unexposed cohort is used to estimate the frequencies of disease and/or injury expected in the absence of the exposure of interest.

Another way to think about comparability is that comparability means that the members of the unexposed cohort are *similar* to the members of the exposed cohort in their distributions of exposures that cause/prevent the health outcomes of interest except for the exposure under study. Comparability does not mean that the members of the unexposed and exposed cohorts need to be *identical* to one another in their distributions of exposures except for the exposure of interest. For example, the unexposed cohort may contain more members who fail to exercise regularly and the exposed cohort may contain more members who are overweight. If exercise and weight have the same effects on the outcome of interest, then the two cohorts are comparable to each other without being identical to each other.

Sometimes, rather than an unexposed cohort, a minimally exposed cohort is established. For example, it would be difficult to identify a cohort of individuals in an urban environment who lack at least some exposure to asbestos. Similarly, because of widespread use and contamination, it probably would not be possible, at least in the United States, to establish a cohort of people who totally lack exposure to at least several pesticides used in agriculture.

Sources of the Unexposed Cohort

As there were for the exposed cohort, there are two primary approaches for establishing an unexposed cohort. In the first approach, people who lack the exposure of interest are identified and specifically enrolled in the study. In the second approach, a group of people is enrolled in the study and their exposure levels determined after enrollment; subjects who are determined to be unexposed form the unexposed cohort.

A third approach for establishing an unexposed cohort sometimes is used. This approach entails comparing the frequency of disease or injury for the exposed cohort with the corresponding frequencies for the **general population** (usually all residents of a certain state or residents of the entire United States), as calculated from routinely collected local, state, and/or national data. This approach is the least expensive of the three approaches but offers little opportunity for collecting detailed information about individual subjects. As a minor concern, because the proportion of the general population that is exposed often is small, data for exposed individuals typically will be included among the data for the majority of the general population who are unexposed.

How Are Data Collected?

After the exposed and the unexposed cohorts are established, data about demographic characteristics, other risk factors for disease and injury, and health outcomes are collected in a comparable manner from each subject. That information can be obtained from a variety of sources, and, depending on the particular study, the different sources of data are more or less useful. Table 10.2 lists some of the more commonly used sources of data and their advantages and disadvantages.

TABLE 10.2
Commonly Used Sources of Data and Some of Their Advantages and Disadvantages

Source of Data	Advantages	Disadvantages
Personal interviews with subjects or their friends and relatives	Usually high-quality data, especially interviews with subjects	Expensive
Mail questionnaires	Less expensive	Potential for low response rate; little opportunity to clarify responses
Telephone interviews	Opportunity to clarify responses	Not all people have telephones; "busy" people are harder to reach by phone
Death certificates	Death certificate filed for every death in the United States; National Death Registry exists	Listed cause of death may be incorrect; may need to follow up with review of medical records
Physician or hospital records	High-quality data	Access to records may be difficult to obtain, especially with the HIPAA* regulations that went into effect on April 19, 2003
Population-based disease or injury registries	Inexpensive because data already have been collected	Quality of data varies among registries; may be little opportunity to obtain useful supplemental data
Prepaid medical plans	High-quality data	Access to data may be difficult to obtain
Direct physical examination, including biologic samples	High-quality data	Expensive
Occupational records	Data from environmental samples may be available to establish exposure levels	Access to data may be difficult to obtain; need to negotiate right to publish study findings upfront without company's right to approve/censure findings

*HIPAA is the Health Insurance Portability and Accountability Act, issued by the U.S. Department of Health and Human Services, Office for Civil Rights. See www.os.dhhs.gov/ocr/hipaa/.

The choice of a data collection plan involves developing efficient procedures that provide data of equally high quality for both the exposed and the unexposed cohorts. Vigorous data quality-control procedures must be undertaken early and repeatedly during data collection to ensure that the data accurately reflect the exposures, health outcomes, and other characteristics of the study participants.

How Do Investigators Follow Up on Participants?

One of the largest potential sources of error in cohort studies is **lost-to-follow-up.** Lost-to-follow-up is the inability of the study investigator to collect information about all study subjects throughout the duration of the study. Lost-to-follow-up can be a serious threat to the accuracy of a study, because subjects who become lost-to-follow-up may differ from subjects who are not lost in ways that are related to the health outcomes and exposures under investigation. For example, a serious error in comparing disease frequencies between an exposed and an unexposed cohort would result if members of the exposed cohort (but not members of the unexposed cohort) became lost-to-follow-up when the health outcome of interest occurred. That type of error might occur, for example, in an occupational health study in which members of the exposed occupational cohort left employment upon becoming ill and could not be followed.

Lost-to-follow-up creates a substantial error only when the consequences of lost-to-follow-up differ between the cohorts. That the consequences of lost-to-follow-up differ between the cohorts may be suggested by **differential lost-to-follow-up;** that is, the percentage of subjects who are lost-to-follow-up is substantially higher in one cohort than in the other. Even similarity in the percentage lost in each cohort, however, does not guarantee that the consequences of the loss are the same. Sometimes, an investigator will undertake an especially vigorous effort to locate a sample of the subjects in each cohort who were lost. The goal of that effort is to determine whether the disease and/or injury experiences of the lost subjects are similar to the health experiences of the cohort members who were not lost-to-follow-up.

How Are Data Analyzed?

Establishing a plan for data analysis is part of the overall study design. Importantly, this plan is a part of the *initial planning stages* for the study rather than an effort undertaken solely at the end of the study, after the data have been collected. The plan for data analysis corresponds closely with the plan for data collection in that both plans focus on the variables for which data will be collected for each subject. The data analysis plan, in addition, outlines the approach that will be used for controlling any confounding bias not prevented in the design of the study. Data analysis will be discussed in more detail in Chapter 11.

EXAMPLES OF COHORT STUDIES

THE NURSES' HEALTH STUDY

The Nurse's Health Study was one of the first large-scale prospective cohort studies focused specifically on the health of women. The initial study, designed in the mid-1970s with data collection beginning in 1976, enrolled approximately 120,000 married female nurses between the ages of 30 and 55 years at the start of the study who were registered in any of eleven states in the United States (Belanger et al. 1978). Nurses were selected for study because of their ability to respond accurately to clinical questions about their medical conditions. In addition, the investigators thought nurses' interest in health-related matters would increase follow-up over the anticipated long duration of the study. The original objective of the study was to evaluate the long-term effects, if any, of oral contraceptive use. Data provided on the baseline questionnaire were used to categorize the nurses into cohorts according to their levels of oral contraceptive use and according to their levels for other exposures of interest. Follow-up questionnaires were mailed at two-year intervals to update exposure information and to obtain data on health outcomes. The response rate for each of those questionnaires has been approximately 90 percent.

The study was expanded in 1980 by including a food-frequency questionnaire to allow evaluation of the effects of nutrition on disease. In addition, the participating nurses provided samples of toenail clippings and blood, enabling the investigators to analyze exposure to minerals and identify hormone levels and genetic factors that may be related to disease.

The Nurses' Health Study II was initiated in 1989 to study the effects of oral contraceptive use, diet, and lifestyle risk factors among women who were somewhat younger (25 to 42 years) than were the women enrolled in the initial study. Many of these women were not married at the time of entry into the study, making follow-up more challenging if women changed their surnames at the time of marriage. Nevertheless, response rates to the questionnaires mailed to the cohort every two years have been approximately 90 percent.

The Nurses' Health Study (parts I and II) has been and continues to be a rich source of information about risk factors for chronic diseases and other health outcomes among women. Publications based on the study data are listed at www.channing.harvard.edu/nhs.

CORONARY HEART DISEASE AMONG WORKERS EXPOSED TO CARBON DISULFIDE

Two cohorts of workers were enrolled in a prospective cohort study in 1967 (Hernberg, Nurimen, and Tolonen 1973). The exposed cohort was comprised on 343 men who had been exposed to carbon disulfide while working in a viscose rayon plant for at least five years. The unexposed cohort was comprised on 343 paperworkers from the same town who were frequency-matched to the exposed subjects on age, district of birth, and similarity of work activities. Frequency matching is the selection of comparison subjects who have the same or similar characteristics as the exposed subjects with respect to demographic variables such as age, gender, and ethnic or racial identification. Frequency matching is performed as a strategy to prevent confounding by the frequency-matched variables, as described more fully later in this chapter.

At the end of the 5.5-year period of follow-up, the mortality rate from coronary heart disease was 5.2 times higher in the exposed cohort than in the unexposed cohort. A second comparison was made between the 5.5-year coronary mortality between the exposed population and the coronary heart disease mortality rate in the general male population of Finland of similar ages. In this comparison, the rate among the viscose rayon workers was 2.1 times the rate in the general population. Thus, although the coronary heart disease mortality rate among the viscose rayon workers was higher than expected in each comparison, the choice of the unexposed cohort affected the magnitude of the increase.

One possible explanation for the difference in the relative mortality rates of coronary heart disease is the **healthy worker effect,** an apparent decrease in mortality (or of morbidity) among workers compared with the general population that comprises both workers and nonworkers. The effect occurs because people must have obtained and then maintain a certain level of health to remain in the workforce; workers who become ill leave the workforce but still are part of the general population until death. Thus, there is a selection process that removes people who are ill from the workforce. In this study, workers in the unexposed cohort of paper workers may be healthier than the general population in part because of the healthy worker effect, resulting in a lower mortality rate from coronary heart disease.

CASE/CONTROL STUDIES

A case/control study is made up of **cases** (people who have the disease or injury of interest) and **controls** or comparison subjects (people who do not have the disease or injury of interest). The exposure history for each case and each control is determined, for example, by interview, mail survey, or review of preexisting records (see Table 10.2), and then the exposure histories of the cases are compared with the exposure histories of the controls. The comparison of past exposures provides data about which exposures may have resulted in the current health outcome of interest. In other words, exposure histories that differ in frequency between the cases and the controls may be causes or preventives of the disease or injury under investigation.

The hypotheses in a case/control study are the same as the hypotheses in cohort studies, namely, that the presence of certain exposures may increase or decrease the frequency of disease or injury relative to the frequency of these health outcomes among unexposed people. Also, like hypotheses for cohort studies, a hypothesis will be specific with respect to the population to whom the hypothesis applies, to the time- and dose-responses, and to other variables reflective of person, place, and time.

The study design of a case/control study is considerably different from the design of a cohort study. In a case/control study, subjects are enrolled in the study on the basis of their health status and not on the basis of their exposure status, as occurs in a cohort study. Data about the relative frequencies of the disease or injury of interest among exposed and unexposed people are derived from a comparison of the cases' and controls' exposure histories and not from a direct comparison of the disease or injury frequencies in exposed and unexposed cohorts. The data analysis plan for case/control studies is discussed in Chapter 11. For now, the important point to appreciate is that information about the *relative* but not the *absolute* rates of the health outcome of interest *in the exposed cohort compared with the unexposed cohort* can be gained by comparing exposure histories in the case and control groups. For example, an investigator may discover that the incidence rate of disease is twice as high in the exposed cohort

TABLE 10.3
Questions to Consider When Designing a Case/Control Study

Question	Choices/Objectives
Who is a case?	Strict diagnostic criteria to ensure a homogeneous disease entity; select incident (newly diagnosed) cases rather than prevalent cases.
What are the sources for cases?	Hospital or other clinical setting versus identification of cases from the general population.
Who is a good control?	Select people who do not have the disease under study, do not have another disease that is caused or prevented by the exposure under study, and are comparable to the case group.
What are the sources for controls?	Hospital controls, community (general population) controls, special groups such as relatives or co-workers.

as in the unexposed cohort but will not know the actual magnitude of the disease incidence rate in either cohort. Symbolically, the investigator will know the value of ($IR_{exposed\ cohort}/IR_{unexposed\ cohort}$) but will not know the magnitudes of $IR_{exposed\ cohort}$ or $IR_{unexposed\ cohort}$.

Sometimes case/control studies are referred to as "retrospective studies" or "retrospective case/control studies," because case/control studies "look back" at the past exposures of cases and of controls. This nomenclature may be confusing or at least redundant because, unlike cohort studies, all case/control studies compare past exposure histories for groups of cases and controls.

Table 10.3 summarizes several of the salient questions to consider when designing a case/control study. In addition to the questions listed in Table 10.3, the initial study design for a case/control study includes plans for the selection of subjects, for data collection, and for data analysis.

IMPORTANT QUESTIONS TO CONSIDER WHEN DESIGNING CASE/CONTROL STUDIES

Who Is a Case?

A case is a person who meets the medical criteria for having the disease or injury whose etiology is under investigation and who satisfies other study enrollment criteria, such as age, gender, and/or place of residence. The medical criteria must be stringent to ensure that a homogeneous disease entity makes up the case group. As an example, enrolling "cases of Hodgkin's disease" into a case/control study is insufficient to ensure a homogeneous disease entity. The epidemiologic and etiologic features of Hodgkin's disease differ by age, with the disease in people under the age of about 40 years resembling an infectious disease and the disease in older people resembling a noninfectious disease. Because the ultimate goal of most case/control studies is elucidation of disease or injury etiology, the criteria for enrolling cases ideally should define a pathologic entity that is caused by the same etiologic pathway rather than being a collection of different pathologic entities that have different etiologies.

Breast cancer in women provides a second example of a disease that probably has several different etiologies, with breast cancer in young women differing from breast cancer in older women with respect to etiology. Worldwide, women in some countries develop breast cancer primarily as young women, whereas in other countries women develop breast cancer primarily as older women. Women in the United States develop both types of breast cancer. The **age incidence rate curve** (incidence rate by age) of breast cancer among women in the United States is **bimodal** (having two modes or peaks), with one mode among women approximately 40 years of age and a second mode that increases steadily with age. Women and their offspring who migrate from countries having low breast cancer incidence to countries having high breast incidence rapidly (usually within one or two generations) acquire the breast cancer incidence rate of their new host country (Figure 10.2).

Cases enrolled in a case/control study should be **incident cases** (newly diagnosed cases) rather than **prevalent cases** (cases diagnosed at some point in the past). The timing of disease diagnosis depends upon variables such as access to medical care, insur-

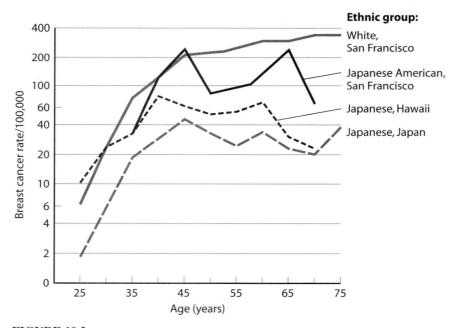

FIGURE 10.2

Incidence rate of breast cancer in Japanese women in Japan, Hawaii, and San Francisco and in White women in San Francisco.

Source: K. McPherson, C. M. Steel, and J. M. Dixon, Breast Cancer—Epidemiology, Risk Factors, and Genetics, *British Medical Journal* 321, no. 7261 (September 9, 2000): 624–28. (September 9, 2000): 624–28. Reproduced with permission from the BMJ Publishing Group.

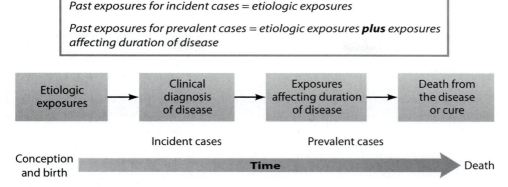

> Past exposures for incident cases = etiologic exposures
>
> Past exposures for prevalent cases = etiologic exposures **plus** exposures affecting duration of disease

Etiologic exposures → Clinical diagnosis of disease → Exposures affecting duration of disease → Death from the disease or cure

Incident cases   Prevalent cases

Conception and birth ——— Time ——→ Death

FIGURE 10.3
Etiologic exposures and exposures affecting disease duration.

ance status, and attitude about seeking medical care. Nevertheless, the strategy for enrolling cases usually is to enroll cases as soon as possible after diagnosis rather than enrolling cases that have been diagnosed in the past, especially for diseases or injuries that are life threatening. The reason for that strategy resides in the relationship among the incidence rate of disease, the prevalence of disease, and its average duration, discussed in Chapter 5. Prevalence $= (IR \times D)/(1 + (IR \times D))$ where IR is the incidence rate of disease or injury and D is the average duration of the disease or injury. A case/control study that enrolls prevalent cases, and then queries about past exposures, usually will not be able to separate exposures that may be related to disease etiology from exposures that may affect a case's ability to survive with the disease, that is, from exposures that affect the disease's duration (Figure 10.3). For that reason, ideally only incident cases should be enrolled into a case/control study, especially if the primary study objective is to identify exposures that may be related to disease etiology.

Sources of Cases

Where does an epidemiologist find cases to include in a case/control study? One source is a hospital or some other clinical setting. Medical records or logs can be searched to identify patients who meet the study enrollment criteria. This approach for identifying cases, though convenient, may not yield a representative group of cases in some situations. For example, some people may not have access to clinical facilities either because of geographic isolation, lack of medical insurance, or for some other reason. Thus, those individuals may not be represented among a case group identified from clinical records. This potential problem is more likely to occur for diseases or injuries that do not require medical treatment, such as minor illnesses or health conditions for which treatment is elective. For those conditions, identifying cases from the general (nonhospitalized or hospital-identified) population may be preferred. For a discussion of geographic information systems in identifying cases, see Box 10.1.

BOX 10.1

ETHICS MATTERS: GEOGRAPHIC INFORMATION SYSTEMS

GINA LEGAZ

"Geographic Information Systems (GIS) are the most widely used technological applications in municipal government" (Esnard 1998). GIS also are being used more often in public safety, administration, finance and tax, public works, and the social and health sciences (Esnard 1998). Epidemiological studies are using GIS to identify high-prevalence areas of a disease of interest as well as risk assessment in geographically identified areas. The technology available to researchers is increasing and spreading to other specialties within public health, such as health promotion. Along with the increasing technological advances and abilities of GIS come ethical questions concerning GIS uses and abuses, most specifically surrounding individual and community privacy.

In a 2005 journal article titled "Geographic Identification of High Gonorrhea Transmission Areas in Baltimore, Maryland," by Jennings et al., investigators attempted to identify significant clusters and sexual transmission networks of neighborhoods with high prevalence of gonorrhea persisting after adjustment for racial/ethnic composition using GIS. The implications of identifying a transmission network are significant for a reduction in STIs as well as the cost-effectiveness of public health prevention programs. However, at what price do those advancements come? Researchers have the ability to identify the neighborhoods that core transmitters live in and in some instances even the block they live on. Of course, STI prevention aimed solely at the specific core of individuals spreading the disease is more time- and cost-efficient than an STI intervention targeting the entire city or community; however, what privacy do we afford these communities and individuals within them? Recent increases in the availability of fine-scaled, geocoded data bring concerns about the confidentiality of blocks, neighborhoods, and communities (Elliott and Wartenberg 2004). The right to privacy becomes even more profoundly important when dealing with identification of specific, defined geographic areas and individual networks concerning diseases with a stigma, such as STIs (Curry 1997). An investigation may take place in a city; ask yourself what might have been the ethical implications if it had taken place in an unicorporated geographic location? Such a location would make it remarkably simple to locate specific individuals compared with more densely populated locations. As health promotion investigators, epidemiologists, and government public health agencies use GIS to identify areas of high prevalence to target interventions and prevention programs, GIS is redefining ethical considerations for researchers as well as issues involving individual rights to privacy. There is a current move to reconceptualize one's individual right to privacy. Previously, privacy was frequently seen as a right to be left alone; now it needs to be seen as a right to control the passage of information in society (Curry 1997).

In addition to ethical considerations of breaches in individual privacy concerning the use of GIS, there are the misuses of GIS, such as data profiling, the use of inaccurate data, and the evolving question of where to draw the line with community and

Box 10.1 continued

neighborhood right to privacy, especially concerning the misrepresentation of data. "The ability to identify with a particular place or group is fundamental to the development of a sense of identity, and a sense of privacy is a critical element in that identity; defining neighborhoods in terms that render that relationship statistical and contingent undercuts the role of individual privacy, and hence its power" (Curry 1997). Dealing with stigmatized diseases, such as STIs, certainly has consequences for neighborhoods as well as individuals. If an area is misclassified as a prevalent area of a stigmatized disease, the community can be directly affected in many ways. For example, property values may decrease. We must start asking to what extent, if any, a community of individuals is entitled to a right to privacy. The right to privacy, at least in the United States, has always been a function of the individual; GIS technologies, and specifically data profiling, have been used to apply to clusters of households, neighborhoods, states, and nations (Curry 1997). The permissive ethical considerations for research need to evolve alongside technology rather than lag behind it. Without that continuity, there will certainly be ethical abuses within the field. In addition to ethical considerations concerning GIS, there needs to be a reevaluation of what privacy is, and a rethinking of who or what can have a right to privacy (Curry 1997).

REFERENCES

Curry, M. 1997. Digital people, digital places: Rethinking privacy in a world of geographic information. *Ethics and Behavior* 7 (3): 253–63.

Elliott, P., and Wartenberg, D. 2004. Mini-monograph. *Environmental Health Perspectives* 112 (9): 997–1008.

Esnard, A. M. 1998. Cities, GIS, and ethics. *Journal of Urban Technology* 5 (3): 33–45.

Jennings, M., F. Curriero, D. Celentano, and M. Ellen. 2005. Geographic identification of high gonorrhea transmission areas in Baltimore, Maryland. *American Journal of Epidemiology* 161 (1): 73–80.

Another potential difficulty associated with using a clinical setting as the source of cases pertains to specialty hospitals, which have a reputation for offering especially high-quality care for certain health conditions. These hospitals tend to attract patients from a wide geographic area. Such patients typically are not a representative group of all patients with the disease or injury of interest but instead are either people with unusual (and so perhaps medically interesting) symptoms or people who have the economic means to seek treatment at a specialty facility. These cases may not represent the typical person with the disease or injury and can make assembling a comparable control group difficult.

Who Is a Good Control?

A good control group comprises people who satisfy at least three criteria: They do not have the disease or injury of interest (although they may have some other medical condition); they do not have a health condition that is either caused or prevented by the exposure(s) under evaluation; and they are comparable to the case group. As an example of the second criterion, in the evaluation of a hypothesis related to the causes of lung cancer, people who have emphysema, heart disease, bladder cancer, throat cancer, or any of a number of other health conditions should not be included in the control group, because each of those diseases, like lung cancer, is caused by tobacco smoking. Including in the control group people who have a health condition caused by smoking would increase the prevalence of smoking in the control group relative to the prevalence that would have been observed if the control group had been comprised of people who did not have a tobacco-related health condition. Thus, the comparison of tobacco smoking histories between the cases and the controls would be biased, yielding a comparison that underestimated the magnitude of association between smoking and lung cancer.

As in selecting an unexposed group for a cohort study, **comparability** between the cases and the controls is of paramount importance. In a case/control study, comparability between the case and control groups means that, in the absence of an effect of the exposure(s) of interest on the health outcome of interest (i.e., being a case), the proportion of cases that are positive for exposure history will equal the proportion of controls that are positive for exposure history. In other words, the study will find that there is no association between the exposure(s) and the health outcome of interest if no association exists. As an example, a case group made up of subjects who are older than the subjects in the control group probably will not yield an unbiased estimate of the association between an exposure and the case disease. Age is related to many exposures and to many diseases and injuries. Failure to take that association into account either in the study design or in the data analysis may undermine the comparability between the cases and controls.

Although the three criteria for being a "good control group" are clear in theory, there can be difficulties in determining whether an actual control group meets those criteria. For example, because many of the causes of ill health are not known, it may not be possible to determine whether the subjects in a control group have a disease or an injury that is caused or prevented by the exposure(s) under evaluation. To address that difficulty, investigators sometimes enroll in the control group people having a variety of diseases and injuries; in that way, an error in the selection of a portion of the controls will not seriously undermine the validity of the study.

Sources of Controls

There are several possible choices for the source of the controls in a case/control study. One choice, which may be appropriate for case/control studies in which the cases are identified from clinical records, is to select controls from among the patients treated at the same clinical facilities from which the cases were identified. One advantage of this approach is that the same selection factors that brought cases to a particular clinical facility probably brought controls to the same clinical facility. Thus, the cases and the controls would be comparable to each another, at least in that respect. A second advantage of this approach is that the mind-set of the cases and the controls will tend to be the same: Because both the cases and the controls are ill, they may be wondering what they might have done to cause their illness. For that reason, the cases' and controls' abilities to recall past events that may be related to their present health condition will tend to be equal.

A disadvantage of using controls identified from clinical records is that the controls are ill. The exposures that caused the controls' ill health may be the same exposures that caused the cases' ill health, tending to make the cases and the controls unduly similar with respect to their exposure histories. For example, the prevalence of tobacco use, being overweight, and infrequent exercise typically are higher among people seeking inpatient care at a hospital than among people who remain well, because those exposures cause so many diseases and injuries.

A second choice for the source of a control group is the general population of people in good health. An advantage of this choice is the lower probability that the controls have a health condition that is caused or prevented by the exposure(s) under evaluation. A disadvantage is that busy schedules or lack of interest in participating in the study may make it difficult to enroll in the study people who are in good health. In addition, people who are in good health usually differ from people in ill health with respect to their ability to recall past exposures. Finally, identifying population-based controls usually costs more in time and money than does identifying controls from clinical records.

A third possible choice for the control subjects is the selection of friends, relatives, co-workers, or neighbors of the cases. The advantage of this choice is the general willingness of acquaintances to participate in a study in which they know the case. The large disadvantage of this choice for the source of controls is the tendency for acquaintances to be overly similar to the cases in terms of their past and present exposures. For instance, people who smoke tobacco and drink alcoholic beverages tend to have as friends people who also smoke and drink alcoholic beverages. The term **overmatching** describes this "oversimilarity" between cases and controls. Overmatching is undesirable in an epidemiologic study because it makes the cases and the controls unduly similar in their prevalences of exposure(s). Consequently, acquaintances of the case group rarely are selected as the source for the control group.

Unlike overmatching, **frequency matching** often is employed in the selection of control subjects. The objective of frequency matching is to enroll in the study a control group that is similar to the case group with respect to variables, often demographic variables that are related to disease and injury frequency. As an example of frequency matching, if a male White case aged 50 years old is enrolled in the study, an attempt will be made to enroll a male White control who is about 50 years old. Frequency matching is used to prevent confounding by the variables that were frequency-matched. Lack of bias hopefully occurs because those variables occur in equal frequencies among the cases and the controls. The mere fact that certain etiologic factors are present in similar percentages among the case and control groups, however, does not guarantee that there is no confounding by those factors, as demonstrated in Table 10.4. The underlying assumptions in Table 10.4 are that only two factors, alcohol and tobacco smoking, are potential confounding factors in the study and that those two factors occur in equal proportions in both the case and the control groups. An additional assumption is that the effect(s) of alcohol *plus* tobacco smoking differs from the effects of the sum of their individual effects, such as occurs with the incidence of laryngeal cancer.

The ultimate choice for the source of the control group in any given case/control study involves weighing the advantages and the disadvantages of each possible source, given the particular hypothesis under investigation, and making a decision based on the perceived merits of each possible choice.

TABLE 10.4

Demonstration of Two Potential Confounding Factors That Occur in the Same Proportion in Case and Control Groups with Residual Confounding by Those Factors *

Confounding Factor	Cases (% of cases)	Controls (% of controls)	Total (= cases + controls)
Alcohol	0	*100 (20%)*	100
Tobacco smoking	0	*100 (20%)*	100
Alcohol and tobacco smoking	*100 (20%)*	0	100
Neither alcohol nor tobacco smoking	400	300	700
Total	500	500	1,000

*There are 100 alcohol users (20%) and 100 tobacco smokers (20%) in each group. If the combined effects of alcohol *plus* tobacco use in an individual are more or less than the individual effects of alcohol *or* tobacco use, the fact that there are 100 alcohol and 100 tobacco users in each the case and control group will not prevent confounding by alcohol and tobacco use.

EXAMPLES OF CASE/CONTROL STUDIES

ESOPHAGEAL CANCER AND GREEN TEA CONSUMPTION

All esophageal cancer cases or cases of pancreatic, colon, or rectal cancer aged 30–74 years who were diagnosed between October 1, 1990, and January 31, 1993, in the urban area of Shanghai, People's Republic of China, were eligible for the study. Cases were identified from the records of the Shanghai Cancer Registry. The study focused on cases of esophageal cancer, a subset of all the cases (Gao et al., 1994).

Of the 1,016 esophageal cases identified, 902 participated in the study (83 cases died before interview, 18 moved away from Shanghai, and 13 refused to participate in the study). The control subjects were 1,552 people frequency-matched to the esophageal cases, or to the other cases, for age and gender. All control subjects were selected from the Shanghai Resident Registry. Information about demographic characteristics, diet history, and other risk factors was obtained by personal interview with each subject.

The study findings demonstrated a strong protective association between drinking green tea and esophageal cancer, particularly among women and nonsmokers. Drinking scalding hot liquids (green tea or other beverages) was associated with a large increase in the risk of esophageal cancer. The protective effect of green tea was observed only when the tea was consumed as a warm but not scalding hot beverage.

SMOKING AND CARCINOMA OF THE LUNG

Probably the most famous case/control study is Doll and Hill's landmark study of smoking and carcinoma of the lung (1950). This study of 709 lung carcinoma cases and 709 noncancer controls, frequency-matched for age and gender, was conducted in the greater London area in the late 1940s. The study is one of the first investigations of a chronic disease using the case/control design approach and is an outstanding example of a carefully designed and executed study.

The comparison of smoking histories between the cases and the controls revealed that a greater proportion of cases smoked than did controls and that among those who did smoke, the cases smoked more cigarettes per day on average than did the controls. The study found that a larger proportion of smokers among the controls inhaled while smoking than among the cases. This anomalous finding could not be explained.

Box 10.2 summarizes a case/control study designed to elucidate the interaction among genetic factors, environmental and behavioral information, clinical data, psychological indexes, lung-tissue markers, and functional enzyme activities in viable mononuclear cells in the etiology of lung cancer and smoking (the GELCS study). Figures 10.4 and 10.5 complement Box 10.2 by outlining the study's management approach (Figure 10.4) and plan for data collection (Figure 10.5). These figures illustrate the complex but necessary coordination of efforts that can be required in conducting an epidemiologic study. The figures also outline the data collection and data management strategies needed to ensure that the study data are accurate and that data collection methods are standardized among the fourteen participating hospitals.

BOX 10.2

THE GENETIC EPIDEMIOLOGY OF LUNG CANCER AND SMOKING (GELCS) STUDY

Maria Teresa Landi, M.D., Ph.D.

GELCS is a population-based case/control study designed to integrate genetic factors, environmental and behavioral information, clinical data, psychological indexes, lung-tissue markers, and functional enzyme activities in viable mononuclear cells, in a comprehensive evaluation of the etiology of lung cancer and smoking. We are recruiting 2,000 incident lung cancer cases from fourteen hospitals in Lombardy region, Italy, and 2,000 age- and gender-matched controls from population registers. Hospital-based personnel identify eligible cases by verifying eligibility and nonduplications in the database, and abstract medical charts, draw blood, interview cases via Computerized Assisted Personal Interview (CAPI), and collect tissue specimens and self-administered questionnaires. Controls are randomly selected from the same population of the cases, and interviews, blood specimens, and self-administered questionnaires are collected at home or in hospitals. Several incentives, such as involvement of family physicians, gas coupons, establishment of a toll-free phone line for questions, media advertisement, and mailing of material describing the study, are adopted to increase participation rates.

Biospecimens are processed in a central laboratory within four hours of collection, and whole blood, buffy coats, cryopreserved lymphocytes, red blood cells, granulocytes, plasma, serum, fresh frozen tissue, paraffin-embedded tissue blocks, and slides are stored in liquid nitrogen, in $-80°C$ and $-20°C$ freezers, and at room temperature

Box 10.2 continued

according to specimen type and future use. All documents and vial labels are scanned, and data are transmitted to a data processing center via a relational database on a Microsoft SQL server. Computerized data are transmitted to the principal study investigators weekly, and synthetic weekly reports are automatically generated. Biospecimens are shipped according to the ITAS regulation semiweekly.

COHORT VERSUS CASE/CONTROL STUDIES

What are the relative strengths and limitations of the cohort and case/control study designs? In general, the strengths of one study design are the weaknesses of the other design. Those strengths and weaknesses are summarized in Table 10.5. The table is organized by first listing the questions that often are asked when deciding which study design is preferable for studying a particular exposure-outcome relation. Then, the table presents the advantages and the disadvantages of the case/control, retrospective cohort study, and prospective cohort study in response to each question.

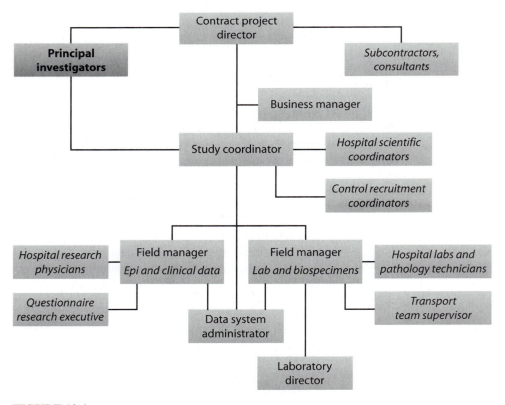

FIGURE 10.4
Management approach for the GELCS study.
Source: Maria Teresa Landi, M.D., Ph.D.

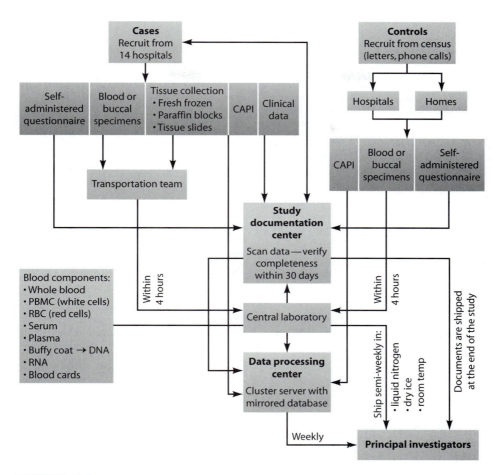

FIGURE 10.5
Plan for data collection smoking GELCS study.
Source: Maria Teresa Landi, M.D., Ph.D.

SUMMARY

The analytic observational studies are the primary study designs used to evaluate causal associations in epidemiology. Because these studies lack the random allocation of exposures, they are more prone to bias than are the intervention studies. Nevertheless, because of ethical constraints, observational studies often are the only types of designs available to evaluate the possible causal associations between certain exposures and health outcomes.

The goal of observational studies is clear, namely, to determine the human health effects of exposures and the etiologies of human disease or injury. Nevertheless,

TABLE 10.5
Strengths and Weaknesses of Case/Control and Cohort Studies

Question	Case/Control Study	Retrospective Cohort Study	Prospective Cohort Study
How rare or common is the exposure under study?	Good only for common exposure unless exposure causes a large percent of the disease	Especially good for rare exposure	Especially good for rare exposure
How rare or common is the health outcome under study?	Especially good for rare disease	Good only for common health outcome unless the exposure causes a high rate of the health outcome	Good only for common health outcome unless the exposure causes a high rate of the health outcome
How many exposures or health outcomes are of interest?	Good for one disease but many exposures	Good for one exposure but many health outcomes	Good for one exposure but many health outcomes
How much time and money are available to complete the study?	Shorter time period and less money	Shorter time period and less money	Longer time period and more money
Are records and information on exposure available?	If no records are available, may be a problem collecting accurate information on exposure	If no records are available, may be a problem identifying the exposed cohort	Usually not a problem because data are collected prospectively
Is the temporal pattern between exposure and outcome clear?	May be a problem to determine temporal pattern	Usually not a problem	Usually not a problem
How probable is bias?	Most prone to bias because both the health outcome and the exposure already have occurred when the study is initiated	Moderately prone to bias because both the exposure and the health outcome already have occurred at the time the study is initiated	Least prone to bias because data are collected prospectively using methods specifically designed to ensure comparability
How probable is lost-to-follow-up?	Not a large problem	Potentially a large problem	Potentially a large problem
What ethical constraints are present?	Varies, but typically not as many constraints as intervention trials have	Varies but typically not as many constraints as intervention trials have	Varies but typically not as many constraints as intervention trials have
Can disease frequency be calculated?	Usually not	Yes	Yes

observational studies often are "blunt" measuring tools, being able to distinguish among exposures that protect against disease or injury, have no health effects, slightly or moderately increase the rate of disease or injury, or have large effects in causing disease or injury. The lack of precision in measuring associations between exposures and health outcomes can be frustrating to the student embarking on his or her first epidemiologic investigation. That frustration can be particularly troublesome if the student comes from an academic background, such as a "wet" laboratory science, in which precise findings are commonplace. The antidote to that frustration comes from the record of success epidemiology has had in determining causes of disease and injury, even if only imprecisely. Most if not all of the known causes of cancers and of birth defects as well as of other diseases were first discovered either by epidemiologists and/or by clinicians studying human populations. As epidemiologists' abilities to accurately measure pathophysiologic amounts of exposures and early stages of health outcomes increases, the findings from epidemiologic studies will become more precise, lending themselves more readily to positive scrutiny by scientists used to viewing precise study findings. It is in the field of improved measurement that are seen part of the future of epidemiology and its promise for improving the public's health.

REVIEW QUESTIONS

1. Define "analytic observational study." List, define, and differentiate between the main types of analytic observational studies.
2. Define "cohort." How does a "dynamic cohort" differ from a true cohort?
3. What hypothesis is under investigation in a cohort study?
4. In what ways does a prospective cohort study differ from a retrospective cohort study?
5. How is exposure measured in a cohort study?
6. What are possible sources of exposed subjects for a cohort study?
7. What is meant by "the primary concern in establishing an unexposed cohort (for a cohort study) is *comparability* with the exposed cohort"?
8. What are the possible sources of unexposed subjects for a cohort study?
9. List possible sources of information about exposures, health outcomes, and other characteristics of people and their environments that may be used in an observational study.
10. Define "lost-to-follow-up." Why is lost-to-follow-up potentially a large problem in cohort studies?
11. What hypothesis is under evaluation in a case/control study?
12. What criteria are used in determining "who a case is" for a case/control study?
13. List possible sources for cases in a case/control study.
14. What criteria are used in determining a good control group for a case/control study? What does it mean for the control group to be "comparable" to the case group?
15. List the possible sources for control subjects. Then list the advantages and the disadvantages of each source.
16. Define "overmatching." How does overmatching occur? Why is overmatching an undesirable feature of an epidemiologic study?
17. Define "frequency matching." What is the primary benefit of employing frequency matching in an epidemiologic study?
18. Compare case/control prospective cohort studies and case/control retrospective cohort studies with respect to each study design's strengths and weaknesses.

## CHAPTER 11

Simple Analysis of Epidemiologic Data: Effect Measures

Epidemiologic studies generate data that are analyzed to yield the study findings. After data have been collected and entered into a computer file, an epidemiologist works with those data in four activities: **data editing, data reduction, data analysis,** and **data interpretation.** Sometimes data entry occurs as part of the process of data collection rather than occurring as a separate stage in data analysis.

This chapter will focus on the **simple analysis** of epidemiologic data. Simple analysis is an analysis of the data based on the least complicated arrangement of data. This arrangement is one in which all the data are contained in a single data table. Once the data have been placed in a single table, the data are analyzed.

Data analysis consists of two activities: **hypothesis testing** (measuring the consistency between the data and the null hypothesis of no association between the exposure and the heath outcome) and **estimation.** Estimation has two components: **point estimation** and **interval estimation** of the **effect measure(s)** of interest. An effect measure quantifies the size of association between an exposure and a health outcome. A point estimate is the best single "guess" for the size of an effect measure. An interval estimate (also referred to as a "confidence interval estimate") is a range of values for the effect measure taking random variation into account. Figure 11.1 summarizes the steps in data analysis.

A complete discussion of data analysis is beyond the scope of this text. Instead, the discussion will focus on point estimation for the simple analysis of data from cohort studies and from case/control studies. Chapter 12 (under the heading "Precision") contains additional information about several aspects of data analysis, and especially about methods to quantify the amount of random error associated with an effect measure. In addition, Box 11.1 discusses the differences between hypothesis generation and hypothesis evaluation.

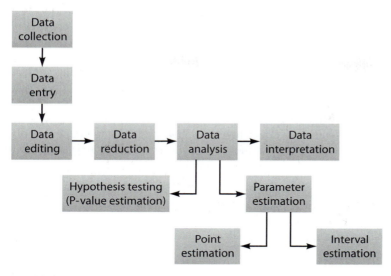

FIGURE 11.1
Steps in data analysis.

BOX 11.1

ETHICS MATTERS: HYPOTHESIS GENERATION VERSUS HYPOTHESIS EVALUATION

Data management and analysis is an art as well as a technical skill, requiring multi-dimensional thinking and organizational skills. It is a talent best learned by practice-analyzing data from an actual epidemiologic study and/or by participating in the design phase of an epidemiologic study and following through to the data collection and analysis, and write-up of the study results.

Typically, data analysis begins with inspection of the crude effect measures and then proceeds through more complicated displays of the data, such as presenting the data in a series of strata to assess the presence of effect modification or confounding. Different approaches to data analysis may at times lead to contradictory results, even for the same set of data. Those differences may occur for a variety of reasons, including differences in recognizing and reporting effect modification or controlling for confounding factors.

Another reason data analyses from the same set of data may differ pertains to *hypothesis generation versus hypothesis evaluation*. It may be tempting to look at a data set, find an interesting exposure-outcome association, and then evaluate the

Box 11.1 continued

exposure-outcome hypothesis with the same data set used to generate the hypothesis. This approach is inappropriate because the probability of finding what already is known to exist (from inspection of the data) is 100 percent. The same reasoning applies to stratifying data into different strata to evaluate the presence of effect modification or to identify and control for confounding bias. There should be some a priori reason *why* the data should be stratified into certain strata. This reason cannot be based on inspection of the data but should come from reviewing the results from other epidemiologic studies on the same exposure-outcome association or from other reasons from the scientific literature. This point is illustrated in Table 1.

TABLE 1
Illustration of How Different Data Layouts Yield Different Study Findings

Crude Table	HYPOTHETICAL DATA FROM A CASE/CONTROL STUDY	
	Exposed	Not Exposed
Cases	230	70
Controls	145	110
	EOR* = 2.49	

DATA STRATIFIED INTO TWO OF THREE POSSIBLE LEVELS
OF A POTENTIAL EFFECT MODIFIER OR CONFOUNDING FACTOR

Interpretation: No effect modification and no confounding of the crude EOR

	LEVEL ONE		LEVELS TWO PLUS THREE	
	Exposed	Not Exposed	Exposed	Not Exposed
Cases	50	10	180	60
Controls	40	20	105	90
	EOR = 2.50		EOR = 2.57	

DATA STRATIFIED INTO ALL THREE LEVELS OF A POTENTIAL EFFECT MODIFIER OR CONFOUNDING FACTOR

Interpretation: Effect modification between Level One, and Levels Two and Three

	LEVEL ONE		LEVEL TWO		LEVEL THREE	
	Exposed	Not Exposed	Exposed	Not Exposed	Exposed	Not Exposed
Cases	50	10	80	10	100	50
Controls	40	20	80	40	25	50
	EOR = 2.5		EOR = 4.0		EOR = 4.0	

*See pages 236–238 for a discussion of the exposure odds ratio (EOR).

In the example given in Table 1, a data analyst who did not stratify the data into all three levels of the potential effect modifier or confounding factor would have missed the effect modification between Level One, and Levels Two and Three. In other words, effect modification between Level One, and Levels Two and Three, would not have

Box 11.1 continued

been detected if the data for Levels Two and Three were added together, as they were in the second example (EOR = 2.57, not very different from the EOR for level one (EOR = 2.5) or from the crude EOR (EOR = 2.49)). If the presence of effect modification were recognized, the final analysis would report the EOR for Level One (EOR = 2.5) and, separately, the EOR (= 4.0) for Levels Two and Three. Whether it is *appropriate* to stratify the data into three strata, however, depends upon whether there was an a priori reason to do so (that is, a preexisting hypothesis pertaining to how the data should be stratified) and not a result of inspecting the data (hypothesis generation). The same reasoning pertains to hypotheses that are evaluated in an epidemiologic study. The hypothesis must be based on preexisting data and not formed as a result of inspecting the study data.

DATA EDITING

Before data analysis can begin, the data are **edited** for completeness and quality. Editing means looking for errors in the data. Computer programs are useful in editing data, especially for finding inconsistencies in the data. For example, multiple questions querying alcohol use should yield answers that are consistent with one another; a person who does not drink alcoholic beverages should not list a "preferred alcohol beverage." Missing data are sought, and data that seem implausible are verified.

Data quality control, though part of the data analysis process, also proceeds concurrently with data collection. Vigorous data quality-control procedures are followed during the development and pilot testing of the data collection process and instrument, at the start of data collection, and then periodically throughout the period of data collection. Errors in the accuracy or the completeness of data are more easily corrected if identified soon after they occur, rather than at the end of the study during data editing.

DATA REDUCTION

Once the data have been edited, they are **reduced** into one or more tables of numbers on which the actual data analyses are conducted. Data reduction means taking the often thousands of pieces of data collected as part of the study and organizing them into a series of data tables. Sometimes epidemiologic analyses are performed based on multivariate or other statistical models rather than on a series of data tables. The overall objectives and principles of data analysis remain the same regardless of the complexity of the approach used for data analysis.

DATA ANALYSIS

The objective of epidemiologic analysis is to estimate an **unbiased measure of effect(s),** taking random error into account. **Bias** refers to systematic error. Bias means that the point estimate of the effect measure is either too large or too small as a result of systematic error(s) in how subjects were selected for study, how and which data were collected, and/or how the data were analyzed

Random error is unsystematic error and thus differs from bias. Random error occurs because epidemiologists enroll only a small proportion of all eligible subjects in each study rather than all subjects. Estimates of effect measures for the same exposure-outcome association vary from study to study because the particular subjects enrolled in each study vary. Bias and random error are discussed in greater detail in Chapter 12.

EFFECT MEASURES

Effect measures (also referred to as **measures of effect**) quantify the size of association between an exposure and a health outcome. These measures can be either **ratio measures** (usually incidence rate ratios, cumulative incidence ratios, or exposure odds ratios) or **difference measures** (usually incidence rate differences or cumulative incidence differences).

Each effect measure is a ratio or a difference of two measures of disease frequency. For example, an **incidence rate ratio** is the ratio of two incidence rates:

$$\text{Incidence rate ratio} = \frac{(\text{\# new cases divided by the person-time in the exposed population})}{(\text{\# new cases divided by the person-time in the unexposed population})}$$

$$\text{In other words, an } \textit{incidence rate ratio (IRR)} = \frac{IR \text{ in the exposed population}}{IR \text{ in the unexposed population}}$$

An **incidence rate difference** is the difference between two incidence rates:

$$\textit{Incidence rate difference (IRD)} = (\text{\# new cases divided by the person-time in the exposed population}) \text{ minus } (\text{\# new cases divided by the person-time in the unexposed population})$$

$$\text{In other words, an } (IRD) = (IR \text{ in the exposed population} - IR \text{ in the unexposed population})$$

By convention, the measure of disease frequency in the exposed population is placed in the numerator of the ratio effect measure, and the measure of disease frequency in the unexposed population is placed in the denominator of the ratio. Similarly, for the difference effect measure, by convention, the measure of disease frequency in the unexposed population is subtracted from the measure of disease frequency in the exposed population. Ratio measures are calculated more often than are difference measures, especially when the etiology of a health outcome is of interest. In addition, only ratio measures and not difference measures can be estimated in case/control studies, as discussed below.

COHORT STUDIES

For the purposes of data analysis, there are two kinds of cohort studies: cohort studies with **count denominators** (denominators that consist of numbers of people) and cohort studies with **person-time denominators** (denominators that consist of person-time, usually person-years). The analysis for each type of cohort data is the same whether the cohort study is prospective or retrospective.

Cohort Studies with Count Denominators

Cohort studies that enroll and follow people without calculating person-time generate data from which the cumulative incidence (or attack rate) in the exposed and unexposed cohorts can be estimated. Cohort studies with count denominators yield two measures of effect: the **cumulative incidence ratio,** often referred to as the **risk ratio,** and the **cumulative incidence difference,** sometimes called **attributable risk.** The data layout for a cohort study with count denominators is shown in Table 11.1.

The cumulative incidence ratio (CIR) is estimated as $(a/N_1)/(b/N_0)$. This quantity is the cumulative incidence (CI) in the exposed population divided by the CI in the unexposed population.

The cumulative incidence difference (CID) is estimated as $(a/N_1) - (b/N_0)$. This quantity is the cumulative incidence (CI) in the exposed population minus the CI in the unexposed population.

The CIR and the CID are **point estimates** because each is the best *single* estimate for the size of the association between an exposure and a health outcome, on their respective scales of measurement (CIR on the ratio scale and CID on the difference scale). The range of possible values for the CIR is 0 to positive infinity (0 to $+\infty$). The range of possible values for the CID is -1 to $+1$.

TABLE 11.1
Data Layout for a Cohort Study with Count Denominators

Subjects	Exposed	Not Exposed	Total
New cases	a	b	$M_1 = a + b$
Noncases	c	d	$M_0 = c + d$
Total	$N_1 = a + c$	$N_0 = b + d$	$T = a + b + c + d$

NUMERICAL EXAMPLE OF HOW TO ESTIMATE THE CIR AND THE CID

TABLE 11.2
Numerical Example of the CIR and the CID

Subjects	Exposed	Not Exposed	Total
New cases	124	61	185
Noncases	218	146	364
Total	342	207	549

The CIR = (124/342)/(61/207) = 1.2.

The CID = (124/342) − (61/207) = 0.068 or 6.8%.

What is the interpretation for each of these point estimates? The CIR of 1.2 means that the CI in the exposed population is 1.2 *times* the CI in the unexposed population. In other words, the CI is 20% higher in the exposed population than in the unexposed population. (If the CI in the exposed population were equal to the CI in the unexposed populations or 0% higher, the CIR would equal 1.0.) The CID of 0.068 means that the CI in the exposed population is 0.068 *more* than the CI in the unexposed population. CIDs often are converted into percentages. (In this example, 0.068 is expressed as 6.8%.)

The values for the CIR and the CID if the CI in the exposed and unexposed populations are identical would be 1.0 for the CIR, as just mentioned, and 0 for the CID. These values are called **null values.** "Null" refers to a value for an effect measure when, in the hypothesis relating an exposure to a health outcome, there is no association between the exposure and the health outcome. Null values are used to establish the "null hypothesis," which is used as a benchmark to test other hypothesis (discussed in more detail in Chapter 12). Values for a CIR that are larger than 1.0 indicate a larger CI among the exposed population than among the unexposed population. A CIR larger than 1.0 *may* indicate that the exposure causes the health outcome. A CIR less than 1 *may* indicate that the exposure prevents the health outcome.

Similarly, a CID larger than 0 indicates that the CI in the exposed population is larger than the CI in the unexposed population; thus, the exposure under study *may* cause the health outcome. A CI less than 0 indicates that the CI in the exposed population is less than the CI in the unexposed population; thus, the exposure *may* prevent the health outcome. The word "may" is italicized to emphasize the fact that there could be many possible explanations for why a CIR is different from 1.0 or a CID is different from 0 other than a causal relation between the exposure and the outcome under study. Other possible explanations include random error and any of a number of kinds of biases, as discussed in greater detail in Chapter 12.

Cohort Studies with Person-Time Denominators

Table 11.3 shows the data layout for a cohort study with person-time denominators. Effect measures that can be estimated from a cohort study with person-time denominators are the **incidence rate ratio** (IRR) and the **incidence rate difference** (IRD). The range of possible values for the IRR is 0 to positive infinity (0 to $+\infty$). The range of possible values for the IRD is negative infinity to positive infinity ($-\infty$ to $+\infty$).

TABLE 11.3
Data Layout for a Cohort Study with Person-Time Denominators

	Exposed	*Not Exposed*	*Total*
New cases	a	b	$M_1 = a + b$
Person-time	N_1	N_0	$T = N_1 + N_0$

The IRR is estimated as $(a/N_1)/(b/N_0)$. The IRR equals the IR in the exposed population divided by the IR in the unexposed population.

The IRD is estimated as $(a/N_1) - (b/N_0)$. The IRD equals the IR in the exposed population minus the IR in the unexposed population.

NUMERICAL EXAMPLE OF HOW TO ESTIMATE THE IRR AND THE IRD

The data on which the IRR and the IRD are based are the numbers of exposed and unexposed cases, and the numbers of exposed and unexposed *person-years,* not the total numbers of exposed and unexposed *individuals.*

TABLE 11.4
Numerical Example of the IRR and the IRD

	Exposed	*Not Exposed*	*Total*
New cases	23	19	42
Person-years	550	1,080	1,630

The IRR = (23/550 P-Y)/(19/1,080 P-Y) = 2.2. The IR in the exposed population is 2.2 *times* the IR in the unexposed population, or, equivalently, 120% higher. The IRD = (23/550 P-Y) − (19/1,080 P-Y) = 2.3/100 P-Y. The IR in the exposed population is 2.3/100 P-Y *more* than the IR in the unexposed population. The unit of person-time in the denominator (in this example, person-years) is retained when an IRD is calculated; that is, the unit of person-time is not "lost" when one IR is subtracted from another IR.

IRRs less than 1.0 indicate that the exposure *may* prevent the health outcome. For example, an IRR equal to 0.8 indicates that the IR in the exposed population is 0.8 *times* the IR in the unexposed population, or, equivalently, 20% lower. IRDs less than 0 indicate that the IR in the exposed population is less than the IR in the unexposed population; thus, the exposure *may* prevent the health outcome.

Like the CIR and the CID, the null values for the IRR and the IRD are 1.0 and 0, respectively. These are the values for the IRR and the IRD under a null hypothesis of "no association between the exposure(s) and the health outcome(s) under study," that is, when the IR in the exposed population is equal to the IR in the unexposed population.

Note that the number of new cases of a health outcome and the number of person-years (or some other measure of person-time) cannot be added together to try to estimate a quantity that resembles a CI estimate. For example, using the data from the previous IR example, 23 cannot be added to 550 to yield an effect measure that is equal to 23/(23 + 550). New cases of disease cannot be added to a measure of person-time to yield an interpretable quantity.

RATIO MEASURES VERSUS DIFFERENCE MEASURES

The *direction* of ratio measures and the direction of difference measures are related to each other. In other words, if a ratio measure from a cohort study is greater than 1, then the difference measure calculated from the same set of data will be greater than 0 (both measures indicating a direction toward a causal association between the exposure and the health outcome under study). Likewise, if a ratio measure is less than 1, the corresponding difference measure will be less than 0 (both measures indicating a direction toward a preventive association between the exposure and the health outcome under study).

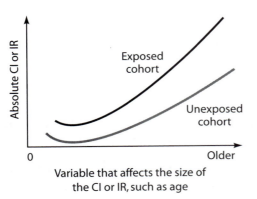

The *relative magnitudes* of ratio and difference measures depend on the absolute magnitude of the rate measure in the exposure cohort relative to the absolute magnitude of the rate measure in the unexposed cohort, as illustrated in Figure 11.2.

FIGURE 11.2
Absolute versus relative magnitudes of rates and differences.

In Figure 11.2, the magnitude of the ratio measure is *larger* when the absolute rate is close to 0 and *smaller* when the absolute rate is farther from 0. In contrast, the difference measure is *smaller* when the absolute rate is close to 0 and *larger* when the absolute rate is farther from 0.

CASE/CONTROL STUDIES

Unlike cohort studies, the case/control study has only one effect measure that can be estimated: the **exposure odds ratio (EOR),** often referred to simply as an **odds ratio (OR).** There is no difference measure such as an "exposure odds difference" or an "odds difference."

An **odds** is an expression of the form $(a/(a + b))$ compared with $(b/(a + b))$, which, mathematically, is equivalent to (a) compared with (b). An example of an "odds" occurring at a betting arena might be a gambler who believes that the odds that his or her horse will win the race are 3 to 2. (Out of 5 chances to win, the horse will win 3 times and lose 2 times.) In case/control studies, the odds of interest are the odds of having a positive exposure history. For example, in Table 11.5, the odds of a case's having a positive exposure history are 5 to 3 (500/800 compared with 300/800).

TABLE 11.5
Example of Data that Yield an Exposure Odds of 5 to 3 for a Case's Being Exposed

Subjects	Exposed	Not Exposed	Total
Cases	500	300	800

An EOR is equal to the odds of exposure among the cases divided by the odds of exposure among the controls. *The EOR is numerically equivalent to an incidence rate ratio (IRR) calculated in a cohort study with person-time denominators, as long as incident rather than prevalent cases are enrolled in the study.* If the control group comprises people who are ill (with an illness other than that of the cases), then those illnesses must be incident as well. Because an EOR = IRR, data from a case/control study can be used to estimate the *relative magnitude* of the incidence rates in the exposed and unexposed populations even though the *absolute* incidence rates in those populations are not known.

Whereas the effect measures calculated in cohort studies make sense intuitively, because each is a ratio or a difference of two measures of disease frequency, the EOR is less intuitively obvious. Nevertheless, because case/control studies are commonly conducted, it is essential to understand what EORs are and how they are interpreted.

In a case/control study, because subjects are enrolled in the study on the basis of their disease or injury statuses (that is, on the basis of their being a case or a control), usually no measure of disease frequency (incidence rate, prevalence, or cumulative incidence) can be estimated. Instead, case/control studies provide data on the percentages of cases and controls that have a positive exposure history on certain factors. Although information about the exposure percentages of cases and controls is somewhat interesting, information concerning measures of disease frequency is substantially more useful. Table 11.6 shows the data layout for a case/control study. This data layout is referred to as a **fourfold table** or a **2 × 2 table** because of the four cells (*a, b, c,* and *d*) in the table.

The data layout for a case/control study, at first glance, looks like the data layout for a cohort study with count denominators. The apparent similarity does not extend to the measures of effect that can be estimated in these two different types of studies. In a cohort study with count denominators, subjects are enrolled in the study on the basis of their exposure statuses, and then their disease/injury frequencies are measured and compared. In other words, in a cohort study, N_1, the number of exposed subjects, and N_0, the number of unexposed subjects, are enrolled in the study. For that reason, the quantities (a/N_1) and (b/N_0) are meaningful.

In contrast, in a case/control study, because subjects are enrolled in the study on the basis of their health statuses (that is, M_1 and M_0 subjects are enrolled in the study), (a/N_1) and (b/N_0)) have no meaning. Thus, neither the CIR nor the CID can be estimated from case/control data.

The EOR is calculated as $(a/b)/(c/d)$, which algebraically is equivalent to (ad/bc). To reiterate, an EOR equals the odds of a case's having a positive exposure history divided by the odds of a control's having a positive history. With a little algebra (not

TABLE 11.6
Data Layout for a Case/Control Study

Subjects	Exposed	Not Exposed	Total
Cases	*a*	*b*	$M_1 = a + b$
Controls	*c*	*d*	$M_0 = c + d$
Total	$N_1 = a + c$	$N_0 = b + d$	$T = a + b + c + d$

shown), it can be demonstrated, as stated previously, that the EOR is equal numerically to the IRR, as long as the case/control study enrolled incident cases and, if the controls comprise individuals who are ill, incident control illnesses. The interpretation of an EOR is the same as the interpretation of an IRR.

As an example, an EOR equal to 1.8 means that the IR of disease in the exposed population is 1.8 *times* the IR in the unexposed population, or, equivalently, 80% higher. An EOR equal to 0.7 means that the IR in the exposed population is 0.7 *times* the IRR in the unexposed population, or, equivalently, the IR in the exposed population is 30% lower. The EOR estimates the IRR even though neither the IR in the exposed population nor the IR in the unexposed population can be calculated from data collected in a case/control study. Like the IRR, the range of possible values for an EOR extends from 0 to +infinity (0 to $+\infty$), and the null value is 1.0.

NUMERICAL EXAMPLE OF HOW TO ESTIMATE AN EOR

TABLE 11.7
Numerical Example of the EOR

Subjects	Exposed	Not Exposed	Total
Cases	82	30	112
Controls	21	12	33
Total	103	42	145

The EOR is equal to $(82 \times 12)/(30 \times 21) = 1.6$. An EOR equal to 1.6 means that the IR of the health outcome of interest in the exposed population is 1.6 times the IR of the health outcome in the unexposed population, or, equivalently, 60% higher.

SUMMARY

The simple analysis of epidemiologic data is a straightforward process of estimating the effect measures that are appropriate given the type of study that generated the data. In a full analysis of epidemiologic data, often the data are arranged into a series of strata (a series of tables) and the data analyzed based on that arrangement. The effect measures that can be estimated from a set of data remain the same whether the data analysis is simple or based on a more complex arrangement of the data. In addition, the interpretation of the effect measures is the same; that is, an EOR estimated from simple analysis has the same interpretation as does an EOR estimated from a more complex arrangement of the data. Similarly, an incidence rate difference estimated from a series of strata has the same interpretation as does an incidence rate difference estimated from a simple analysis.

A goal in analyzing data is to obtain one or more effect measures that are unconfounded. Given that an effect measure is unconfounded, the simpler the analysis the better, because simple analyses are more easily understood than are more complex analyses. In addition, there typically is less random error associated with effect measures estimated from a simple data analysis than with effect measures estimated from more complex analysis.

How and whether effect measures are put into practice usually depends on the extent to which the effect measures lend themselves to public health programming and to effective strategies for disease and injury prevention. (See Boxes 11.2 and 11.3, and the special case study on the effects of the 1996 National Welfare Reform Act, PRWORA.) The usefulness of effect measures in improving the public's health also depends on the distribution of exposure statuses in the population targeted for disease or injury prevention. As an example, a large incidence rate ratio associated with an exposure-outcome association does not necessarily translate into the opportunity to substantially reduce disease or injury in a targeted population: It may be that few people in the targeted population have the exposure; thus, a prevention program can at most improve the health of only a few people. In contrast, a small incidence rate ratio, if causal, may translate into many improved lives if the exposure in the targeted population is common. An example of this situation is alcohol consumption (a common habit) and certain injuries such as traffic-related injuries, drownings, and burns in the United States.

Similarly, a small exposure-outcome association may translate into a larger public health benefit than does a large association. For example, the incidence rate ratio associated with (an average amount of) tobacco smoking and lung cancer is approximately 10.0, a large ratio, whereas the incidence rate ratio associated with smoking and coronary heart disease is approximately 1.4, a small ratio. Reduction of smoking in the United States would have a larger impact on the numbers of cases of coronary heart disease than on cases of lung cancer, however, because the incidence rate of coronary heart disease is so much higher than is the rate of lung cancer.

BOX 11.2

PROGRAM EVALUATION

Although the majority of epidemiologic research is directed toward identifying the causes, preventives, and effective treatments of human disease, epidemiologic methods also are used to evaluate public health programs, such as screening programs (discussed in Chapter 5). In the evaluation of public health programs, the primary question of interest is whether the program prevented more cases of disease or injury than ongoing programs and, if so, at what monetary and human costs. Related questions concern in what groups of people, defined by age, gender, ethnic heritage and/or other variables, the program was most effective.

Typically, program evaluation involves **process evaluation** as well as **outcome evaluation. Process evaluation** summarizes the practical aspects of the program, such as how many people were exposed to the program, how many educational materials were distributed (in an educational program), and how readily program participants joined the program and maintained their participation in the program. Taken together, process measures document what the program comprised so that, if successful, the

Box 11.2 continued

program may be replicated in other populations. It is a serious error, however, to confuse process evaluation with outcome evaluation. For example, just because program participants enjoyed the program does not mean that their enjoyment translated into public health benefits from participation. **Outcome evaluation** measures the magnitude of any changes in the incidence, morbidity, or mortality rates of disease or injury attributable to the program, and thus is the primary means for evaluating the effectiveness of the program together with the cost of developing and delivering the program.

Special considerations often need to be taken into account when designing and implementing a preventive program for vectorborne diseases such as West Nile fever, St. Louis encephalitis, or malaria, each transmitted by mosquitoes. One primary challenge concerns the counterintuitiveness of the control strategies. For pest control, such as the control of mosquitoes, programs are designed to reduce the number of mosquitoes by, for example, the elimination of breeding sites. For mosquitoborne disease control, however, reduction in the number of mosquito vectors typically results in an *increase* in disease transmission. This idea is explored further in Box 11.3.

BOX 11.3

RONALD ROSS'S MODEL OF MALARIA TRANSMISSION

PHILIPPE A. ROSSIGNOL, PH.D.

PROFESSOR, DEPARTMENT OF FISHERIES AND WILDLIFE, OREGON STATE UNIVERSITY

Ronald Ross (1857–1932) was one of the giants of infectious disease epidemiology. His best-known accomplishment was elucidating the life cycle of malaria, proving that mosquitoes were obligatory vectors of the parasite. That study, the subject of his doctoral degree, earned him the second Nobel Prize in Medicine awarded (in 1902), a knighthood, and lifelong recognition.

His most lasting contribution, however, still lay ahead of him. In 1915, he published the first of two mathematical models that were to revolutionize infectious disease epidemiology and malariology. Those models, which he called a "theory of happenings," appear to have preceded slightly Volterra's model of the predator-prey relationship. Lotka, in 1924, wrote an extensive mathematical study of Ross's model, ensuring its wide acceptance. The malaria model was "popularized" (for a technical audience) in the 1950s by George Macdonald. The model then was used as a theoretical justification for the World Health Organization's (WHO's) malaria eradication campaign, as well as for practical tools in evaluating the impact of insecticides in the field. Few other models have had such a long and powerful impact, and still are the subject of ongoing study.

Box 11.3 continued

The Model: An Algebraic Derivation

Ross devised the model to answer a specific question. Having gained the knowledge that mosquitoes are vectors of malaria, he wished to know whether mosquito eradication was a prerequisite for malaria eradication. That question was most worrisome because it was known even at that time that mosquito eradication was unrealistic on a broad scale.

Ross's model calculates the basic reproduction rate (R_0) of malaria. The basic reproduction rate is defined as the average number of infective secondary cases of malaria generated by a primary case over the average duration of the disease. The derivation can be achieved a number of ways. Here, I share the algebraic derivation devised by Macdonald.

Assuming that hosts and vectors for malaria are uniformly distributed and that no case currently exists, the number of cases that a primary case would generate can be calculated. First, assume a relative number of vectors, m, the number of vectors divided by the number of hosts. Given that female mosquitoes (males do not blood-feed) bite only once per period of egg development (the oogonic cycle) and that only a certain proportion of female mosquitoes will bite a human host when they do bite, only a proportion, a, the biting habit, will bite a person on a given day. In other words, a is the proportion of female mosquitoes that bite humans divided by the length of the oogonic cycle. The product, ma, is the number of mosquitoes biting one person per day, and is called the "human-biting rate." Once a female mosquito acquires the malaria parasite, the parasite must undergo a long extrinsic period of incubation, of duration n days, before the mosquito vector can infect a human host. The duration of the extrinsic incubation period is substantial and often is longer than the average life expectancy of the mosquito vector. On any day, therefore, only a proportion, p, of vectors survive, and thus only a proportion, p^n, of mosquitoes will survive the extrinsic incubation period of the malaria parasite. These infective vectors still bite at a daily rate, a, for $-\log_e(p)^{-1}$ days. The efficiency of transmission, b, is the number of human cases generated per day of host infection. Then b is multiplied by the average duration of infection, r^{-1}, where r is the recovery rate. (If a disease is in a steady state, the average duration of disease equals (1/recovery rate)).

The product of those parameters is the **basic reproduction rate** of malaria, namely,

$$R_0 = \frac{ma^2p^nb}{r(-\log_e(p))}$$

The basic reproduction rate must equal 1 for malaria to maintain itself, must be larger than 1 to expand, and must be less than 1 for extinction to occur. Given that none of the parameters' basic reproduction rate is equal to 0, it can be seen that the number of vectors, m, need not be 0 for a malaria eradication to be successful.

Three interesting and counterintuitive properties emerge from the model. First, there is a nonzero threshold for all parameters. In other words, absolute efficiency is

Box 11.3 continued

not required from a practical perspective: All parameters (the relative number of mosquito vectors, life expectancy, and biting habit) are reasonable targets for control. Second, the parameters are related hierarchically to the basic reproduction rate: m is related linearly to R_0, a is related to R_0 as a squared variable, and p is related exponentially to R_0. Third, it is possible to use basic reproduction rate as a practical tool for evaluating malaria control programs. Garrett-Jones proposed an abbreviated form of Ross's model that he termed **vectorial capacity,** namely,

$$VC = \frac{ma^2 p^n}{-\log_e(p)}$$

This model is a linearly proportional estimate of the basic reproduction rate. Vectorial capacity can be used to estimate the risk of malaria transmission in the absence of the parasite because it relies solely on entomological parameters. In short, Ross's model was nothing short of extraordinary. It provided a theoretical basis for understanding malaria transmission, pointed to specific methods of measurements and estimation of field parameters. For those reasons, Ross's model has remained a source of theoretical study and the basis for practical applications in malaria control to this day.

REFERENCES

Garrett-Jones, C. 1964. Prognosis for interruption of malaria transmission through assessment of the mosquito's vectorial capacity. *Nature* 204:1173–75.

Lotka. Alfred J. 1923. Contributions to the analysis of malaria epidemiology. *American Journal of Hygiene* 3. (Suppl. no. 1): S1–S121.

Macdonald, George. 1957. *The epidemiology and control of malaria.* London: Oxford University Press.

Ross, Ronald. 1915. Some *a priori* pathometric equations. *British Medical Journal* 1:546–47.

REVIEW QUESTIONS

1. List and define the four activities involved in data processing.
2. Define "simple analysis."
3. List and define the two procedures involved in data analysis. Then, differentiate "point estimation" from "interval estimation."
4. What is the primary objective of epidemiologic data analysis?
5. List and define each measure of effect for both types of cohort studies and for case/control studies. What is the interpretation for each measure of effect? What is the range of possible values for each effect measure?
6. Define "null value." How are null values used? What is the null value for each effect measure?
7. Define "odds" as in "exposure odds ratio" or "odds ratio."
8. Although data from a cohort study with count denominators and data from a case/control study seem similar at first glance, the data analyses for these two types of studies are not similar. Explain in your own words why these data analyses differ.

REVIEW EXERCISES

1. The following data come from a study of the effects of passive smoking on young infants' respiratory health in Shanghai, PRC (Jin and Rossignol 1993). Using these data, calculate the 18-month CIRs and 18-month CIDs of respiratory disease for boys, for girls, and overall. Use the "none" category of "cigarettes consumed per day" as the referent category.

Data Table

# Cigarettes Smoked per Day in Household	# New Cases of Respiratory Disease	# Children in Cohort	Cumulative Incidence (CI)	Cumulative Incidence Ratio (CIR)	Cumulative Incidence Difference (CID)
Boys					
None	19	151			
1–9	24	140			
10–19	25	118			
20–39	27	116			
Total	95	525			
Girls					
None	14	143			
1–9	17	134			
10–19	18	109			
20–39	20	96			
Total	69	482			
Boys/Girls					
None	33	294			
1–9	41	274			
10–19	43	227			
20–39	47	212			
Total	164	1,007			

2. The following data come from a study of burn injuries before and after a burn-prevention educational intervention program (MacKay and Rothman 1982). The intervention program had three components: a school-initiated intervention, a community-initiated program, and a media campaign. In addition, burn incidence rates were monitored in an area in which no intervention was implemented (the control site). The investigators collected data on burn incidence rates for four years before the implementation of the intervention program, for the eight months during which the program was implemented, and for one year after the end of the intervention program.

   The effectiveness of each intervention was evaluated by comparing burn incidence rates before and after the interventions within each community in which the intervention was implemented. For example, the school-initiated intervention, which was implemented in Lynn, Massachusetts, compared burn IRs in Lynn before, during, and after implementation of the intervention program. Because of the seasonal variation in burn IRs, burn IRs during the eight-month period during which the programs were implemented were compared with the four eight-month-periods before the program; the twelve-month period after implementation of the program was compared with the entire four-year preprogram (baseline) period.

Given that synopsis of the burn-prevention program, complete the following table comparing burn IRs during and after the intervention programs with their respective preintervention burn IRs.

Data Table

Type of Intervention	Four 8-Month Baseline IR*	8-Month Program Implementation IR*	IRR and IRD*	4-Year Baseline IR*	1-Year Postprogram Period IR*	IRR and IRD*
School-initiated (Lynn, MA)	35.2	35.8		38.7	41.1	
Community-initiated (Quincy, MA)	16.6	13.7		18.0	16.9	
Media campaign (Salem and Saugus, MA)	22.0	25.5		26.3	27.0	
No intervention (Holyoke and South Hadley, MA)	21.2	20.3		22.2	21.7	

*Number of burns per 10,000 person-years.

   a. Which, if any, of the intervention programs were effective in reducing burn IRs?
   b. What effect, if any, did the differing baseline burn IRs have on the study results?
3. Estimate the appropriate effect measures (ratio and/or difference measures) for each of the following sets of hypothetical data.
   a.

	Smokers	Nonsmokers
Lung cancer cases	217	57
# person-years	13,278	11,702

   b. These hypothetical data come from a cohort study.

	Alcohol Use	No Alcohol Use
Cases of liver disease	221	573
No liver disease	944	4,991
Total	1,165	5,564

c. These hypothetical data come from a case/control study.

	Exercise	*No Exercise*
Cases	218	654
Controls	759	1,233

d.

	Pesticide Exposure	*No Pesticide Exposure*
Cases of tremor	82	13
# person-years	1,063	874

4. Analyze the following hypothetical data first as a cohort study (with count denominators) and then as a case/control study.

Subjects	*CS_2 Exposure*	*No CS_2 Exposure*
New cases of heart disease	165	433
No heart disease	746	3,878
Total	911	4,311

See selected answers for exercises 1–4 on page A–6.

■ **SPECIAL CASE STUDY:**

Truly a Success? The Effects of the 1996 National Welfare Reform Act on Children's Health in the United States

Benjamin Harrison, M.S.

In 1996, the United States Congress passed into law the Personal Responsibility and Work Opportunity Reconciliation Act (PRWORA). The stated goal of the legislation was to help families leave the welfare program and enter the workforce, thus moving out of poverty and reducing the strain of the welfare programs on the national and state budgets. The welfare reform legislation reduced spending into the welfare programs and gave great freedom to states in setting up new regulations on how the welfare program would be administered.

Three years after the inception of the legislation, lawmakers nationwide were calling the program a startling success. Large declines in welfare caseloads and an increase in employment among former recipients were cited (Lawson et al. 1999). Welfare recipient rolls were cut by 57 percent, their lowest levels in thirty-two years (Mann et al. 2002). As often is the case, however, little attention was given to the health aspects of these programs. The legislation itself fundamentally reduced the level of access to Medicaid, thus reducing the availability of health care to poorer families and, in particular, to single-mother families.

Because of these observations, several key questions need to be answered before Congress revisits renewing the welfare law in the upcoming years. Is simply looking at the number of people receiving welfare a good way to quantify the success of a program such as welfare? Has access for families that truly need assisted health care been changed? What is the effect of poverty on health, in particular with respect to children? Are mothers' welfare and health related to their children's health?

Truly a Reduction in Poverty?

If we look at sheer numbers, PRWORA does indeed appear to be a great success. Many factors, however, were not considered when the evaluative numbers were being collected. What do the claims of these great caseload decreases truly mean? Are people really much better off? Many reports contend that substantial numbers of families who no longer are enrolled in the welfare program probably should be, but because of the newly imposed regulations and the reduction in funds available, they no longer have access to the assistance they need. The lack of access is particularly true for women, where it is estimated that between 50 and 74 percent of PRWORA leavers are living in poverty (Mann et al. 2002). In addition, because of work requirements, many jobs former recipients take pay minimum wage or less, and are temporary positions; only about 35 to 40 percent of former recipients work consistently over a year (Mann et al. 2002). Because those jobs cannot sustain families with children, most former recipients return to the program within one year. There also is debate concerning what constitutes poverty in the United States. The income ceiling for poverty for a family of three is $13,738 per year. According to that rate, 36.4 million people in the United States are poor. Of that number, 5.8 million are children under the age of 6 years, which accounts for 24 percent of all children in this age group (Aber et al. 1997). To be eligible for Medicaid, a family cannot earn more than 133 percent of the poverty line ($18,271), and many states have imposed even lower requirements (Aber et al. 1997). With the rising cost of living and health care, adequate health care for a family of this size often is not possible.

Health-Related Aspects of Welfare Reform and the Effects on Accessibility

When designing the new welfare reform legislation, Congress did not intend for the reform to affect health-care coverage (Mann et al. 2002). Many significant changes, however, occurred relating to the availability of health care. PRWORA set work participation requirements, time limits, and eligibility restrictions on assistance (Lawton et al. 1999). States were given great leeway in placing recipients into jobs, and most states set minimum hours of work per week for recipients (Lawton et al. 1999). There also was a five-year cap placed on benefits, and, again, states were given the leeway to shorten that period (Lawton et al. 1999). States also were given financial incentives to move people into jobs quickly.

The most dramatic effects might have been seen, however, on the restrictions placed directly on children. Children born to mothers who were receiving assistance no longer were assured assistance. Many states set up programs in which receiving benefits was contingent upon paternity identification and cooperation in child support programs (Lawton et al. 1999). In addition, there was a five-year restriction on receiving assistance placed on immigrants, adults and children alike, even if they were in the country legally or were naturalized citizens (Lawton et al. 1999). Thus, children moving to this nation from abroad no longer are eligible for national assistance, and rarely qualify for state assistance.

Effects on Women

There have been substantial negative effects upon women's health as a result of PRWORA. This fact is particularly important because nine out of ten adults receiving welfare are mothers caring for their children, and their ability to care for their children is influenced heavily by their own health and access to health care (Breslau et al. 1994). As of 2000, the number of uninsured mothers had risen from 21 percent in 1994 to 37 percent, and that percentage appears to be rising still (Mann et al. 2002). Looking more closely at the effects of PRWORA shows that although more poor mothers are now employed than in 1995, the vast majority of these jobs have no employer-based health-care coverage. Compounded with the reduced eligibility standards for Medicaid, it has become extremely difficult for mothers to find insurance for their children, much less for themselves. Only 39 percent of poor mothers with children are enrolled in Medicaid, and 40 percent of poor women reported having no insurance for their children (Mann et al. 2002). To further compound those difficulties, poorer women are more likely to experience health problems, reporting poor health three times as frequently as women living above the poverty line (Mann et al. 2002). Many of those health problems are related to a lack in access to health services; this point is illustrated by the fact that poorer and uninsured women are far less likely to receive preventive care such as Papanicolaou tests and breast exams (Mann et al. 2002). The combination of those factors appears to have a direct and significant adverse effect on children's welfare, since in most cases the mother is the main or sole provider.

Direct Impact on Children's Health

It is clear that poverty has numerous significant, deleterious effects on childhood health and welfare. Poverty has been associated with increased neonatal and post-neonatal mortality rates, greater risks of injuries resulting from "accidents" or physical abuse/neglect, higher risk of asthma, and lower developmental scores in a range of tests (Aber et al. 1997). In the United States, as stated previously, 24 percent of all children under the age of 6 years are living in poverty, and thus are susceptible to those effects. Lower birth weights, which are associated with many lasting neurological effects as well as with increased infant mortality, are more frequent among poor children (Mann et al. 2002). Poorer children also exhibit higher general morbidity, which researchers attribute to two main factors: lower odds of early intervention and increased risk of injuries and illness (Aber et al. 1997).

From August 1998 through December 2000, a multisite study was conducted in six urban medical centers in six U.S. cities to evaluate the health of poorer children since the passage of PRWORA. The goal of the study was to examine associations of loss or reduction in welfare benefits with food security and health outcomes among children aged 36 months or younger at urban hospitals and clinics (Cook et al. 2002). At hospital clinics and emergency departments, investigators interviewed 2,718 children aged 36 months or younger whose households received welfare or had lost welfare through sanctions (Cook et al. 2002). The study found that children in families who had lost benefits because of changes in the welfare policy experienced higher rates of food insecurity and that those insecurities were not offset by food stamp programs. In addition, these children also experienced more frequent hospitalizations, which often is an indication of inadequate primary care. Thus, the loss of previous benefits had placed many children at risk by removing accessibility to adequate medical and preventive care.

Conclusions

Welfare reform has had a considerable impact on many families. Since welfare reform in 1996, the number of recipients nationally has decreased significantly. Although some families probably are doing well, the fact that 24 percent of children under the age of 6 years still are living in poverty indicates the persistence of poverty as a major public health problem in the United States. In the upcoming year (2003), there will be many significant decisions made about the health and welfare of poor populations in our country. Congress again will revisit the application of PRWORA, and many states that are operating in deficit will look for ways to reduce spending. Hopefully, legislators (and others) will look back at the welfare reform act of 1996 and examine closely what really happened to poor families as a result of this reform. With the gift of hindsight and an ethical and respectful view of people, these legislators, before claiming success in 1996, should look at the 24 percent of young children still living in poverty in this country and realize that this percentage is far too high.

REFERENCES

Aber, J. L., N. G. Bennet, D. C. Conley, and J. Li. 1997. The effects of poverty on child health and development. *Annual Review of Public Health* 18:463–83.

Breslau, N., J. E. DelDotto, G. G. Brown, S. Kumar, S. Ezhuthachan, K. G. Hufnagle, and E. L. Peterson. 1994. A gradient relationship between low birth weight and IQ at age 6 years. *Archive of Pediatric and Adolescent Medicine* 148 (4): 377–83.

Cook, J. T., D. A. Frank, C. Berkowitz, M. M. Black, P. H. Casey, D. B. Cutts, A. F. Meyers, N. Zaldivar, A. Skalicky, S. Levenson, and T. Heeren. 2002. Welfare reform and the health of young children: A sentinel survey in 6 U.S. cities. *Archive of Pediatric and Adolescent Medicine* 156 (7): 678–84.

Lawton, E., K. Leiter, J. Todd, and L. Smith. 1999. Welfare reform: Advocacy and intervention in the health care setting. *Public Health* 114 (6): 540–49.

Mann, C., J. Hudman, A. Saganicoff, and A. Folsom. 2002. Five years later: Poor women's health care coverage after welfare reform. *Journal of American Medical Women's Association* 57 (1): 16–22.

## CHAPTER 12

Accuracy

Epidemiologic studies can be thought of as measuring tools in which the measurements of interest are the sizes of associations between exposures and health outcomes, that is, of effect measures (discussed in Chapter 11). Those measurements can be in error for a variety of reasons, many of which arise from the observational nature of most epidemiologic studies. For example, observational studies are prone to *bias,* because they lack the random allocation of exposure/treatment that forms the essence of the design of intervention studies.

Other sources of error arise from statistical considerations, such as random error (often referred to as "chance") or violations of the statistical model or statistical assumptions underlying the data analysis. Still other reasons pertain to limitations in available methodology for estimating exposures, including confounding factors, and for identifying pathophysiologically meaningful preclinical disease states.

The term **accuracy** is used to refer to any of the ways in which an epidemiologic study can be in error. Accuracy has two components, **precision** and **validity.** Those

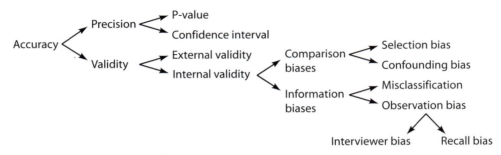

FIGURE 12.1
Primary components of accuracy.

components and their primary subcategories are summarized in Figure 12.1 and will be discussed individually. There are other types of bias, not listed, that can occur depending on the particular type of epidemiologic study being conducted and/or on the hypothesis being evaluated. For example, several of the biases related to screening programs, such as lead-time bias, were discussed in Chapter 5.

PRECISION

Precision refers to the amount of **random error** (nonsystematic error or "chance") in a study and largely is a function of the number of subjects included in a study and the amount of statistical information that can be obtained from each subject. The amount of information that can be obtained from each subject is called **efficiency.**

Precision is summarized by a **p-value** (the "p" stands for probability) or by a **confidence interval.** A full discussion of how to estimate p-values and confidence intervals is beyond the scope of this text. Nevertheless, it is important to appreciate what those terms mean and how each is used in epidemiologic research to critically read and interpret the epidemiologic literature. There are three basic ideas to understand about precision.

P-Value

First, a p-value is the probability that an effect measure observed in an epidemiologic study, or an effect measure more extreme in size than that observed, could have occurred by random error, given that there is *no association* between the exposure and the health outcome. P-values convey information about how probable it is that the study results could have occurred simply by random variation in the exposure levels and health outcomes for the subset of all eligible subjects included in a study. P-values, like all probabilities, range in magnitude from 0 to 1 (or, equivalently, 0% to 100%). P-values are obtained by performing tests of statistical significance (such as a chi-square test or t-test) assessing how consistent the study data are with the **null hypothesis** that there is no association between the exposure and the health outcome under study. The null hypothesis is the hypothesis of "no effect" and is the hypothesis that is tested by calculating a p-value. The hypothesis of "some effect" or, equivalently, of some association between the exposure and the health outcome under study is called the **alternative hypothesis.** By convention, p-values less than 0.05 usually are considered **statistically significant;** that is, p-values less than 0.05 are interpreted as meaning that the observed association between the exposure and the health outcome probably did not occur simply because of random error. The **cutoff point** of p less than or equal to 0.05 is called alpha, α. For the **simple analysis** of case/control data, one approach for testing whether the size of association between an exposure and a health outcome is statistically significant involves the calculation of a χ-statistic, as shown in Table 12.1. Simple analysis means that all the data being analyzed are placed into one table, or **stratum,** of numbers. If the data are arranged in a series of tables (more than one stratum), the data analysis is called **stratified analysis.**

TABLE 12.1
Data Layout (= Fourfold Table or 2 × 2 Table) for the Simple Analysis of Case/Control Data: Calculation of χ_{1DF}

	History of Exposure	*No History of Exposure*	*Total*
Cases	a	b	$M_1 (= a + b)$
Controls	c	d	$M_0 (= c + d)$
Total	$N_1 (= a + c)$	$N_0 (= b + d)$	$T (= a + b + c + d)$

Null hypothesis: EOR = 1.0; that is, there is no association between the exposure and the health outcome under study. (There is no difference measure for case/control data.)

Alternative hypothesis: EOR $\neq$ 1.0

Hypothesis test: $\chi_{1DF} = (a - (M_1 N_1 / T)) / (((M_1 M_0 N_1 N_0)/(T^2 (T-1)))^{1/2}$

χ with one **degree of freedom** (χ_{1DF}) is equal to the statistic Z (the standard normal deviate). For that reason, a p-value associated with χ_{1DF} can be determined from the probability table for Z-scores. In the present context, degrees of freedom indicate how many variables in the table may vary before the values for the rest of the variables are determined, assuming that the numbers in the margins are fixed. If the values for N_1, N_0, M_1, and M_0 are given, then knowing the value for the a cell *or* the b cell *or* the c cell *or* the d cell will allow determination of the other cell values. The χ statistic associated with this table has one degree of freedom because knowing only one cell value determines the value for each of the other three cell values.

In calculating the χ_{1DF} statistic, it is necessary to assume an underlying probability model for the arrangement of the data in the fourfold table. Fourfold tables, as indicated previously, also are referred to as **2 × 2 tables** (two possible values for the columns, case and control, and two possible values for the rows, exposed and not exposed). The underlying probability model describes the behavior of the *a, b, c* or *d* cell under the null hypothesis of no effect. The underlying probability model for a fourfold table is the **hypergeometric distribution.** This distribution also underlies the arrangement of data for the simple analysis of cohort data having count (rather than person-time) denominators, because the data arrangement for the simple analysis of cohort studies with count denominators is identical to the data arrangement for the simple analysis of case/control data. The effect measure(s) that can be estimated from each type of study differ, as discussed in Chapter 11. The underlying probability distribution for a cohort study with person-time denominators is the **binomial distribution,** as shown in Table 12.2. More in-depth discussions of probability models may be found in most textbooks on biostatistics or in more advanced textbooks on epidemiologic methodology.

TABLE 12.2
Data Layout for the Simple Analysis of Cohort Data with Person-time Denominators

	Exposed	*Unexposed*	*Total*
Incident cases	a	b	M_1
Person-time	N_1	N_0	$T = N_1 + N_0$

Null hypotheses: IRR = 1.0 and IRD = 0; that is, there is no association between the exposure and the health outcome under study.

Alternative hypotheses: IRR $\neq$ 1.0 and IRD $\neq$ 0.

Hypothesis test: $\chi_{1DF} = (a - (M_1N_1/T)) / ((M_1N_1N_0)/T^2))^{1/2}$

As with all χs with one degree of freedom (Z-score), a χ_{1DF} expresses the *difference* between what was *observed* (a number of exposed cases) and what was *expected* to be observed *under the null hypothesis of no effect* (M_1N_1/T) in **standard deviation** or in **standard error units** $((M_1N_1N_0)/T^2))^{1/2}$. A standard deviation or a standard error is the square root of the variance of a variable and is estimated by the underlying probability model.

The above notwithstanding, the essential point to understand about p-values, after learning how to calculate them, is how they should be interpreted. P-values measure the degree of consistency between the data in a study and the null hypothesis that there is no association between an exposure and a health outcome. If the p-value is small, typically less than 0.05, then the interpretation centers on the belief that the data are not very consistent with the null hypothesis of no effect. In other words, there is an association between the exposure and the outcome in the study data that is not easily explained by random error. If the p-value is 0.05 or larger, then the interpretation centers on the belief that the data are consistent with the null hypothesis of no effect. In other words, there probably is no association between the exposure and the outcome that cannot be explained by random error.

Tests of statistical significance in general offer dichotomous interpretations of data: The data either *are* or *are not* consistent with the null hypothesis. That dichotomy may be too rigid. For example, the difference between a p-value equal to 0.051 (the data are consistent with the null hypothesis) from one study and a p-value equal to 0.049 (the data are not consistent with the hull hypothesis) from a second study may be due to the inclusion of a few more subjects in the second study. Thus, the magnitude of the p-value may have little "real-world" significance. In addition, p-values do not provide information about the magnitude of an effect measure, only about the amount of random error associated with the effect measure.

Confidence Intervals

The second fundamental idea about precision is that *confidence intervals* summarize the amount of random error in a study's findings by providing a *range of values* for the effect measure of interest, taking random error into account. The amount of **confidence** for an interval must be specified. Possible values for confidence extend from 0 to 100 percent. *A 0 percent confidence interval is the point estimate of an effect measure.* A 100 percent confidence interval contains all possible values for an effect measure. Table 12.3 defines confidence $(1-\alpha)$, **Type I error** (alpha, α), **statistical power** (beta, β), and **Type II error** $(1-\beta)$.

TABLE 12.3
Definitions of Confidence, Power, Type I Error, and Type II Error

| | | "REALITY" = TRUE IN FACT | |
		Null Hypothesis Is True	*Null Hypothesis Is False*
RESULTS OF THE HYPOTHESIS TEST	Data are consistent with the null hypothesis	Confidence or $(1 - \alpha)$	Type II error or β
	Data are *not* consistent with the null hypothesis	Type I error or α	Power or $(1 - \beta)$

Confidence intervals are bounded by the upper and lower **confidence limits.** As an example of a confidence interval and confidence limits, the point estimate for the EOR in a case/control study might equal 1.6, and the 95 percent confidence interval around the point estimate might extend from 1.4 to 1.9. In this example, 1.4 is the lower confidence limit, and 1.9 is the upper confidence limit. One approach for estimating confidence intervals around EORs in a case/control study uses the following formulae.

$$\text{Upper confidence limit} = \text{EOR}^{1+(Z_\alpha/Z_p)}$$
$$\text{Lower confidence limit} = \text{EOR}^{1-(Z_\alpha/Z_p)}$$

In these formulae, EOR is the point estimate for the EOR, Z_α is the Z-score corresponding to the desired level of confidence $(1 - \alpha)$, and Z_p is the Z-score (χ_{1DF}) calculated from the hypothesis test.

The interpretation of the confidence interval centers on the idea of what values for the EOR are consistent with the study data, taking random error into account. In the example just provided, an EOR as small as 1.4 or as large as 1.9 is consistent with the data at the 95 percent level of confidence. In other words, the effect of the exposure on the health outcome of interest may be as small as 1.4 or as large as 1.9, even though the "best guess" for the size of the effect is 1.6, the point estimate. The width of the interval for any effect size generally is larger when the data contain more random error and narrower when the data contain less random error.

Confidence intervals, like other **random variables,** follow **probability distributions** that depict the probability that the confidence interval will have certain limits for a given set of data and a given level of confidence. A random variable is a factor whose values follow a probability distribution. The idea that confidence intervals follow probability distributions emphasizes an essential component in the interpretation of a confidence interval. The interpretation of a 95 percent confidence interval, for example, means that 95 percent of all 95 percent confidence intervals for a given set of data will contain the "true" effect measure. *The theoretical underpinnings of a confidence interval include the idea of replicating an identical study infinitely many times to determine a confidence interval's probability distribution.* A 95 percent confidence interval *does not mean* that an investigator can be 95 percent sure that the true effect measure lies within the interval. For any given study, a 95 percent confidence interval (or any other percent confidence interval) either does or does not contain the true effect measure.

Unlike p-values and statistical tests, a confidence interval does not convey the idea of a dichotomous interpretation (that is, an interpretation that the data either are or are not statistically significant). What is important is the width of the interval and where the interval stands in relation to an effect size of 1 for the ratio scale, and 0 for the difference scale (that is, to the values of no association between an exposure and a health outcome). A 95 percent confidence interval that contains the value of either 1 or 0 for the ratio and difference scales, respectively, corresponds to a statistical test yielding a result of "no statistically significant association between an exposure and a health outcome" (a p-value greater than 0.05). If an α-value equal to 0.05 is the cutoff value for deciding whether an effect measure is or is not statistically significant, a statistical test yielding a p-value equal to 0.05 will result in a corresponding confidence interval that has "one" as a confidence limit for the ratio measure and, for cohort studies, "zero" as a confidence limit for the difference measure.

The Mathematical Relationship

The third fundamental idea about precision is that p-values and confidence intervals are mathematically related to each another, as suggested in the preceding paragraph. Logically, these measures must be related, because each gauges the amount of random error associated with an epidemiologic effect measure. The choice of whether to report p-values or confidence intervals when reporting the results of an epidemiologic study is somewhat a matter of personal preference. Confidence intervals provide not only information about the amount of random error associated with a particular effect measure but also the range of magnitudes for the effect measure that is consistent with the study data, taking random error into account. For that reason, confidence intervals convey additional, pertinent information that p-values cannot convey. Because a majority of epidemiologic research focuses on the magnitude of effect measures (and not only on whether the study findings are statistically significant), presenting confidence intervals rather than p-values may be the preferred approach for summarizing the amount of random error associated with an effect measure.

As a final point regarding p-values, p-values associated with effect measure estimates are either one-sided or two-sided. The usual choice is to present two-sided p-values that correspond to a "two-sided" null hypothesis such as IRR = 1.0. The alternative hypothesis, IRR $\neq$ 1, means that an IRR larger than 1.0 *or* smaller than 1.0 may be associated with a p-value less α. P-values are one-sided when the null hypothesis is "one-sided," such as IRR $\leq$ 1.0 or IRR $\geq$ 1.0 (IRR is less than or equal to 1.0 or greater than or equal to 1.0, respectively). When reporting a p-value, it is helpful to add a subscript to the p-value indicating whether the p-value is one-sided ($P_{(1)}$) or two-sided ($P_{(2)}$) so the reader has that information to aid in interpreting the study findings.

VALIDITY

Validity refers to the amount of bias or systematic error in a study, in contrast to precision, which quantifies the amount of random error. There are two general types of validity: **external validity,** which refers to the generalizability of a study's findings to people who were not participants in a study, and **internal validity,** which refers to the amount of bias within a study.

External Validity

External validity or **generalizability** refers to the extent to which the results of an epidemiologic study apply to people who were not included in the study. For example, if a study includes only a subset of all young men living in California, do the study results apply to the other young men living in California? Do the results apply to young men living in states other than California? Do the results apply to women? Do the results apply to older men?

Results that cannot be generalized have little scientific merit. In other words, results that apply *only* to the particular people included in a study usually cannot advance epidemiologic knowledge or contribute meaningfully to a better understanding of the theoretical basis of human disease etiology.

To be generalizable, an epidemiologic study need not include all the many types of people to whom the investigator wishes to apply the results. Many excellent epidemiologic studies have employed **restriction** (enrolling people in a study based on their sharing a narrow range of certain characteristics such as age, gender, or some other potential confounding factor or **effect modifier**) in the selection of subjects. Restriction may allow the study to have statistically meaningful (precise) results for at least the type of people included in the study instead of only imprecise results for subsets of subjects sharing certain characteristics. For example, if an investigator has the resources to study only two hundred people, restricting the subjects to one gender and to a narrow range of age might be preferable to enrolling people regardless of their gender or age. Using restriction by gender and age is particularly important if the presumed effect of the exposure on the outcome of interest varies according to age and gender, that is, if age and gender are effect modifiers. In that situation, unless restriction is employed, the data analysis may entail dividing the overall study into subsets such as young males, older males, young females, and older females, thus reducing the number of subjects available for estimating the effect measure(s) for each category of gender and age. That reduction may markedly reduce the precision of each estimated effect measure and thus affect the accuracy of the study.

A related issue pertains to the concept of external validity as the term is used in epidemiology. In epidemiology, the populations to whom study results can be generalized *may* extend beyond the source population from which the subjects were selected. For instance, data showing a large association between tobacco smoking and the incidence rate of lung cancer were available for men long before comparable data were available for women. Nonetheless, a reasonable person might well have generalized to women the results of the effects of the smoking and lung cancer studies conducted among men. Such generalization would be based on the fact that there are few reasons to believe a woman's reactions to tobacco smoke in the lung are materially different from a male's reactions to tobacco smoke in the lung.

Broader generalizations may not be valid in other situations. For example, epidemiologic studies have demonstrated that women develop liver disease in response to alcoholic beverage consumption more quickly and at lower levels of consumption than do men. Generalizing to women the results from alcohol studies conducted among males would result in bias. The reverse, generalizing to men the results of alcohol studies conducted among women, also would result in bias.

Decisions regarding those to whom the results of an epidemiologic study can be generalized are based on current knowledge about how and why a certain exposure might cause a particular health outcome. Extant knowledge in medicine and biology, pathology, toxicology, epidemiology, and related fields is used in the decision-making process to arrive at a "best guess" about the appropriateness of generalizing study findings to types of people who were not included in a study.

External validity in epidemiology differs from the concept of generalizability as used in classical statistics. In classical statistics, generalizability refers to inferring properties about a population (for example, its average value for some variable, or the variance of that variable) from properties of a sample selected at random from that population. There is little notion of having the properties of a sample generalizable to any population other than the population from which the sample was randomly selected. According to classical statistical thinking, the results of an epidemiologic study conducted among subjects selected at random from women residing in New York City could be generalized only to the female population of New York City. That difference in the concept of generalizability may reflect the practical underpinnings of epidemiology, an engaged science that attempts to solve real-life problems in health and illness, and so actively seeks appropriate applications of its studies' findings. In addition, all samples of people selected for inclusion in an epidemiologic study are restricted by calendar time and geography and so are not random samples in the classical statistical sense.

Internal Validity

Internal validity refers to the amount of bias within an epidemiologic study. If an epidemiologic study lacks internal validity, it cannot have external validity: A study containing a large amount of bias has no valid findings to generalize to any other group of people. The reverse, however, is not necessarily true. A study can be internally valid but not generalizable. As noted previously, such a study usually has little scientific merit.

Internal validity has two general components: **comparison biases,** which pertain to how comparisons between cases and controls or between exposed and unexposed subjects are made, and **information biases,** which pertain to the methods used to collect epidemiologic data and the quality of the collected data. Within those two broad categories of bias are several specific types of bias, each of which will be discussed in turn.

Comparison Biases

There are two types of comparison biases: selection bias and confounding bias.

Selection bias.   **Selection bias** is a systematic error that is introduced into a study when knowledge of potential subjects' exposure *and* disease statuses determine to some extent which particular subjects are enrolled in a study. Study subjects selected on the basis of their exposure and disease statuses are not representative of their source population with respect to their exposure and disease. Such subjects, as a group, may have a higher or a lower prevalence of the exposure and/or disease of interest.

Selection bias can occur *only* when knowledge of exposure *and* disease statuses to select subjects for study is used *differentially* between the groups to be compared. In a case/control study, knowledge of exposure status(es) must be used differentially to select particular cases and controls for study, as depicted in Table 12.4. In a retrospective cohort study, knowledge of the health outcome(s) of interest must be used differentially to select the particular exposed and unexposed subjects for study. Selection bias cannot occur in a prospective cohort study or in an intervention trial, because the health outcome of interest is not known at the time that participants are enrolled in the study.

TABLE 12.4
Example of Selection Bias in a Case/Control Study

	ENTIRE POPULATION*		
Subjects	*Exposed*	*Not Exposed*	*Total*
Cases	A	B	$M_1 = A + B$
Controls	C	D	$M_0 = C + D$
Total	$N_1 = A + C$	$N_0 = B + D$	$T = A + B + C + D$

Population EOR = (AD/BC)

*The "entire population" is a census of all possible subjects that could be included in an epidemiologic study. The EOR calculated from the entire population is the *true EOR* that an epidemiologic study wishes to estimate by selecting a sample (subset) of individuals belonging to the entire population.

	EPIDEMIOLOGIC STUDY = SAMPLE OF THE ENTIRE POPULATION: EOR IF THERE IS NO SELECTION BIAS		
Subjects	*Exposed*	*Not Exposed*	*Total*
Cases	k_1A	k_1B	$M_1 = k_1A + k_1B$
Controls	k_2C	k_2D	$M_0 = k_2C + k_2D$
Total	$N_1 = k_1A + k_2C$	$N_0 = k_1B + k_2D$	$T = k_1A + k_1B + k_2C + k_2D$

Note: EOR = $(k_1A\ k_2D/k_1B\ k_2C) = (k_1k_2/k_1k_2)/(AD/BC)$, in which k_1 is the sampling fraction for cases and k_2 is the sampling fraction for controls. "Sampling fraction" refers to the proportion of subjects selected from among all potential subjects in each of the A–D cells. Whenever the ratio of sampling fractions $(k_1k_2/k_1k_2) = 1.0$, the EOR based on a sample of the entire population will equal the true population EOR; there is no selection bias in this situation because knowledge of exposure did not alter the magnitude of the sampling fraction among cases or among controls. The sampling fractions for cases and for controls *do not* have to be equal. Usually the sampling fraction for exposed cases must equal the sampling fraction for unexposed cases, and the sampling fraction for exposed controls must equal the sampling fraction for unexposed controls, for selection bias to be absent. Typically, k_1 is larger than k_2 because there are more potential controls (people without the disease of interest) in the population than there are people with the disease of interest.

	EPIDEMIOLOGIC STUDY = SAMPLE OF THE ENTIRE POPULATION: EOR IF THERE IS SELECTION BIAS		
Subjects	*Exposed*	*Not Exposed*	*Total*
Cases	k_1A	k_2B	$M_1 = k_1A + k_2B$
Controls	k_3C	k_4D	$M_0 = k_3C + k_4D$
Total	$N_1 = k_1A + k_3C$	$N_0 = k_2B + k_4D$	$T = k_1A + k_2B + k_3C + k_4D$

Note: EOR = $(k_1A\ k_4D/k_2B\ k_3C) = (k_1k_3/k_2k_3)/(AD/BC)$, in which k_1 is the sampling fraction for exposed cases, k_2 is the sampling fraction for unexposed cases, k_3 is the sampling fraction for exposed controls, and k_4 is the sampling fraction for unexposed controls. Unless by good fortune $(k_1k_4/k_2k_3) = 1.0$, the EOR estimated from the sample of the entire population will not equal the true population EOR; in other words, there will be selection bias in the study. It is not necessary for both k_1 to differ from k_2, and for k_3 to differ from k_4 for selection bias to occur.

Once selection bias has occurred in a study, the groups to be compared remain forever noncomparable, and no amount of statistical or epidemiologic analysis can remove the bias. Selection bias, when present, is an intractable problem. For that reason, one goal of epidemiologic study design for case/control and for retrospective cohort studies is to develop a plan to *prevent* selection bias.

AN EXAMPLE OF SELECTION BIAS: ORAL CONTRACEPTIVES AND EMBOLISMS

In the 1970s, in the United States and elsewhere, women who used oral contraceptives (OCs) were at increased risk of developing emboli. As the knowledge of the association between OCs and emboli became known among clinicians, women who presented at clinicians' offices with leg pain, a common symptom of an embolism in the leg, were asked whether they were using OCs. Women who answered that question affirmatively were more apt to be referred for follow-up tests to determine whether an embolism was present than were women who responded negatively. Women not using OCs may have been told to "go home, rest, and take aspirin" in the hope that the leg pain would improve. If these women did have emboli, the emboli sometimes resolved with rest at home and so never were diagnosed.

The difference in the clinical protocol between women who responded affirmatively to the question of whether they were taking OCs and women who responded negatively resulted in an overabundance of women who were OC users among women diagnosed as having an embolism. In other words, the difference in the probability of diagnosing the presence of an embolism among OC users compared with OC nonusers resulted in a nonrepresentative group of women with respect to their OC use among women whose emboli were diagnosed.

Selection bias would occur if an epidemiologist, unaware of the differential probability of diagnosing an embolism among OC users and nonusers, were to conduct a case/control or retrospective cohort study of OC use and emboli relying on clinicians' diagnoses of the presence of an embolism. The study would find a stronger association between OC use and emboli than actually existed, because the clinicians' knowledge that a woman used OCs was part of the process leading to the diagnosis (Figure 12.2).

In this example, the knowledge concerning OC use that led to selection bias was not an error on the part of the epidemiologist conducting the study. The situation that led to selection bias was "set up" beforehand by the process that resulted in a woman being diagnosed with an

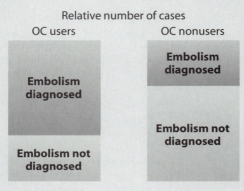

FIGURE 12.2
Example of selection bias: Oral contraceptives (OC) and emboli.

embolism. For that reason, an investigator may not be aware that selection bias has occurred in a particular epidemiologic study. To prevent selection bias, an investigator could have enrolled OC users and nonusers in a prospective cohort study in which the process of making the diagnosis of "having an embolism" was standardized for both OC users and OC nonusers. In that way, the answer to the question "Do you use OCs?" would not affect the probability of diagnosis.

Confounding bias.   The second type of comparison bias is confounding bias, usually referred to simply as "confounding." Confounding was addressed previously in the discussion regarding the benefits of randomly allocating exposure in intervention studies (Chapter 9) and in the discussion of observational versus intervention studies (Chapters 9 and 10). **Confounding** bias occurs when a variable that is an **independent cause of the health outcome under study** (a variable that is a cause of the health outcome of interest even in the absence of the exposure of interest) occurs more or less frequently among exposed persons than among unexposed persons. The observed size of the association between the exposure and the health outcome is biased, because the size of the effect measure results in part from the effect of the confounding factor on the health outcome of interest (Figure 12.3).

As an example, tobacco smoking may be a confounder in studying the association between coffee consumption and the incidence rate of myocardial infarction (MI). Smoking often occurs more frequently among those who consume high amounts of coffee than among those who consume no coffee or low amounts of coffee, and smoking is an independent cause of MI. To be an independent cause, smoking must be a cause of MIs even among those who consume no coffee. Because smoking does cause MIs among that group, the causal pathway between smoking and MIs must differ from the causal pathway, if any, between coffee and MIs.

If an epidemiologic study were conducted assessing the association between coffee consumption and MIs, without taking into account the confounding effect of tobacco, the observed association between coffee and MIs would be biased toward a

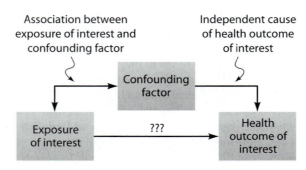

FIGURE 12.3
Pictorial representation of confounding.

larger association than in fact exists. The bias would occur because the study measured not only the effect, if any, of coffee on MIs but also, in part, the effect of tobacco on MIs.

Only factors that vary (can have different values) can be confounders, because only those factors can have different frequencies between the groups to be compared. *"Making a factor not vary" is the basis for all approaches to prevent confounding during the design of the study or to control confounding in the data analysis.*

Sometimes, confounding variables themselves are not independent causes of the outcome under study but instead are **risk indicators** of the outcome. A risk indicator is a variable that is correlated with an independent cause of the outcome under study and so serves as a marker for its presence. The presence of the risk indicator means that the independent cause also is present. As an example, the habit of always carrying matches or a lighter is a risk indicator for tobacco smoking, because in most circumstances only smokers and not nonsmokers carry matches or lighters. A study that took into account "carrying matches or a lighter" in effect would be taking most of the effects of tobacco smoking into account.

Prevention and control of confounding. Detection and control of confounding is the main data analysis problem in epidemiology. Confounding also can be prevented from occurring in an epidemiologic study by the way a study is designed.

Prevention of confounding. **Prevention of confounding** means designing an epidemiologic study in such a way that confounding by one or more factors does not occur. There are three approaches for preventing confounding: random allocation of exposure, matching (frequency matching and individual matching), and restriction.

As discussed in Chapter 9, randomly allocating exposure to the groups whose health outcomes will be compared almost always prevents confounding by both known and unknown factors, especially if the number of subjects studied is large. Randomly allocating exposure to the groups prevents confounding by removing the association between the confounding variable(s) and the exposure under investigation. For that reason, intervention studies, unlike observational studies, typically do not contain a large amount of confounding bias.

Restriction also can prevent confounding. Restriction prevents confounding by narrowing the range of values for the potential confounding factor to such a point that the factor no longer is a variable; that is, the factor no longer assumes a wide enough range of values to exert a differential effect on the health outcome. For example, in an epidemiologic study that enrolls only women, gender could not be a confounding factor because gender would not vary.

Matching, either frequency matching or individual matching, can prevent confounding by the variables on which the cases and controls (in a case/control study) or the exposed and unexposed subjects (in a cohort study) are matched. In general, matching means that the subjects being compared are selected for study because of their similarity on certain variables that the investigator anticipates will be confounders in a study.

In cohort studies, **frequency matching** means that the unexposed subjects are selected for study on the basis of their similarities to the exposed for common demographic features such as their ages, genders, and racial and/or ethnic identification. The matching is performed on a "group basis"; that is, no individual unexposed subject is matched to any particular exposed subject(s). It is the groups in their entirety that are similar. In case/control studies, the cases and the controls are selected for study on the basis of the similarity of their demographic profiles. The rationale for frequency matching is that because the distributions of the frequency-matched variables are so similar for the compared groups, confounding by those variables may not occur. Frequency matching is a common part of the plan to prevent confounding in epidemiologic studies.

In **individual matching,** usually employed only in case/control studies, the cases and the controls are matched not only on common demographic variables but also on potential confounding variables that otherwise would rarely be similar among the cases and the controls. Such complex, nominal scale variables typically have many possible values. Examples of variables for which individual matching might be performed are large number of siblings, work environment, and neighborhood. In individual matching, each case is matched individually to a particular control or controls, and these case/control pairs, triplets, or quartets remain together throughout the data analysis, each set forming its own stratum in the data analysis.

Although discussion of the analysis of individually matched case/control studies is beyond the scope of this text, it nonetheless is important to appreciate that individual matching introduces selection bias into a study. The selection bias thus introduced *can* be removed during data analysis and ordinarily is the only situation in which selection bias can be removed from a study. A review of Figure 12.3 shows why selection bias is introduced by individual matching in case/control studies. In Figure 12.3, only potential confounding variables are those for which individual matching is performed. Matching on those variables tends to match also on the exposure(s) under study, making the cases and the controls unduly similar with respect to those exposures. Thus, "knowledge of exposure" via knowledge of the confounding factors is used in part to select specific cases and controls for study.

Control of confounding. Three approaches are used to control confounding during the data analysis phase of the study: standardization, stratification, and multivariate analysis. Each approach is a method that prevents the distribution of the confounding factor from varying in making comparisons between cases and controls in a case/control study or between exposed and unexposed subjects in a cohort study.

In **standardization,** the distribution of a confounding factor(s) is made similar between the groups to be compared by selecting a standard distribution for the confounders. For example, in a hypothetical cohort study, the exposed population may have 25 percent males and 75 percent females, and gender may be a confounding factor. An unexposed population that has a gender distribution different from that of the exposed population may result in a comparison that is confounded by gender. Using standardization, the gender distribution of the unexposed population is made identical to that of the exposed population "artificially." The identical distribution is accomplished by comparing the disease or injury frequency in the exposed population with what the disease or injury frequency would have been in the unexposed population if the unexposed population had a gender distribution of 25 percent male and 75 percent female. Table 12.5 and the discussion that follows provide a numeric exam-

TABLE 12.5
Numeric Example of Standardization

Gender	EXPOSED		UNEXPOSED	
	Number of Cases	*Number of People*	*Number of Cases*	*Number of People*
Male	25	250	200	2,000
Female	30	750	40	1,000
Total	55	1,000	240	3,000

Note: The crude cumulative incidence (CI) of disease in the exposed population is $55/1,000 = 0.055 = 5.5\%$. The crude CI of disease in the unexposed population is $240/3,000 = 0.080 = 8.0\%$.

The cumulative incidence ratio (CIR) for the exposed population relative to the unexposed population is $0.055/0.080 = 0.69$, suggesting that the CI of disease in the exposed population is 0.69 times the CI in the unexposed population, a 0.31 (31%) decrease in the CI of disease.

The exposed and unexposed populations can be standardized for gender using the formula $(\Sigma_i W * (CI_i)/ \Sigma W_i)$, where W is the standard or "weight" for gender category "i."

For the exposed population, standardizing for gender using the gender distribution in the exposed population as the standard yields $(250 * (25/250) + 750 * (30/750))/(250 + 750) = (25 + 30)/(250 + 750) = 55/1,000 = 0.055$ or 5.5%. Because the distribution of gender in the exposed population was used as the standard, the CI standardizing for gender is equal to the crude CI. In this example, 250 and 750 are the standard values for men and for women, respectively.

For the unexposed population, standardizing for gender using the gender distribution in the exposed population as the standard yields $(250 * (200/2,000) + 750 * (40/1,000)/(250 + 750)) = (25 + 30)/(250 + 750) = 55/1,000 = 0.055$ or 5.5%.

The standardized CIR comparing the exposed with the unexposed populations is $0.055/0.055 = 1$, demonstrating that the CIs in the two populations are equal after controlling for the confounding effect of gender.

Why did standardization for gender result in identical CIs? The CI for males in the exposed population is $25/250 = 0.10$ or 10%. The CI for males in the unexposed population also is 0.10 or 10% (200/2,000). The CI for females in the exposed population is $30/750 = 0.040$ or 4.0%. The CI for females in the unexposed population also is 0.040 or 4.0% (40/1,000). Because the gender-specific CIs are the same in each population, any set of standards would result in a CIR = 1.0.

ple of standardization based on confounding by gender with the distribution of gender in the exposed population of 25 percent male and 75 percent female.

In the numeric example given in Table 12.5, the standards or weights for gender were selected to equal the distribution of gender in the exposed population. When the distribution of standardized variable(s) equals the distribution of the variable(s) in the exposed population, the resulting standardization is called **indirect standardization.** When a different standard is selected, the resulting standardization is called **direct standardization.** The only difference between indirect and direct standardization is the choice of the standard used.

In performing standardization, an investigator may select any standard he or she wishes to select. Most often, however, the distribution of the confounder in the exposed population, the age and gender distribution in the United States in 2000 (if age and gender are the variables standardized), or some other well-recognized standard is used. Using well-recognized standards facilitates comparisons among different epidemiologic studies because using the same standard results in analyses that are comparable to one another.

In utilizing **stratification** to control confounding, investigators use different values of the confounder to form groups (strata) of subjects that have the same or nearly the same values for the confounding factor. Measures of effect are calculated for each stratum, and then **pooled** (combined according to the amount of statistical information in each stratum) into one overall measure of effect. Stratification is based on making comparisons within strata containing data for subjects with nearly the same values of the confounding factor. Because those values do not vary within each stratum, the stratification factor cannot confound. Tables 12.6 and 12.7 provide numeric examples of stratification to control confounding and a contrasting example demonstrating the difference between confounding and effect modification. Effect modification, sometimes called synergy or antagonism, may be thought of as an interaction between exposures that produces a larger or smaller effect than the sum of the exposures' individual effects.

TABLE 12.6
Numeric Example of Stratification to Control Confounding in a Case/Control Study

CRUDE DATA (ALL THE DATA IN ONE TABLE, AS IN SIMPLE ANALYSIS)

	Diet A	*Diet B*	*Total*
Stomach cancer cases	80	220	300
Controls	180	420	600
Total	260	640	900

EOR = (80 * 420)/(220 * 180) = 0.85, suggesting a protective effect of Diet A on stomach cancer.

DATA STRATIFIED BY AGE, A CONFOUNDING FACTOR

	Young Age				*Older Age*		
	Diet A	*Diet B*	*Total*		*Diet A*	*Diet B*	*Total*
Stomach cancer cases	20	180	200	Stomach cancer cases	60	40	100
Controls	10	190	200	Controls	170	230	400
Total	30	370	400	Total	230	270	500

$EOR_{Young\ Age} = (20 * 190)/(180 * 10) = 2.1$ $EOR_{Older\ Age} = (60 * 230)/(40 * 170) = 2.0$

In Table 12.6, stratifying by age changes the EOR from 0.85 (a protective effect) to 2.1 and 2.0 for young-age and for older-age people, respectively, suggesting a causal effect of Diet A on stomach cancer. A pooled estimator of the EOR based on the stratified data would produce a value for the EOR that is between the stratum-specific EORs of 2.1 and 2.0. The difference between the crude EOR of 0.85 and the pooled estimate for the EOR is due to confounding by age.

In Table 12.7, stratifying by tobacco use resulted in stratum-specific EORs that differ substantially from each other (2.1 versus 81). This difference occurs because tobacco use is an effect modifier: The effect of asbestos in causing lung cancer is different for tobacco users than for nonusers. When effect modification is present, the stratum-specific EORs should be reported. The crude EOR, 6.4, is not relevant because it applies neither to the effect of asbestos on lung cancer among tobacco users nor among nonusers.

TABLE 12.7
Numeric Example of Effect Modification in a Case/Control Study

CRUDE DATA (ALL THE DATA IN ONE TABLE, AS IN SIMPLE ANALYSIS)

	Exposed to Asbestos	*Not Exposed to Asbestos*	*Total*
Lung cancer	110	190	300
Controls	50	550	600
Total	160	740	900

EOR = (110 * 550)/(190 * 50) = 6.4.

DATA STRATIFIED BY TOBACCO USE, AN EFFECT MODIFIER

	Tobacco Use				*No Tobacco Use*		
	Asbestos Exposed	*Not Asbestos Exposed*	*Total*		*Asbestos Exposed*	*Not Asbestos Exposed*	*Total*
Lung cancer	20	180	200	Lung cancer	90	10	100
Controls	10	190	200	Controls	40	360	400
Total	30	370	400	Total	130	370	500

EOR $_{\text{Tobacco Use}}$ = (20 * 190)/(180 * 10) = 2.1   EOR $_{\text{No Tobacco Use}}$ = (90 * 360)/(10 * 40) = 81.

In **multivariate analysis,** a statistical model is adopted to explain the relation between the exposure, confounding variable(s), the health outcome, and sometimes effect modifier(s). Comparisons are made within categories of potential confounding factors in which the values for a confounder do not vary substantially. For example, a logistic model might be adopted for the analysis of case/control data. In this model, the natural log of the odds of disease is the dependent variable and is predicted by the exposure, confounding factors, and effect modifiers as follows:

$$\ln(Y/1-Y) = a + \Sigma\, b_i x_i$$

Y is the probability of disease, a is the y-intercept, and the b's are the coefficients for the "x's" (the exposure(s), confounding factors, and effect modifiers). The EORs are estimated by: e^x. A thorough explanation of multivariate analysis in epidemiologic research, beyond the scope of this text, can be found in Rothman and Greenland 1998 as well as in other textbooks on biostatistics or on epidemiologic analysis.

AN EXAMPLE OF CONFOUNDING BIAS: HORMONE REPLACEMENT THERAPY (HRT) AND CORONARY HEART DISEASE

Over the past several decades, many observational studies consistently demonstrated a 40% to 50% reduction in the risk of coronary heart disease among women taking hormone replacement therapy (HRT). That large reduction in the risk of heart disease was viewed as a major benefit associated with the use of HRT.

In 1998, reports from a randomized clinical trial of HRT comparing an estrogen/progestin combination with an inert placebo raised serious doubts about the benefits of HRT in the prevention of recurrent heart events. The trial, the "Heart and Estrogen-Progestin Replacement Study," or "HERS," was conducted among 2,762 postmenopausal women with preexisting coronary disease. Women were enrolled in the trial from any of seventeen participating clinical centers in the United States. After an average follow-up period of 4.1 years, the trial reported a slight increase in coronary heart events during the first year of the trial among women randomly allocated to the HRT group compared with women taking the placebo, and a slight decrease in coronary events between years 3 and 5 of follow-up. The temporal pattern of the findings led to the hope that HRT would reduce coronary events when taken over long periods of time.

After an additional 2.7 years of follow-up, however, the trial (HERS-II) reported that women taking HRT had a slightly increased risk of a recurrent coronary event compared with the women taking the placebo (Grady et al. 2002). The trial results, at least in regard to the prevention of a secondary coronary event, differed materially from the results of the preceding observational studies of HRT and coronary events.

Why did the observational studies consistently find a 40% to 50% reduction in coronary events among women taking HRT, whereas the results from the HERS and HERS-II clinical trials found essentially no significant effects, either preventive or causal, on recurrent coronary events? The most plausible explanation for the difference in the findings is confounding bias.

Confounding bias could have produced the large observed reductions in the risk of coronary events if women who were taking HRT differed substantially from women who were not taking HRT in terms of their other risk factors for coronary heart disease. When data were collected concerning which women were taking HRT, it was discovered that HRT users were women who had greater access to health services than did comparably aged women who were not taking HRT, higher income levels, and fewer risk factors for coronary heart disease such as tobacco use, uncontrolled high blood pressure, and low HDLs. These other favorable risk factors for coronary heart disease confounded the apparent beneficial effect of HRT on coronary events. This confounding can be shown pictorially as follows:

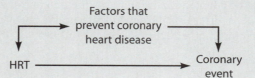

In addition, during many of the years the observational studies were conducted, the advice given in the *Physicians' Desk Reference,* a standard reference for clinicians, was that estrogen should not be prescribed for women who had heart disease, diabetes, or hypertension. Because of that advice, women who had heart disease or who were at higher risk of developing heart disease selectively were removed from the population of women for whom estrogen or estrogen-progestin might be prescribed.

Several questions remain concerning the effects, if any, of HRT on coronary health. For example, the HERS trials did not evaluate the health effects of unopposed estrogen (estrogen without progestins), nor did the trials evaluate the effects of HRT on women without preexisting heart disease. The ongoing Women's Health Initiative (WHI) may help to resolve these remaining questions (Prentice et al. 1996). The WHI is a randomized clinical trial involving 27,438 women who are receiving estrogen replacement therapy, either with or without progestins, or a placebo. The planned follow-up period is nine years. The results of this trial should be available about 2005.

Information Biases

Information biases occur when epidemiologic data are collected differentially from the groups to be compared. There are two kinds of information bias: misclassification and observation bias. Observation bias has two types: interviewer bias and recall bias.

Misclassification. **Misclassification** occurs when exposed people are classified as unexposed, or vice versa, when the dose of exposure is incorrect, or when cases are classified as noncases, or vice versa. The presence, absence, or dose of a confounding factor or an effect modifier also can be misclassified. Misclassification can occur as a result of errors in disease diagnosis, medical-record entries, exposure-level records, instruments to measure exposure, or for a wide variety of other reasons.

Misclassification can be a major problem in an epidemiologic study. Large errors can occur from the accumulated effects of measurement errors in a study in which many variables are measured for each subject. Typically, the magnitude of the accumulated effects on the study findings is unknown, although sometimes a general idea of the effects of misclassification can be gleaned (Rockett and Thomas 1999). In some studies, however, not even the direction of the effects of misclassification on the findings (an increase or decrease in observed effects measures) may be known.

Part of the explanation for why the size of estimated exposure-outcome associations in epidemiology tend to be small probably reflects difficulties in accurately measuring exposure levels. As an example, even for an "easily measured" exposure such as tobacco smoking, it is not clear how to quantify the "physiologically and/or pathologically meaningful amount of lifetime smoking." The challenge in measuring lifetime smoking results, for example, from changes in the levels of smoking over time, changes in the content of the smokes from different brands of cigarettes, degree of inhaling, age at smoking initiation, and effects of nonsmoking (quitting) intervals. It is challenging for an epidemiologist to decide which people have experienced the same physiologically and/or pathologically relevant dose of exposure and so should be grouped together during data analysis. An innovative method for collecting accurate information on complex occupational histories is presented in Box 12.1.

Observation bias. The second kind of information bias is observation bias. Observation bias is divided into two types: recall bias and interviewer bias.

Recall bias. **Recall bias** occurs when information, based on subjects' memories of past events, is obtained from subjects whose abilities to recollect past exposures and events differ. The quality obtained or the completeness of information collected differs between the groups, resulting in data that are noncomparable (Infante-Rivard and Jacques 2000).

As an example, in a case/control study, data obtained directly from women who recently gave birth to children with major birth defects may not be comparable to data obtained from mothers of healthy newborns. Mothers who recently gave birth to children with major birth defects may be asking themselves what they might have "done"

BOX 12.1

PRACTICAL EPIDEMIOLOGY IN A PUBLIC HEALTH SETTING: AN ALTERNATIVE METHOD FOR COLLECTING COMPLEX OCCUPATIONAL HISTORIES

SHELIA HOAR ZAHM, SC.D.

DIVISION OF CANCER EPIDEMIOLOGY AND GENETICS,

NATIONAL CANCER INSTITUTE, NIH, DHHS

In studies of the effects of workplace exposures, the starting point is usually the collection of a detailed occupational history. The traditional epidemiologic method of obtaining an occupational history involves asking about the first job/task, then the next job/task, and repeating for the life span. When subjects have lengthy, complex job histories, accurate recall is difficult, and the traditional method quickly become extremely tedious, causing subjects to become frustrated and to lose interest in providing the full details of their occupational histories.

An alternative method of collecting occupational histories from migrant and seasonal farmworkers who frequently change jobs and geographic locations, sometimes up to hundreds of times over a working lifetime, has been developed by the University of Washington. The method, which was pilot-tested by the National Cancer Institute and the Farmworker Epidemiology Research Group for use in epidemiologic studies, uses a visual approach, called a life events/icon calendar, to obtaining a subject's work history. In this method, icons (pictures on sticky labels) are applied to a calendar to represent the subject's important life events, crops, and work activities (Zahm et al. 2001).

The life events/icon–calendar method of collecting occupational histories uses a calendar covering the years from the subject's first job to the present (Figure 12.4). Each year is divided into months and weeks. Information is entered on the calendar by a combination of written notations and small pictures, or "icons," of life events, crops, tasks, and protective clothing or equipment. Interviewers use a supply of computer-generated colored pictures on sticky labels to symbolize significant life events, such as country flags and state maps to indicate geographic moves, a bride and groom to symbolize marriage, a red cross to symbolize a major illness or injury, babies for the birth of a child, cars for the purchase of a first automobile, and planes for a first plane ride. Icons representing historical events, such as major hurricanes or government changes, could also be used. The labels are affixed to the calendar at the beginning of the interview and used as chronological "anchors" around which the subject might more easily recall his or her work history.

Icons of crops, farm tasks (for example, harvesting/picking, weeding/hoeing, planting, thinning), and common nonfarm jobs (for example, construction) also are used to record the work history. Three rows are provided to record up to three crop/task combinations per time period. The names of farms, orchards, or ranches and their locations are written on the calendar. The names of crops, farm tasks, and nonfarm jobs for

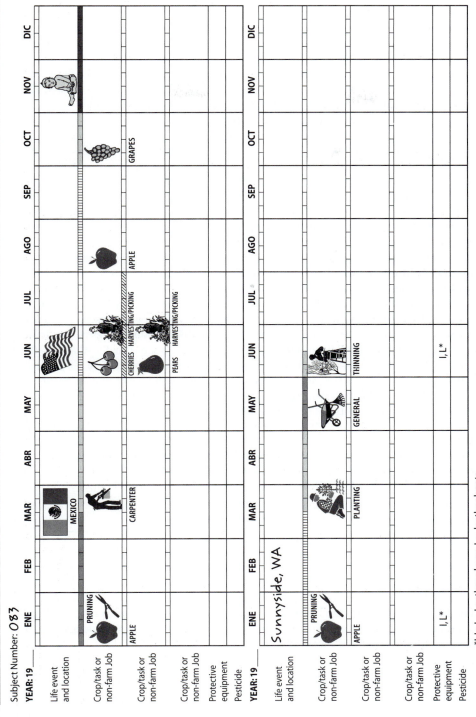

Subject Number: 083

YEAR: 19___

	ENE	FEB	MAR	ABR	MAY	JUN	JUL	AGO	SEP	OCT	NOV	DIC
Life event and location			MEXICO									
Crop/task or non-farm Job	PRUNING / APPLE		CARPENTER			CHERRIES HARVESTING/PICKING		APPLE		GRAPES		
Crop/task or non-farm Job						PEARS HARVESTING/PICKING						
Crop/task or non-farm Job												
Protective equipment												
Pesticide												

YEAR: 19___   Sunnyside, WA

	ENE	FEB	MAR	ABR	MAY	JUN	JUL	AGO	SEP	OCT	NOV	DIC
Life event and location												
Crop/task or non-farm Job	PRUNING / APPLE		PLANTING		GENERAL	THINNING						
Crop/task or non-farm Job												
Crop/task or non-farm Job												
Protective equipment	I, L*					I, L*						
Pesticide												

*I, L: I = Leather gloves, L = leather boots.

FIGURE 12.4

Two-year sample of life events/icon calendar for collecting occupational histories from farmworkers.

269

Box 12.1 continued

which no icons are available also are written on the calendar. The last two rows of the calendar are used to record protective clothing or equipment and pesticide names. The narrow lines between the rows are filled in with colored markers or pencils to denote the dates and duration of each job (unique crop/task combination) (the color changed at the start of a new job) or periods of unemployment (black color). The colorful icons serve as memory aids to help the subjects place the jobs in time and to recall crops and tasks they might have forgotten. Generally, the work history is recorded starting with the most recent job and moving backward in time. If the subject is unable to recall certain periods despite the memory aids and interviewer prompting, those periods are left blank on the calendar. After the rest of the calendar has been filled in, the interviewer and the subject together review the missing periods in case the subject's memory of past work history has been triggered by the reporting of other jobs.

This approach to collecting work histories is extremely effective, as evidenced by the greater number of jobs reported and more work time accounted for than when using traditional interview methods to obtain occupational histories in a pilot study (Table 12.8) (Engel et al. 2001). The median total job count reported by subjects was 23 (range: 3–97) using the icon-calendar questionnaire compared with 9 (1–26) using the traditional questionnaire. The total number of work months accounted for in the icon-calendar questionnaire (160.3 [range: 1.9–370.7]) was much greater than in the traditional questionnaire (47.3 [0.1–190.9]). In addition, the reliability of the life events/icon–calendar questionnaire was demonstrated by interviewing a group of farmworkers twice, 8–14 months apart, and by comparing occupational histories self-reported by farmworkers with those reported by their spouses.

TABLE 12.8
Number of Jobs and Working Months Reported By Migrant Farmworkers* Using a Traditional Occupational History Approach and a Life Events/Icon Calendar

	TRADITIONAL	LIFE EVENTS
Median (Range)	*Occupational History*	*Icon Calendar*
Working months	47.3 (0.1–190.9)	160.3 (1.9–370.7)
Number of jobs	9 (1–26)	23 (3–97)

*89 farmworkers (48 men, 41 women).

The life events/icon method is well suited for people with long occupational histories, particularly if those workers are semiliterate or illiterate, and produces a more complete picture of a person's work history.

Box 12.1 continued

REFERENCES

Engel L. S., M. C. Keifer, and S. H. Zahm. 2001. Comparison of a traditional questionnaire with an icon/calendar–based questionnaire to assess occupational history. *American Journal of Industrial Medicine* 40:502–11.

Zahm S. H., J. S. Colt, L. S. Engel, M. C. Keifer, A. J. Alvarado, K. Burau, P. Butterfield, S. Caldera, S. P. Cooper, D. Garcia, C. Hanis, E. Hendrikson, N. Heyer, L. M. Hunt, M. Krauska, N. Mac-Naughton, C. J. McDonnell, P. K. Mills, L. D. Mull, D. L. Nordstrom, B. Outterson, D. P. Slesinger, M. A. Smith, L. Stallones, C. Stephens, A. Sweeney, K. Sweitzer, S. W. Vernon, and A. Blair. 2001. Development of a life events/icon calendar questionnaire to ascertain occupational histories and other characteristics of migrant farmworkers. *American Journal of Industrial Medicine* 40:490–501.

during the pregnancy to cause the defects. In contrast, mothers of healthy newborns may not be reliving the events of their pregnancies. The difference in the mind-sets of the two groups of mothers may make the data based on their recall noncomparable. More recent data suggest that recall bias in that situation may not be as large as previously thought.

Another example, which continues to be controversial, is the apparent association between breast cancer and having had an abortion: Is that association causal, or does it result from recall bias? In general, the opportunity for recall bias arises in situations in which "sensitive" data are desired and can be obtained only from direct questioning of the subjects themselves without independent verification. Independent data may be available from, for example, routinely collected medical data or from other written files such as lists of prescription drug dispensed, occupational air quality data, or some other previously recorded information.

Interviewer bias. **Interviewer bias** occurs when an investigator uses different methods to collect data from the groups to be compared. For example, in a case/control study, if an investigator collects information from cases through personal interviews but data from controls through a mail survey, the resulting data most likely would not be comparable. The quality and the completeness of data obtained through personal interviews almost always are superior to data collected through mail surveys.

An interesting example that may result in interviewer bias is the study of domestic violence in lesbian relationships (Box 12.2). Preconceived ideas about what the study results "should be" and/or how the data "should be interpreted" might affect the internal validity of studies on this topic.

BOX 12.2

ETHICS MATTERS: DOMESTIC VIOLENCE IN LESBIAN RELATIONSHIPS

RITA SAWYER AND TAMARA ADKINS-BATES, M.P.H.

A review of studies on violence in lesbian relationships in the United States reveals a prevalence between 25 and 33 percent, similar to that found in the heterosexual community. In most public education campaigns about domestic violence, however, same-sex couples are invisible.

Homophobia becomes another weapon of power and control over the victim. Victims often report that their abusers threaten to "out" them (reveal them to others as homosexual) if they do not comply with the abuser, and keep the violence secret. Being "outed" could cost the victim her job, her family, her friends, even custody of her children. One survivor, disowned by her family, writes, "My family used the abuse to justify their belief that lesbians are 'sick'" (Broaddus and Merill, 1998).

For victims who do decide to come forward and seek help, the studies reflect the difficulty in finding a responsive and sympathetic party. Among friends in the lesbian community, the victim might suffer a lack of support grounded in a collective reluctance to acknowledge that the male-privilege analysis of domestic violence is inadequate and that women can batter, too. One battered lesbian described her friend's nonsupportive response: "Maybe a good fist fight would clear the air."

The medical system routinely makes heteronormative assumptions, and in a survey of GLBT health-care practitioners, 72 percent report having witnessed lesbian clients being denied care by their colleagues on the basis of their sexual orientation.

Turning to the judicial system may be impossible. Many states still criminalize consensual, private, adult homosexual activity. The ability to petition for a restraining order or other forms of institutional protection also is limited explicitly in many states to heterosexual couples.

Counselors may not be a helpful resource, either. Wise and Bowman (1997) analyzed the responses of graduate psychology/counseling students, at both the master's and the doctoral level, to a written scenario describing intimate-partner abuse. Two versions of the same scenario were drafted, differing only in the gender of the hypothetical perpetrator. Students were randomly assigned to reading either the heterosexual scenario or the lesbian scenario. Following the reading, the students were asked to give treatment recommendations. For the heterosexual partners, the students felt that the victim should call the police, charge him with assault, and seek assistance at the women's shelter. When the perpetrator was female, most respondents simply recommended couples counseling.

Just as in heterosexual couples, racism, poverty, and other forms of discrimination can leave women in same-sex abusive relationships more vulnerable to exploitation. Scherzer (1998) found that race did not play a significant role in the prevalence of abuse, but more research is needed on the role of intersecting oppression in isolating and silencing victims.

Box 12.2 continued

REFERENCES

Beathea, Angela R., Kathryn R. Rexrode, Alexandra C. Ruffo, and Syreeta D. Washington. Violence in lesbian relationships: A narrative analysis. www.employees.csbsju.edu/jmakepeace/perspectives2k/f05Bethea.jmm.html as (accessed on March 4, 2003).

Broaddus, Toni, and Gregory Merill. 1998. Annual report on lesbian, gay, bisexual, transgender domestic violence, 1998. Available from the National Coalition of Anti-Violence Programs. www.vaw.umn.edu/Final Documents/glbtdv.htm (accessed January 26, 2003).

Burke, Leslie K., and Diane R. Follingstad. 1999. Violence in lesbian and gay relationships: Theory, prevalence, and correlational factors. *Clinical Psychology Review* 19 (5): 487–512.

Scherzer, Teresa. 1998. Domestic violence in lesbian relationships: Findings of the Lesbian Relationships Research Project. *Journal of Lesbian Studies* 2:29–47.

Wise, Amy J., and Sharon L. Bowman. 1997. Comparison of beginning counselors' responses to lesbian vs. heterosexual partner abuse. *Violence and Victims* 12 (2), 127–35.

Concluding Remark about Bias

The fact that errors are made in subject selection or data collection does not necessarily result in bias. Bias can occur only when there is a process that acts differentially on the groups whose exposures or outcomes are compared. A difference must exist with respect to how data are collected, in the criteria by which subjects are enrolled in a study, or in how comparisons are made.

When reading the epidemiologic literature, it is essential to assess the probability that certain types of bias may be present in a study. A study's authors may suggest areas in which bias may have entered the study, but it is incumbent upon the reader to make an independent assessment of whether bias was introduced into the study and not controlled for in the data analysis and, if so, how much. When critiquing an epidemiologic study, make a list of possible sources of error. Are these the same kinds of errors that arose in similar studies? Did the authors take care to try to prevent the bias from entering the study? If yes, how? Were the authors successful in doing so? How did other authors address the need to prevent or control these biases in similar studies on the same topic? Gauging the likely magnitude of bias in a study is difficult except in the most obvious of situations (for example, studying lung function and neglecting to ask questions about history of tobacco use). It is, nevertheless, a task that should be undertaken rigorously and dispassionately. It also is a time to reflect upon the large numbers of studies conducted, for example, on HRT and adverse coronary events in women, in which the overwhelming number of studies reached the same conclusion (in this case, that HRT prevented adverse coronary events) but the conclusion was in error. In general, the fact that many studies on the identical or similar topics reach the same conclusions is no guarantee that the studies, taken in their entirety, are unbiased.

REVIEW QUESTIONS

1. List and define the two components of accuracy in epidemiologic studies.
2. Define and differentiate between "p-value" and "confidence interval." What kind of information does each measure convey? How are the p-value and the confidence interval mathematically related to each another?
3. Define "null hypothesis" and "statistically significant." What does it mean for the findings of an epidemiologic study to be "statistically significant"?
4. Define and differentiate between "external validity" and "internal validity."
5. In what way(s) does the concept of external validity differ between epidemiology and classical statistics?
6. Define "restriction." What are the benefits of employing restriction in the selection of subjects for an epidemiologic study?
7. List and define the two main components of internal validity.
8. Define "selection bias." How does selection bias occur? Provide examples of studies in which selection bias may have occurred. (These can be hypothetical studies.)
9. Define "confounding." What is the primary difference between "preventing confounding" and "controlling confounding"?
10. Provide examples of studies in which unprevented and uncontrolled confounding may have occurred. (These can be hypothetical studies.)
11. What does it mean that a confounding factor must be "an independent cause" of the health outcome of interest?
12. Why can confounding factors be only factors that vary (can have different values), and why is this idea the basis for the prevention and the control of confounding?
13. Define "risk indicator." Provide several examples of risk indicators.
14. List and define the primary approaches for preventing confounding.
15. List and define the primary approaches for controlling confounding.
16. List, define, and provide examples of each type of information bias.
17. Why, for bias to occur, must there be a process that acts differentially on the groups to be compared?

Engaged Epidemiology

Simply "knowing epidemiology" is not enough in today's complex field of public health. The effects of interacting social, economic, and political systems all need to be taken into account when planning programs that effectively improve public health. An epidemiologist or any other public health professional needs to understand the fundamental principles that underlie epidemiologic methodology and be willing to apply those principles to help solve public health problems. The term "engaged epidemiology" emphasizes the relationship between epidemiology and applied efforts to better society. It takes epidemiology beyond the personal or professional pursuit of knowledge for knowledge's sake and adds a practical, applied dimension.

A fully engaged epidemiologist should challenge the people, agencies, and corporations whose products, technologies, and/or practices contribute to the public's ill health. Because of their interest in disease etiology, epidemiologists may be uniquely educated to function in that advocacy capacity, serving as the sentinel professionals in safeguarding population health and safety. Being engaged means being held accountable for the application of findings from epidemiologic studies in setting national policies and objectives in the fields of health and safety.

As you pursue your career in public health and safety, think how you can incorporate the skills of an engaged epidemiologist in your work. What kinds of questions might an engaged epidemiologist help to answer in your professional field of interest? How might she or he interact with other professionals in identifying aspects of social, economic, and political systems that detract from public health and safety? What are or should be the goals and competencies of engaged epidemiologists with respect to furthering population health?

Sample Answers to Review Exercises

Chapter 4 Review Exercises 1–5

1.

	23 Weeks Pre-Campaign				10 Weeks Post-Campaign		
Age Group (years)	Cases of Aseptic Meningitis	Person-Months	Incidence Rate*		Cases of Aseptic Meningitis	Person-Months	Incidence Rate*
1–3	9	2,658,294	0.34†		15	462,312	3.24
4–8	12	4,531,920	0.26		37	788,160	4.69
9–11	8	3,282,698	0.24		6	570,904	1.05
Total	29	10,472,912	0.28		58	1,821,376	3.18

*Number of aseptic meningitis cases per 100,000 child-months.
†IR for children aged 1–3 years = 9/2,658,294 P-Y = 0.34/100,000 P-Y.

2.

Age (years)	Number of Cases	Number of Person-Years	Incidence Rate*
1	45	1,000	4.5
2	150	3,500	4.3
3	175	2,500	6.8
4	270	4,000	6.5
5	72	1,000	7.2
6	210	2,000	10.5
7	470	4,500	10.4
8	360	3,500	10.3
9	265	2,000	13.2
10	465	3,500	13.3

*Number of cases/100 P-Y.

Age Category (years)	Number of Cases	Number of Person-Years	Incidence Rate*
1–2	195	4,500	4.3
3–5	517	7,500	6.9
6–8	1,040	10,000	10.4
9–10	730	5,500	13.3

*Number of cases/100 P-Y.

3. *In which age categories are the animal bite rates the highest?* Young: Ages 0–4y, 5–9y, and 10–14y. *In which age categories are the animal bite rates the lowest?* Ages 18–19y, 20–24y, and 60 years and older. *In which age categories is the number of animal bites the largest? the smallest? Do you have enough data to answer this question?* No. *Why or why not?* Denominators (i.e, numbers of person-years on which the animal bite rates are based) are not known.

4. The CHD IR is 3 cases/((3 + 7 + 4 + 5 + 2 + 6 + 7 + 7)P-Y = 3/(41 P-Y).
   The CHD MR is 2 deaths/((3 + 7 + 7 +6 +2 + 6 + 7 + 7)P-Y) = 2/(45 P-Y).

5.

	Population A				Population B		
	Males	Females	Both Genders		Males	Females	Both Genders
Number of new cases	600	100	700	Number of new cases	150	800	950
Number of person-years	4,000	1,000	5,000	Number of person-years	3,000	4,000	7,000

a. Crude IR for Population A = 700/5,000 P-Y = 14.0/100 P-Y.
   Crude IR for Population B = 950/7,000 P-Y = 13.6/100 P-Y.

b. The gender-adjusted incidence rates for Populations A and B using the distribution of person-years in Population A as the weights:
   Gender-adjusted IR for Population A = Crude IR = 14.0/100 P-Y, calculated as (((600/4,000 P-Y) * 4,000 P-Y) + (100/1,000 P-Y) * 1,000 P-Y)) / (4,000 P-Y + 1,000 P-Y)
   Gender-adjusted IR for Population B = 8/100 P-Y, calculated as (((150/3,000 P-Y) * 4,000 P-Y) + ((800/4,000 P-Y) * 1,000 P-Y))/ (4,000 P-Y + 1,000 P-Y)

c. The gender-adjusted incidence rates for Populations A and B using the distribution of person-years in Population B as the weights:
   Gender-adjusted IR for Population A = 12.1/1,000 P-Y (((600/4,000 P-Y) * 3,000 P-Y) + ((100/1,000 P-Y) * 4,000 P-Y))/ (3,000 P-Y + 4,000 P-Y)
   Gender-adjusted IR for Population B = Crude IR = 13.6/100 P-Y, calculated as (((150/3,000 P-Y) * 3,000 P-Y) + ((800/4,000 P-Y) * 4,000 P-Y)/ (3,000 P-Y + 4,000 P-Y)

The following table summarizes the answers to question 5.

	Population A	Population B
a. Crude IR	14.0/100 P-Y	13.6/100 P-Y
b. Gender-adjusted IR using the P-Y from Population A as the weights	14.0/100 P-Y	8/100 P-Y
c. Gender-adjusted IR using the P-Y from Population B as the weights	12.1/100 P-Y	13.6/100 P-Y

Chapter 5 Review Exercises 1–4, 6

1.

Industry	Daily Personal Computer Use (hours)	Total # Workers	# Workers with Symptoms	Prevalence*
Both categories of industries				
	0	366	62	0.17
	0.5–3	417	63	0.15
	4–6	250	50	0.20
	7 or more	414	128	0.31
Computer and data processing; public utilities				
	0	188	28	0.15
	0.5–3	183	31	0.17
	4–6	151	29	0.19
	7 or more	321	103	0.32
Banking, communications, and hospitals				
	0	178	36	0.20
	0.5–3	234	33	0.14
	4–6	99	23	0.23
	7 or more	93	25	0.27

*Prevalence = (# workers with symptoms/total # of workers).

Is there a consistent increase or decrease in the magnitude of the prevalence as the number of daily personal computer use (hours) increases? Why, or why not? Yes. In general, as the dose (daily personal computer use) increases, the prevalence increases.

2. a.

Age	Incidence Rate	Average Duration of Disease	Prevalence*
Young	2.3/(100 P-Y)	7 years	0.14
Middle-aged	2.9/(100 P-Y)	2 years	0.05
Older	5.1/(100 P-Y)	1 year	0.05
Oldest	5.4/(100 P-Y)	4 months	0.02

*Prevalence = (Incidence rate * average duration of disease)/(1 + (incidence rate * average duration of disease)).

b. *Are the age-specific prevalences a good indication of the relative magnitudes of the age-specific IRs?* No, at least not as a direct relation. As the IR increases, P decreases.

c. *In general, if data on the prevalence of disease, but not on the IR of disease, are available, what if anything can you conclude about the IR of disease?* Nothing.

3. *If the prevalence of a preclinical stage of cancer is 10 percent and the average duration of the preclinical stage is 3 years, what is the IR of the preclinical stage?* By rearranging the formula for prevalence, $IR = P/((1 - P) D)$. Solving for the IR yields an IR = 3.7/(100 P-Y); that is, $IR = 0.10/((1 - 0.10) * 3Y)$.

4.

Question and Respondent's Age (years)	Boys			Girls		
	Total #	# Smokers	Prevalence* of Smoking	Total #	# Smokers	Prevalence* of Smoking
Ever Tried Smoking						
13–14	1,311	516	0.39	1,303	559	0.43
15–16	1,395	818	0.59	1,391	837	0.60
17–18	1,237	819	0.66	1,212	849	0.70
Current Smoking (daily and occasionally)						
13–14	1,282	108	0.08	1,289	133	0.10
15–16	1,351	278	0.21	1,366	335	0.25
17–18	1,201	323	0.27	1,191	405	0.34
Daily Smoking						
13–14	1,282	58	0.05	1,289	41	0.03
15–16	1,351	132	0.10	1,366	159	0.12
17–18	1,201	182	0.15	1,191	246	0.21

*Prevalence = (# smokers/total #).

6.

		TRUE ("REAL WORLD") SITUATION		
		Positive for Factor	Negative for Factor	Total
SCREENING TEST RESULTS	Positive for Factor	180	1,000	1,180
	Negative for Factor	20	4,000	4,020
	Total	200	5,000	5,200

Sensitivity = 180/200 = 0.9.
Specificity = 4,000/5,000 = 0.8.
Predictive Value Positive = 180/1,180 = 0.15.
Predictive Value Negative = 4,000/4,020 = 0.995.
Only 15 percent of the people who screened positive on the test have the condition that was targeted by the screening program. On the other hand, over 99 percent of the people who screened negative on the test were negative for the condition that was targeted by the screening program.

Chapter 6 Review Exercises 1–3

1.

Age Category (years)	Injury IR	Δt (years)	CI
0–2	273/(2,490 P-Y)	3	0.280
3–9	201/(10,973 P-Y)	7	0.120
10–14	84/(9,714 P-Y)	5	0.042
15–19	151/(11,450 P-Y)	5	0.064
20–24	65/(11,206 P-Y)	5	0.029
25–64	307/(57,924 P-Y)	40	0.19
65 and older	172/(1,469 P-Y)	Unknown	*
All ages	1,253/(105,226 P-Y)	Unknown	*

a. The 65y- (0–64 years) crude CI starting at birth is 0.492, or 49.2%. This CI is based on a crude IR equal to (1,081 injuries/103,757 P-Y) and a Δt equal to 65 years. The corresponding 65y-CI taking the age-specific IRs into account is 0.554, or 55.4%, based on the age-specific IR and Δt for each age category. In this calculation, $\Sigma IR \Delta t = 0.8072$.

b. Can the CIs for the two "*" age categories be calculated? Why, or why not? No, CIs cannot be calculated because the Δts are unknown.

2.

Cohort	# People in the Cohort	# Cases of Disease Over 5 Years	5y-CI
A	752	87	0.116
B	1,189	52	0.044
C	3,009	177	0.059
D	2,667	344	0.129

3. The fact that the average duration of disease is 3 months is not relevant to calculating the 8y-CI; that is, this datum is "extra" information. First approach: 8y-CI = 833/5046 = 0.165, or 16.5%. Second approach: The number of cases = 833. The number of P-Ys = 833 * 4y for people who developed disease (4 years = 0.5 times the 8-year follow-up period; that is, on average, the 833 people who developed disease were followed for about half of the total 8-year follow-up if the cases of disease occurred uniformly throughout the 8-year period). The number of P-Ys = (5,046-833) * 8y for people who did not develop disease. Therefore, the IR of disease over the 8-year period = 833/((833 * 4 P-Y) + (5,046 − 833) * 8 P-Y) = 833/37,036 P-Y. Inserting this IR into the CI formula gives an 8-year CI equal to 0.165 or 16.5% $(1 - e^{-((833/37,036 \text{ P-Y}) * 8Y)})$.

Chapter 11 Review Exercises 1–4

1. Data table and answers for the study of the effects of passive smoking on young infants' respiratory health in Shanghai, PRC.

Data Table

# Cigarettes Smoked per Day in Household	# New Cases of Respiratory Disease	# Children in Cohort	Cumulative Incidence (CI)	Cumulative Incidence Ratio (CIR)	Cumulative Incidence Difference (CID)
Boys					
None	19	151	0.1258	1.0 (ref)*	0 (ref)
1–9	24	140	0.1714	1.36	0.046
10–19	25	118	0.2119	1.68	0.086
20–39	27	116	0.2328	1.85	0.107
Total	95	525	0.1810	N/A	N/A
Girls					
None	14	143	0.0979	1.0 (ref)	0 (ref)
1–9	17	134	0.1269	1.30	0.029
10–19	18	109	0.1651	1.69	0.067
20–39	20	96	0.2083	2.13	0.110
Total	69	482	0.1432	N/A	N/A

# Cigarettes Smoked per Day in Household	# New Cases of Respiratory Disease	# Children in Cohort	Cumulative Incidence (CI)	Cumulative Incidence Ratio (CIR)	Cumulative Incidence Difference (CID)
	Boys/Girls				
None	33	294	0.1122	1.0 (ref)	0 (ref)
1–9	41	274	0.1496	1.33	0.037
10–19	43	227	0.1894	1.69	0.077
20–39	47	212	0.2217	1.97	0.109
Total	164	1,007	0.1629	N/A	N/A

*Ref = reference (unexposed) category.

2. Data table and answers to burn-prevention exercise.

Type of Intervention	Four 8-Month Baseline IR*	8-Month Program Implementation IR*	IRR and IRD*	4-Year Baseline IR*	1-Year Postprogram Period IR*	IRR and IRD*
School-initiated (Lynn, MA)	35.2	35.8	1.02; 0.6	38.7	41.1	1.06; 2.4
Community-initiated (Quincy, MA)	16.6	13.7	0.83; –2.9	18.0	16.9	0.94; –1.9
Media campaign (Salem and Saugus, MA)	22.0	25.5	1.16; 3.5	26.3	27.0	1.03; 0.7
No intervention (Holyoke and South Hadley, MA)	21.2	20.3	0.96; –0.9	22.2	21.7	0.98; –0.5

*Number of burns per 10,000 person-years.

a. *Which, if any, of the intervention programs were effective in reducing burn IRs?* Probably none of the programs was effective, although there was a reduction in the burn incidence rate in Quincy during the eight-month period of program implementation.

b. *What effect, if any, did the differing baseline burn IRs have on the study results?* Unknown, although the results of the interventions may have been different given the different baseline rates of burns.

3. *Estimate the appropriate effect measures (ratio and/or difference measures) for each of the following sets of hypothetical data.*

a.

	Smokers	Nonsmokers
Lung cancer cases	217	57
# person-years	13,278	11,702

IRR = (217/13,278 PY)/((57/11,702 PY) = 3.36.

IRD = (217/13,278 PY) − (57/11,702 PY) = 1.15/100 PY.

b.

	Alcohol Use	No Alcohol Use
Cases of liver disease	221	573
No liver disease	944	4,991
Total	1,165	5,564

CIR = (221/1165)/(573/5564) = 1.84.
CID = (221/1165) − (573/5564) = 0.087.

c.

	Exercise	No Exercise
Cases	218	654
Controls	759	1,233

EOR = (218 × 1233)/(759 × 654) = 0.54.

d.

	Pesticide Exposure	No Pesticide Exposure
Cases of tremor	82	13
# person-years	1,063	874

IRR = (82/1063 P-Y)/(13/874 P-Y) = 5.19.
IRD = (82/1063 P-Y) − (13/874 P-Y) = 6.2/100 P-Y.

4. *Analyze the following hypothetical data first as a cohort study (with count denominators) and then as a case/control study.*

Subjects	CS_2 Exposure	No CS_2 Exposure
New cases of heart disease	165	433
No heart disease	746	3,878
Total	911	4,311

Cohort study
CIR = (165/911)/(433/4311) = 1.8.
CID = (165/911) − (433/4311) = 0.08.

Case/control study
EOR = (195 × 3878)/(433 × 746) = 1.98.

REFERENCES

Abdel-Wahab, M. F., S. S. Zakaria, M. Kamel, M. K. Abdel-Khaliq, M. A. Masbrouk, H. Salama, G. Esmat, D. L. Thomas, and G. T. Strickland. 1994. High seroprevalence of hepatitis C infection among risk groups in Egypt. *American Journal of Tropical Medicine and Hygiene* 51:563–67.

Agar, M. 1996. Recasting the "ethno" in "epidemiology." *Medical Anthropology* 16:391–403.

Alberts, D. S., M. E. Martinez, D. J. Roe, J. M. Guillen-Rodriguez, J. R. Marshall, B. van Leeuwen, M. E. Reid, C. Ritenbaugh, P. A. Vargas, A. B. Bhattacharyya, D. L. Earnest, R. E. Sampliner, and the Phoenix Colon Cancer Prevention Physicians' Network. 2000. Lack of effect of a high-fiber cereal supplement on the recurrence of colorectal adenomas. *New England Journal of Medicine* 342 (16): 1156–62.

Alpha-Tocopherol, Beta Carotene Prevention Study Group. 1994. The effect of vitamin E and beta carotene on the incidence of lung cancer and other cancers in male smokers. *New England Journal of Medicine* 330 (15): 1029–35.

American Cancer Society. 1999. Cancer facts and figures—1999. Atlanta: American Cancer Society.

Angell, M. 2000. Investigators' responsibilities for human subjects in developing countries. *New England Journal of Medicine* 342 (13): 967–69.

Annas, G. J., and M. A. Grodin. 1998. Human rights and maternal-fetal HIV transmission prevention trials in Africa. *American Journal of Public Health* 88:560–63.

Artaud-Wild, S. M., S. L. Connor, G. Sexton, and W. E. Connor. 1993. Differences in coronary mortality can be explained by differences in cholesterol and saturated fat intakes in 40 countries but not in France or Finland. *Circulation* 88:2771–79.

Ast, D. B., S. B. Finn, and I. McCaffrey. 1950. The Newburgh-Kingston Caries Fluorine Study: I. Dental findings after three years of water fluoridation. *American Journal of Public Health* 40:716–24.

Bach, P. B., L. D. Cramer, J. L. Warren, and C. B. Begg. 1999. Racial differences in the treatment of early-stage lung cancer. *New England Journal of Medicine* 341 (16): 1198–1205.

Bayer, R. 1998. The debate over maternal-fetal HIV transmission trials in Africa, Asia, and the Caribbean: Racist exploitation or exploitation of racism? *American Journal of Public Health* 88:567–70.

Belanger, C. F., C. H. Hennekens, B. Rosner, and F. E. Speizer. 1978. The Nurses' Health Study. *American Journal of Nursing* 78:1039–40.

Blendon, R. J., C. M. DesRoches, M. Brodie, J. M. Benson, A. B. Rosen, E. Schneider, D. E. Altman, K. Zapert, M. J. Herrmann, and A. E. Steffenson. 2002. Views of practicing physicians and the public on medical errors. *New England Journal of Medicine* 347 (24): 1993–40.

Boldan, C. F. 1916. Over a century of health administration in New York City. New York City Department of Health. Monograph Service, no. 10:13.

Bonnlander, H. P., and A. M. Rossignol. 1998. Tobacco use among Cuban migrants at Guantanamo Bay, Cuba. *Pan American Journal of Public Health* 3 (2): 131–33.

Boylston, Z. 1726. An historical account of the small-pox inoculated in New England, upon all sorts of persons, whites, blacks, and of all ages and constitutions with some account of the nature of the infection in the natural and inoculated way, and their different effects on human bodies: with some short directions to the unexperienced in this method of practice. London: S. Chandler.

Burke, J. P. 2003. Infection control—A problem for patient safety. *New England Journal of Medicine* 348 (7): 651–56.

Canto, J. G., J. J. Allison, C. I. Kiefe, C. Fincher, R. Farmer, P. Sekar, and S. Person. 2002. Relation of race and sex to the use of reperfusion therapy in medicare beneficiaries with acute myocardial infarction. *New England Journal of Medicine* 342 (15): 1094–1100.

Center for Disease Control and Prevention. 2005. Poliovirus infections in four unvaccinated children—Minnesota, August–October 2005. *Morbidity and Mortality Weekly Report (MMWR)*. www.cdc.gov/mmwr/mmwr_wk.html (accessed October 19, 2005).

Cunin, P., E. Tedjouka, Y. Germani, C. Neharre, R. Bercion, J. Morvan, and P. M. V. Martin. 1999. An epidemic of bloody diarrhea: *Escherichia coli* 157 emerging in Cameroon? *Emerging Infectious Diseases* 5 (2): www.cdc.gov/ncidod/eid/vol5no2/cunin.html.

D'Amico, A. V., M.-H. Chen, K. A. Roehl, and W. J. Catalona. 2004. Preoperative PSA velocity and the risk of death from prostate cancer after radical prostatectomy. *New England Journal of Medicine* 351 (2): 125–35.

Darwish, M., R. Faris, J. D. Clemens, M. R. Rao, and R. Edelman. 1996. High seroprevalence of hepatitis A, B, C and E viruses in residents in an Egyptian village in the Nile delta: A pilot study. *American Journal of Tropical Medicine and Hygiene* 54:554–58.

De Zoysa, I., C. J. Elias, and M. E. Bentley. 1998. Ethical challenges in efficacy trials of vaginal microbicides for HIV prevention. *American Journal of Public Health* 88:571–75.

Doll, R., and A. B. Hill. 1950. Smoking and carcinoma of the lung. *British Medical Journal*, September 30, 739–48.

Dourado, I., S. Cunha, M. G. Teixeira, C. P. Farrington, A. Melo, R. Lucena, and M. L. Barreto. 2000. Outbreak of aseptic meningitis associated with mass vaccination with a urabe-containing measles-mumps-rubella vaccine: Implications for immunization programs. *American Journal of Epidemiology* 151 (5): 524–30.

Dresler, C. M. 1998. The lung cancer epidemic in women. *Women's Health in Primary Care* 1 (1): 85–92.

Drug Strategies. 2000. Millennium hangover: Keeping score on alcohol. Washington, D.C.: Drug Strategies or www.drugstrategies.org.

Elandt-Johnson, R. C. 1975. Definition of rates: Some remarks on their use and misuse. *American Journal of Epidemiology* 102:276–71.

El-Sayed, N., P. J. Gomotos, G. R. Rodier, T. F. Wierzba, A. Darwish, S. Khashaba, and R. R. Arthur. 1996. Seroprevalence survey of Egyptian tourism workers for hepatitis B virus, hepatitis C virus, HIV, and Treponema pallidium infections: Association of hepatitis C virus infections with specific regions of Egypt. *American Journal of Tropical Medicine and Hygiene* 55:179–84.

Evans, A. S. 1978. Causation and disease: A chronological journal. *American Journal of Epidemiology* 108 (4): 1126–95.

Francis, T., Jr., R. F. Korns, R. B. Voight, M. Boisen, F. M. Hemphill, J. A. Napier, and E. Tolchinsky. 1955. An evaluation of the 1954 poliomyelitis vaccine trials. Poliomyelitis Vaccine Evaluation Center, University of Michigan, Ann Arbor, Michigan, April 12. Reprinted as a supplement to the May 1955 issue of the *American Journal of Public Health.*

Frank, C., M. K. Mohamed, G. T. Strickland, D. Lavanchy, R. R. Arthur, L. S. Magder, T. El Khoby, Y. Abdel-Wahab, E. S. O. Ohn, W. Anwar, and I. Sallam. 2000. The role of parenteral antischistosomal therapy in the spread of hepatitis C virus in Egypt. *Lancet* 355: 887–91.

Gamble, T., Jr. 1900. A History of the City Government of Savannah, 1790–1901. In The Mayor's Annual Report, Savannah, 1900, 143.

Gamble, V. N. 1997. Under the shadow of Tuskegee: African Americans and health care. *American Journal of Public Health* 87:1773–78.

Gamblin, S. J., L. F. Haire, R. J. Russell, D. J. Stevens, B. Xiao, Y. Ha, N. Vasisht, D. A. Steinhauer, R. S. Daniels, A. Elliot, D. C. Wiley, and J. J. Skehel. 2004. The structure and receptor-binding properties of the 1918 influenza hemagglutinin. *Science* (February 5), www.sciencemag.org/sciencexpress/recent.shtml.

Gao, Y. T., J. K. McLaughlin, W. J. Blot, B. T. Ji, Q. Dai, and J. F. Fraumeni, Jr. 1994. Reduced risk of esophageal cancer associated with green tea consumption. *Journal of the National Cancer Institute* 86:855–58.

Goldberg, I. J. 2003. To drink or not to drink? *New England Journal of Medicine* 348: 163–64.

Grady, D., D. Herrington, V. Bittner, R. Blumenthal, M. Davidson, M. Hlatky, J. Hsia, S. Hulley, A. Herd, S. Khan, L. K. Newby, D. Waters, E. Vittinghoff, and N. Wenger for the HERS Research Group. 2002. Cardiovascular disease outcomes during 6.8 years of hormone therapy: Heart and Estrogen/Progestin Replacement Study follow-up (HERS II). *Journal of the American Medical Association* 288:49–57.

Graunt, J. 1662. *Natural and political observations made upon the bills of mortality.* London.

Greenwood, M. 1935. *Epidemic and crowd diseases: An introduction to the study of epidemiology.* New York: Macmillan.

Halliday, S. 2000. William Farr: Campaigning statistician. *Journal of Medical Biography* 8:220–27.

Hennekens, C. H., J. E. Buring, and J. E. Manson. 1996. Lack of effect of long-term supplementation with beta-carotene on the incidence of malignant neoplasms and cardiovascular disease. *New England Journal of Medicine* 334:1145–49.

Hennessey, K. A., N. Ion-Nedelcu, M.-D. Craciun, F. Toma, W. Wattigney, and P. M. Strebel. 1999. Measles epidemic in Romania, 1996–1998: Assessment of vaccine effectiveness by case-control and cohort studies. *American Journal of Epidemiology* 150:1250–57.

Herbst, A. L., H. Ulfelder, D. C. Poskanzer, and L. D. Longo. 1971. Adenocarcinoma of the vagina: Association of maternal stilbestrol therapy with tumor appearance in young women. *New England Journal of Medicine* 285:878–81.

Hernberg, S., M. Nurminen, and M. Tolonen. 1973. Excess mortality from coronary heart disease in viscose rayon workers exposed to carbon disulfide. *Scandinavian Journal of Work, Environment, and Health* 10:93–99.

Hill, A. B. 1965. The environment and disease: Association of causation? *Proceedings of the Royal Society of Medicine* 58:295–300.

Holmen, T. L., E. Barrett-Connor, J. Holmen, and L. Bjermer. 2000. Health problems in teenage daily smokers versus non-smokers, Norway, 1995–1997. *American Journal of Epidemiology* 151 (20): 148–55.

Infante-Rivard, C., and L. Jacques. 2000. Empirical study of parental recall bias. *American Journal of Epidemiology* 152 (5): 480–86.

International Agency for Research on Cancer. 2000. www-dep.iarc.fr (accessed February 25, 2000).

International Military Tribunal. 1950. Trials of war criminals before the Nuremberg Military Tribunals under Control Council law no. 10. Washington, D.C.: U.S. Government Printing Office.

Jin, C., and A. M. Rossignol. 1993. Effects of passive smoking on respiratory illness from birth to age eighteen months in Shanghai, People's Republic of China. *Journal of Pediatrics* 123:553–58.

Kohn, L. T., J. M. Corrigan, and M. S. Donaldson, eds. 2000. *To err is human: Building a safer health system.* Washington, D.C.: National Academy Press.

Krug, E. G., G. K. Sharma, and R. Lozano. 2000. The global burden of injuries. *American Journal of Public Health* 90 (4): 523–26.

Levine, S. H., A. M. Rossignol, and M. F. Coleman. 1992. The sale of hazardous consumer products. *Journal of Environmental Health* 55 (2): 20–23.

Liao, Y., D. L. McGee, G. Cao, and R. S. Cooper. 2000. Alcohol intake and mortality: Findings from the National Health Interview Surveys (1988 and 1990). *American Journal of Epidemiology* 151 (7): 651–59.

Little, R. E., S. C. Monaghan, B. C. Gladen, Z. A. Shkyryak-Nyzhnyk, and A. J. Wilcox. 1999. Outcomes of 17,137 pregnancies in 2 urban areas of Ukraine. *American Journal of Public Health* 89:1832–36.

Lurie, P., and S. M. Wolfe. 1997. Unethical trials of interventions to reduce perinatal transmission of the human immunodeficiency virus in developing countries. *New England Journal of Medicine* 337 (12): 853–56.

Lyon, J. L., and J. W. Gardner. 1997. The rising frequency of hysterectomy: Its effect on uterine cancer rates. *American Journal of Epidemiology* 105:439–43.

MacKay, A. M., J. Halpern, E. McLoughlin, J. Locke, and J. D. Crawford. 1979. A comparison of age-specific burn injury rates in five Massachusetts communities. *American Journal of Public Health* 69 (11): 1146–50.

MacKay, A. M., and K. J. Rothman. 1982. The incidence and severity of burn injuries following Project Burn Prevention. *American Journal of Public Health* 72:248–52.

MacMahon, B. 1979. Strengths and limitations of epidemiology. *Current Issues and Studies:* 91–104. Washington, D.C.: National Research Council.

MacMahon, B., and T. F. Pugh. 1970. *Epidemiology: Principles and methods.* Boston: Little, Brown.

McGovern, P. G., J. S. Pankow, E. Shahar, K. M. Doliszny, A. R. Folsom, H. Blackburn, and R. V. Luepker. 1996. Recent trends in acute coronary heart disease. *New England Journal of Medicine* 334 (14): 884–90.

Mokdad, A. H., J. S. Marks, D. F. Stroup, and J. L. Gerberding. 2004. Actual causes of death in the United States, 2000. *Journal of the American Medical Association* 291:1238–45.

MRFIT Research Group. 1982. Multiple risk factor intervention trial. *Journal of the American Medical Association* 248:1465–77.

Mukamal, K. J., K. M. Conigrave, M. A. Mittleman, C. A. Camargo, Jr., M. J. Stampfer, W. C. Willett, and E. B. Rimm. 2003. Roles of drinking pattern and type of alcohol consumed in coronary heart disease in men. *New England Journal of Medicine* 348 (2): 109–18.

National Center for Health Statistics. 2002. *National Vital Statistics Report* 50 (12): 11–14.

———. 2004. *National Vital Statistics Report* 52 (13): 9–13, 19.

Obadia, Y., I. Feroni, V. Perrin, D. Vlahov, and J.-P. Moatti. 1999. Syringe vending machines for injection drug users: An experiment in Marseilles, France. *American Journal of Public Health* 89 (12): 1852–54.

Oregon State University News Service 2005. Aftermath could give rise to disease epidemics. *Corvallis Gazette-Times.* www.gazettetimes.com/articles/2005/09/21/news/community/wedloc 03. prt (accessed September 20, 2005).

Orme-Zavaleta, J., and P. A. Rossignol. 2004. Community-level analysis of risk of vector-borne disease. *Royal Society of Tropical Medicine and Hygiene* 98:610–18.

Pan American Health Organization. www.paho.org (accessed February 17, 2000).

Parker, S. L., T. Tong, S. Bolden, and P. A. Wingo. 1997. Cancer statistics, 1997. *CA: A Cancer Journal for Clinicians* 47:5–27.

Pasternak, D., and P. Cary. 1995. Tales from the crypt. *U.S. News and World Report,* September 18.

Pearce, N. 1996. Traditional epidemiology, modern epidemiology, and public health. *American Journal of Public Health* 86:678–83.

Peto, R., R. Doll, J. D. Buckley, et al. 1981. Can dietary beta-carotene materially reduce human cancer rates? *Nature* 290:201–9.

Prentice, R. L., J. E. Rossouw, S. R. Johnson, et al. 1996. The role of randomized clinical trials in assessing the benefits and risks of long-term hormone replacement therapy. Example of the Women's Health Initiative. *Menopause* 3:71–76.

Raufu, A. 2004. Traditional rulers in Northern Nigeria call for halt to polio vaccination. *British Medical Journal* 328:306.

Ridker, P. M., N. Rifai, L. Rose, J. E. Buring, and N. R. Cook. 2002. Comparison of C-reactive protein and low-density lipoprotein cholesterol in the prediction of first cardiovascular events. *New England Journal of Medicine* 347 (20): 1557–65.

Rivers, T. M. 1937. Viruses and Koch's postulates. *Journal of Bacteriology* 33:1–12.

Rockett, I. R. H., and B. M. Thomas. 1999. Reliability and sensitivity of suicide certification in higher income countries. *Suicide and Life-Threatening Behavior* 29 (2): 141–49.

Rossignol, A. M., and H. P. Bonnlander. 1999. Caffeine-containing beverages, total fluid consumption, and premenstrual symptoms. *American Journal of Public Health* 80 (9): 1106–10.

Rossignol, A. M., H. P. Bonnlander, L. Song, and J. W. Phillis. 1991. Do women with premenstrual symptoms self-medicate with caffeine? *Epidemiology* 2:403–8.

Rossignol, A. M., J. A. Locke, and J. F. Burke. 1989. Burn injuries: An analysis of the risks posed by food preparation. *Journal of Environmental Health* 52 (3): 174–76.

Rossignol, A. M., E. P. Morse, V. M. Summers, and L. D. Pagnotto. 1987. Video display terminal use and reported health symptoms among Massachusetts clerical workers. *Journal of Occupational Medicine* 29 (2): 112–18.

Rossignol, P. A. 1994. Do tropical diseases cause poverty, or does poverty cause tropical diseases? *Epidemiology Monitor* 15:9.

Rothman, K. J. 1976. Causes. *American Journal of Epidemiology* 104 (6): 587–92.

Rothman, K. J., and S. Greenland. 1998. *Modern epidemiology.* Philadelphia: Lippincott-Raven.

Rothman, K. J., and K. B. Michels. 1994. The continuing unethical use of placebo controls. *New England Journal of Medicine* 331:394–98.

Ruffin, J. M., J. E. Grizzle, N. C. Hightower, G. McHardy, H. Shull, and J. B. Kirsner. 1969. A cooperative double-blind evaluation of gastric "freezing" in the treatment of duodenal ulcer. *New England Journal of Medicine* 281 (1): 16–19.

Schatzkin, A., E. Lanza, D. Corle, P. Lance, F. Iber, B. Caan, M. Shike, J. Weissfeld, R. Burt, M. R. Cooper, J. W. Kikendall, J. Cahill, and the Polyp Prevention Trial Study Group. 2000. Lack of effect of a low-fat, high-fiber diet on the recurrence of colorectal adenomas. *New England Journal of Medicine* 342 (16): 1149–55.

Schnyder, G., M. Roffi, Y. Flammer, R. Pin, and O. M. Hess. 2002. Effect of homocysteine-lowering therapy with folic acid, Vitamin B_{12}, and Vitamin B_6 on clinical outcome after percutaneous intervention. The Swiss Heart Study: A randomized clinical trial. *Journal of the American Medical Association* 288:973–79.

Shapiro, S. B., W. Venet, P. Strax, L. Venet, and R. Rueser. 1982. Prospects for eliminating racial differences in breast cancer survival rates. *American Journal of Public Health* 72:1142–45.

Sherburne, H. R., A. M. Rossignol, and B. Wilson. 1977. A bite out of the budget? Costs and characteristics of animal bites in Benton County, Oregon. *Journal of Environmental Health* (April): 13–16.

Shuster, E. 1997. Fifty years later: The significance of the Nuremberg Code. *New England Journal of Medicine* 337:1436–40.

Shyrock, R. H. 1937. The early American public health movement. *American Journal of Public Health* 27:965–71.

Sinclair, U. 1981. *The jungle.* New York: Bantam Books.

Snow, J. 1855. *On the mode of communication of cholera.* London: John Churchill.

Stallones, R. A. 1983. Mortality and the Multiple Risk Factor Intervention Trial. *American Journal of Epidemiology* 117 (6): 647–50.

Steering Committee of the Physicians' Health Study Group. 1988. Preliminary report: Findings from the aspirin component of the ongoing Physicians' Health Study. *New England Journal of Medicine* 318 (4): 262–64.

Struewing, J. P., P. Hartge, S. Wacholder, S. M. Baker, M. Berlin, M. McAdams, M. M. Timmerman, L. C. Brody, and M. A. Tucker. 1997. The risk of cancer associated with specific mutations of BRCA1 and BRCA2 among Ashkenazi Jews. *New England Journal of Medicine* 336 (20): 1401–8.

Susser, M., and E. Susser. 1996a. Choosing a future for epidemiology: I. Eras and paradigms. *American Journal of Public Health* 86:668–73.

———. 1996b. Choosing a future for epidemiology: II. From black box to Chinese boxes and eco-epidemiology. *American Journal of Public Health* 86:674–77.

Sysoyeva, M. 2000. Ukraine has day of mourning for Chernobyl victims: Aftereffects are grimly visible. Associated press release, as reported in the *Corvallis (OR) Gazette-Times.* April 27, sec. A, 9.

Thompson, I. M., D. K. Pauler, P. J. Goodman, C. M. Tangen, M. S. Lucia, H. L. Parnes, L. M. Minasian, L. G. Ford, S. M. Lippman, E. D. Crawford, J. J. Crowley, and C. A. Coltman, Jr. 2004. Prevalence of prostate cancer among men with a prostate-specific antigen level ≤ 4.0 ng per milliliter. *New England Journal of Medicine* 350 (22): 2239–47.

Thun, M. J., R. Peto, A. D. Lopez, J. H. Monaco, S. J. Henley, C. W. Health, and R. Doll. 1997. Alcohol consumption and mortality among middle-aged and elderly U.S. adults. *New England Journal of Medicine* 337 (24): 1705–14.

U.S. Department of Health and Human Services. Health Resources and Services Administration. 2000. Assuring a healthy future along the U.S.–Mexico border: A HRSA priority. Washington, D.C.: U.S. Government Printing Office.

U.S. Department of Health and Human Services. 2003. *Health, United States.* DHHS Publication No. 2003-1232.

Vassilia, K., P. Eleni, and T. Dimitrios. 2004. Firework-related childhood injuries in Greece: A national problem. *Burns* 30:151–53.

Venters, G. A. 2001. New variant Creutzfeldt-Jakob disease: The epidemic that never was. *British Medical Journal* 323:858–61.

Vinten-Johansen, P., H. Brody, N. Paneth, S. Rachman, and M. Rip. 2003. *Cholera, chloroform, and the science of medicine: A life of John Snow.* New York: Oxford University Press.

Wangensteen, O. H., E. T. Peter, D. M. Nicoloff, A. I. Walder, H. Sosin, and E. F. Bernstein. 1962. Achieving "physiological gastrectomy" by gastric freezing: A preliminary report of an experimental and clinical study. *Journal of the American Medical Association* 180:439–44.

World Factbook. 2005. Field listing—HIV/AIDS adult prevalence rate (updated July 14). www.cia.gov/cia/publications/factbook/fields/2155.html.

World Health Organization. 2000. Injury: A leading cause of the global burden of disease. Geneva, Switzerland: World Health Organization. www.cec.gov/diabetes/pubs/facts98.htm (accessed April 26, 2000).

INDEX

9/11 attacks, 17, 53, 155

A

Abdel-Wahab, M. F., 153
Aber, J. L., 247, 248
abruptio placentae, 78
absolute incidence rates, 237
Accreditation Board for Engineering and
    Technology (ABET), 175
accuracy
    defined, 250
    primary components of, 250f
active consent, 110
acute onset diseases, 2
acute onset epidemiology, 23–24, 25
acute onset infectious diseases
    epidemics of in the United States in 1600s,
        1700s, and 1800s, 38–39
    marked seasonal variation in frequency, 36
acute respiratory disease, major cause of morbidity
    and mortality in Afghanistan, 97
Adams, Francis, 20
adenomas, 201
adherence, differential levels of to the treatment or
    exposure protocol, 197
adjusted, 75
Aedes mosquitos, 71
Afghanistan
    average life expectancy, 96
    child mortality, 96
    developmental indicators, 96
    epidemics in, 97
    famine in, 99
    gender-equality issues, 100
    health personnel in, 96
    infectious diseases in, 97–98
    literacy in, 99
    opium in, 100
    public health in, 96–100
    subsistence agriculture, 98
Afghan war, 96
African Americans
    breast cancer mortality rates in women, 65
    cardiac amyloidosis, 24
    infant mortality rate, 36
    limited access to quality health-care services, 77
African trypanosomiasis, 202–3

Agar, M., 4
age, as a strong risk factor for disease, 73
age-adjusted IR, 73–75
age-adjusted mortality rates, 73
age-adjustment, process of, 74–75
age incidence rate curve, 216
age-specific IR, 69, 73
age-specific mortality rates, for screened and
    unscreened populations, 121
age-specific prevalences, 103
aging investigators, 207
alcohol consumption
    deaths from in U.S., 79
    high *vs.* moderate levels of, 10
    prohibitions against, 1
Alexander, Leo, 12
Alpha-Tocopherol Beta Carotene Cancer
    Prevention Study Group 1994, 201
al-Qaeda, 96
alternative hypotheses, 251, 252,
    253, 255
American Academy of Pediatrics, 105
Amish community, and poliovirus, 91
analytic epidemiologic studies, 188–207
    evaluation of causation, 165
    intervention studies, 189–205
    observational studies, 189, 206–7
    study design, 25, 143
Andersson, N., 99
Angell, M., 14
animal models, 10
animal pathogens, "jump species," 44
Annas, G, J., 14
anonymity, of study subjects, 27, 28
antagonism, 264
anthrax, 18, 45
anthropology, 26
antibiotic resistance, of *P. aeruginosa* in Iranian
    burn units, 37
antihypertension drugs, 76
Archer, K., 185
Artaud-Wild, S. M., 159
asbestos, 171
"Asian influenza" pandemic of 1857, 49
aspirin, as a preventive of cardiovascular mortality,
    173, 200
associated, with another variable, 160
Association of State and Territorial Dental
    Directors (ASTTD)

1999 Basic Screening Surveys: An Approach to Monitoring Community Oral Health, 110
"Building Partnerships to Improve Children's Access to Medicaid Oral Health Services," 109–10
Ast, D. B., 199
atherosclerosis, 173
Atmar, M. H., 100
at risk, 46
attack rates
    calculating, 47
    category-specific, 47
    defined, 24, 43, 46, 131
attributable risk. *See* cumulative incidence difference (CID)
Autogen Ltd., 181, 182, 183
autonomy, respect for, 31
"autumnal fevers," 39
average life expectancy, Afghanistan, 96

B

Baby Doe regulations, 104–5
Bach, F., 184, 186
Bach, P. B., 77
Bacille-Calmette-Guerin (BCG), 98
Barber, Caesar, 80, 81
basic reproduction rate, of malaria, 241–42
Bayer, R., 14
BCME (Bis-Chloromethyl Ether), 167
Belanger, C. F., 213
"bell-shaped" curve, 161
Bendectin, 51
beneficence, 31
Bentley, M. E., 14
Benton County Health Department (BCHD)
    after-action report for the August 2003 measles investigation in Corvallis, Oregon, 57–62
    Benton County Child Mental Health Needs Assessment, 150–51
beta-carotene, 165, 200–201
biases (systematic errors), 68
    assessment of, 273
    in comparisons, 36
    defined, 232
    Farr's study of, 21
    in intervention studies, 169
    in observational studies, 167, 191
    versus random errors, 190
    validity and, 255
"bigger is better," 80
bimodal age incidence rate curve, 216
bimodal epidemic curve, 41
bin Laden, Osama, 96

binomial distribution, 252
biocolonialism
    defined, 181
    purchase of human gene pools, 181–83
bioethics, 186
biologic agents, 49
biologic samples analysis, 209
biomedical research, difficulty of conducting on humans, 186
biopiracy, 181
biosafety, 186
bioterrorism, 17, 18, 44, 172
Birmingham, K., 185
birth cohort, 207
birth defects, structural, 55
birth trauma, 78
birth weight
    causes of low in Yemen, 148, 149f
    extremely-low-birth-weight (ELBW) babies, 103, 104–5
    low-birth-weight babies, prevalence of in U.S., 103
Blendon, R. J., 83
body mass index (BMI), 82
Bonnlander, H. P., 157
Bowman, Sharon L., 272
Boyes, M., 181, 182
Brandt, Karl, 12
BRCA1 and BRCA2 genes, 15
breast cancer
    case fatality associated with, 139
    different etiologies, 216
    incidence rate of in Japanese women in Japan, Hawaii, and San Francisco and in White women in San Francisco, 216f
    risk of, 15
breast cancer screening, 122, 123
Breslau, N. J., 247
Broaddus, Toni, 272
bronchogenic carcinoma, 168
Buring, J. E., 165, 201
Burke, J. P., 83
burn injuries
    fireworks-related, 36
    in Iran, 37
Burton, B., 182

C

caffeine-containing beverages, and prevalence and severity of premenstrual syndrome, 157–58
campylobacter, 97
Canadian Pediatric Society, 105
Canadian Public Health Association (CPHA), 185

cancer
  breast, 65, 216f
  deaths in U. S. attributed to dietary risk factors, 82
  esophageal, and green tea consumption, 222
  incidence rate for uterine cancer in U.S., 66
  lung, 38, 79, 239
  mortality rates in women in the U. S., 39f
  stomach, 76, 79
Canto, J. G., 77
carbon disulfide, coronary heart disease among
    workers exposed to, 213–14
cardiac amyloidosis, 24
cardiovascular disease
  becoming a chronic disease, 173
  causation, 172–73
  epidemiology of, 76
carpal tunnel syndrome, 126
carriers, 113
Cary, P., 11
case/control studies, 214–17
  centrality of in modern epidemiology, 33
  versus cohort studies, 206
  data analysis plan, 214
  data layout for, 237t
  demonstrations of two potential confounding
      factors that occur in the same proportion in
      case and control groups with residual
      confounding by those factors, 222t
  design considerations, 214, 215t–217
  estimate of ratio measures, 233
  example of selection bias in, 258t
  examples of, 222–23
  exposure odds ratio (EOR), 236–38
  homogeneous disease entity, 215
  individual matching, 262
  as observational studies, 33, 143
  recall bias, 267, 271
  as "retrospective studies," 215
  selection bias, 258
  sources of cases, 215–16, 217, 219
  sources of controls, 219–22
  strengths and weaknesses of, 226t
case fatality rate, 39, 65, 72–73, 92, 139
case recovery or cure, 92
case reports/case series, 143, 153–57
"cases," 206, 214
category-adjusted IR, 75
category-specific rates, 47, 75
causal webs. See web of causation
causation, 165–87
  and appropriate time-response between
      exposure and health outcome, 167
  consistency in the size of association between
      exposure and health outcome, 166–67
  criteria for evaluating, 169t
  and dose-response relation between exposure
      and health outcome, 167–68
  genetic versus environmental/lifestyle causes of
      disease, 176–77
  and Henle-Koch postulates, 168
  model for disease/injury, 169–71
  strong association between exposure and
      outcome, 166
cell, 114
census data, for measuring person-years, 66–67
Centers for Disease Control and Prevention
    (CDC), 8, 52
  Behavioral Risk Factor Surveillance System
      (BRFSS), 82
  Epidemic Intelligence Service: Training the
      World's "Disease Detectives," 16
certification, 91
chance. See random error
Charles, D., 99
chemical agents, 49
Chernobyl nuclear power plant, 144–45
chest x-rays, for persons with a positive TB skin
    test, 89
chichona tree, 86
chicken influenza, 49
chicken pox, 24
Child Abuse and Treatment Act, 104
child mental health, assessing, 150–51
child mortality
  in Afghanistan, 96
  globally, 77–78
  strong association with living in poverty, 78
children
  dental caries (tooth decay) as top chronic
      disease among, 109
  as study subjects, 28
chimney sweeps, 132
chloroform, 22
chloroquine, 86
cholera, 22–23, 40, 44, 45, 154
chronic disease
  case/control studies of, 33
  causation beliefs, 1
  epidemiology, 26f
  as major public health problem in
      U.S., 72
  most caused by more than one exposure, 169
  temporal and spatial patterns of, 24
chronic fatigue syndrome, 156
cigarettes
  as the ignition source for house fires, 175
  self-extinguishing, 175
classical statistics, 257

clinical epidemiology, example from Burn
    Treatment Units in Iran, 37
clinical (therapeutic) trials
  example of, 201
  intervention seeks to reduce adverse health
      consequences related to a condition, 192
  as intervention studies, 189, 191
cloned pigs, 184–85
Code of Ethics for the Society of Professional
    Journalists, 51
cohort
  defined, 67, 207
  dynamic, 207
  in estimating cumulative incidence, 130
  of interest, 135
  minimally exposed, 210
cohort studies
  versus case/control studies, 224
  with count denominators, 233t–234t, 237
  defined, 67
  examples of, 213–14
  how data are analyzed, 212
  how data are collected, 211–12
  how investigators follow up on participants, 212
  important questions to consider when designing,
      209–12
  as observational studies, 206
  with person-time denominators, 234–35t, 237, 252
  pertinent questions to consider when
      designing, 208t
  prospective versus retrospective, 207, 208f
  relative magnitude of disease or injury
      frequencies, 207
  sources of the exposed cohort, 209–10
  sources of the unexposed cohort, 210–11
  strengths and weaknesses of, 226
  types of, 143
  who is exposed, 209
  who is unexposed, 210
colon cancer screening, 121
colonialism. See biocolonialism
colon polyps, 108, 112–13
colostomy, 121
communicable disease outbreaks, as a local public
    health issue, 61
communicable disease surveillance and response
    (CSR), 44–45
communication systems, 59
community (preventive) trials
  examples of, 199–201
  as intervention studies, 189
  study subjects are free of the health outcome of
      interest, 191
  unit of study, 192

comparability, between cases and controls,
    210, 220
comparison biases
  confounding bias, 260–61
  selection bias, 257–60
comparison group, 153, 155
comparisons, 9–10
comparison treatments, 156
competing causes of lost to follow-up, 135
component causes, 169, 170f, 171f
Computerized Assisted Personal Interview (CAPI),
    52, 223
computer technology, 27
confidence, defined, 254t
confidence interval, 130, 251, 253–55
confidence interval estimate, 228
confidence limits, 254
confidentiality, 27, 28, 31, 62, 218
conflict of interest, 31
confounding bias, 179
  and age adjustment, 74–75
  due to lost-to-follow-up, 197
  hormone replacement therapy (HRT) and
      coronary heart disease, 265–66
  in observational studies, 203, 206
  pictorial representation of, 260f
  pictorial representation of prevented, 191f
  preventing, 189, 190, 261–66
  and random assignment, 169, 196
confounding variables, 162–63f, 221
congestive heart failure, 173
consent
  active and passive, 110
  voluntary, 13
  See also informed consent
consumer products, as causes of death, 174–75
Consumer Product Safety Commission
    (CPSC), 175
Contact Awareness and Referral for Exposure, 30
Contact Tracing, 30
contagion theory, 1–2
controls, 190, 206
  in case/control studies, 214, 219–20
  general population as, 221
  identified from clinical records, 221
  source of, 220–24
Cook, J. T., 248
Cook Islands, 185
coronary bypass surgery, 156
coronary heart disease
  among workers exposed to carbon disulfide,
      213–14
  congestive heart failure, 173
  ischemic, 38

myocardial infarction (MI), 173
    and physical fitness, 168
coronary heart disease mortality
    in relation to cholesterol-saturated-fat index,
        159–160f
    in relation to milk intake, 159–60f
coronaviruses, 18
corporations, ethical stature of, 132
correlational studies, 159–63
correlation coefficient, 161
Corrigan, J. M., 83
Counseling, Testing, Partner Referral and
        Notification, 30
count denominators, 233–34
C-reactive proteins, 76, 173
cross-sectional studies, 103, 143, 157f
crude incidence rate, 69, 73, 74
crude mortality rate, 73, 75
crude prevalence, 103
crude rates, 75
cryptosporidium, 18
culturally appropriate informed consent, 181
cumulative incidence (CI)
    calculating by following a cohort of people over
        time, 131–32
    crude, 263
    difference, 232, 233
    of disease frequency, 130
    estimating from the incidence rate, 133–38
    examples of calculating from the incidence rate,
        136–38
    first approach for estimating, 130–33
    formulae and interpretation, 141
    order of steps in calculating, 137
    pertaining to new cases of death, 133
    risk, 64
    variable that affects the size of, 236
cumulative incidence difference (CID), 234t
cumulative incidence ratio (CIR), 232, 233,
        234t, 263
Curry, M., 218, 219
cutaneous leishmaniasis, epidemic proportions in
        Afghanistan, 98
cutoff point, 115f, 251

D

Darwish, M., 153
da Sousa, C. P., 99
data
    commonly used sources of and their advantages
        and disadvantages, 211t–212
    dichotomous interpretations of, 253
    editing, 228, 231
    interpretation, 228
    profiling, 218
    quality control, 231
data analysis
    objective of, 232
    plan for, 189
    simple analysis, 228–42
    steps in, 222f
data collection, plan for, 189
data layouts, illustration of how different layouts
        yield different study findings, 229, 230t
data reduction, 228, 231
DC-10, 174
DDT, 86
deCODE Genetics, 182–83
deforestation, 44
degree of freedom, 252
dengue and dengue hemorrhagic fever, 55
    as emerging disease, 17, 25, 44
    risk factors affecting morbidity and/or mortality
        from, 72
    serological diagnosis, 71
    surveillance system, 72
    in Thailand, 69–72, 70f
denominator, 64, 65–66
dental caries (tooth decay), top chronic disease
        among children, 109
descriptive studies
    correlational studies, 159–63
    cross-sectional studies, 157–59
    examples of, 144–48
    formulation of epidemiologic hypotheses, 148–53
    major limitations of each type of, 163t
    objectives of, 144
    primary uses of, 144–53
    quantifying variation in exposures and health
        statuses, 144–45, 148
    study-design options, 143
    types of, 153–59
DES (diethylstilbestrol), and adenocarcinoma, 168
desertification, 148
design strategies
    analytic studies, 188–205, 206–7
    descriptive studies, 143–64
De Zoysa, I., 14
diabetes mellitus
    clinical and public health implications, 192–94
    disproportionate effect on certain age and ethnic
        groups, 193
    gestational, 194
    heart disease as the leading cause of death
        among persons with, 193
    two main types of, 193

Diatranz, 185
dietary risk factors, and cancer deaths in the
        United States, 82
difference measures, 232, 236
differential lost-to-follow-up, 212
diptheria, in Afghanistan, 97–98
direct standardization, 263
disability-adjusted life years, 105
disease and injury
    emerging, 43
    interaction of environmental and genetic
            factors, 55
    natural history of, 15
    prevention, 171
    reemerging (resurging), 43
    societal bases for, 50, 53
    variation in frequency, 75–77
disease and injury frequency
    attack rate, 43
    measures of, 24–25, 63, 141
disease causation, prevalent beliefs about until the
        mid-twentieth century, 1–2
"disease detectives," 16
disease duration, etiologic exposures and
        exposures affecting, 217
disease eradication, 85–91
Disease Intervention Specialist (DIS), 30
disease "of interest," 153
Dobson, R., 184
"Doctors Trial," 12
Doll, R., 25, 222
domestic violence in lesbian relationships, bias in
        detecting/studying, 272
Donaldson, M. S., 83
dose-response relation
    between an exposure and a health outcome,
            167–68
    defined, 149, 157
    pictorial representations of, 152f
Dourado, I., 93
drinking-water contamination, 18
drug resistant TB, 54–55
due process, 89
duration of clinically diagnosed disease
    versus distributions of disease durations, 125f
    etiologic exposures and exposures
            affecting, 217
duration of preclinical forms of a
        disease, 124
dynamic cohort, 207
dysentery, 45
dyspnea, 107

E

Ebola, 25, 45
ecological study, 159
ecologic fallacy, 162
economic development, and reduction of tropical
        disease, 85
editing data, 228, 231
effect measure(s), 228, 232–33
    true, 254
    unbiased, 232
effect modification, 264, 265t
effect modifier, 256
efficiency, 251
Elandt-Johnson, R. C., 46
elephantiasis, 84
Elias, C. J., 14
Elliott, P., 218
emerging diseases, 43
encephalitis, St. Louis, 240
endemic area, 84
end-stage kidney disease, 193
engaged epidemiology, 133, 275
Engel, L. S., 270
Enterotoxigenic *Escherichia coli* (ETEC), 97
environmental diseases, 132
environmental epidemiology, 25
environmental factors, 49
Environmental Protection Agency, 17
environmental samples, 209
environmental toxin, 178
epidemic curve, 41–43
    for an acute onset disease from a point exposure
            such as a foodborne bacterium, 41f
    for an outbreak of bloody diarrhea, Cameroon,
            1997-1998, 43, 45f
    for the foodborne outbreak of *Escherichia coli*
            0157 in Lanarkshire in 1996, 41f
    multimodal, 42
    skewed to the left, 41
    skewed to the right, 41
Epidemic Intelligence Service, 16
epidemics
    causes of, 48–50
    cholera in Afghanistan, 97
    cutaneous leishmaniasis in Afghanistan, 98
    defined, 35–36, 38
    of disease associated with eating contaminated
            food, 43
    etiologies of, 55
    lung cancer, 38
    population awareness of, 38–40

and poverty, 49
and public health systems, 55
quantitatively described, 41–48
severe acute respiratory syndrome (SARS), 43
silent, 41
smallpox, 39
in the United States in 1600s, 1700s, and 1800s, 38–39
varying time frames for, 38
See also bioterrorism
epidemiologic data, simple analysis of, 228–42
epidemiologic hypothesis, definition of, 148–49
epidemiologic investigations, questions asked during, 3
epidemiologic methods, development of, 21
epidemiologic studies
critical evaluation of, 47–48
example of, 8–9
epidemiologic triad, 2
epidemiologist, as forensic scientist, 178–79
epidemiology
acute onset versus chronic disease, 23–25
application to health-care-management decision making, 55
and business, 132–33
change in, 1
in clinical settings, 17
comparisons, 9–10
defined, 2, 3–9
development of as a science, 25–33
development of computer technology, 27
as a dynamic science, 172
engaged, 133, 275
ethical considerations, 11
future advances, 33–34
generalizability, 256
genetic, 177
in health services research, 17
historical development of, 20–23
and managerial sciences, 27
modern, 25
news reporters and, 51
nutritional, 25
objectives of, 15–17
population-based, 10–11, 14–15, 25
in a public health setting, 29–32, 52
and social sciences, 26
Epstein-Barr virus, 18
ergonomic-related disability, theoretical web of causation for, 134f
error
sources of, 273

Type I, 253, 254t
Type II, 189, 253, 254t
See also biases (systematic errors); random error
Esnard, A. M., 218
esophageal cancer, and green tea consumption, 222
estimation, 228
Estonia, plans for a national data bank, 182–83
ethical considerations, 11
associated with extremely low birth weight (ELBW), 103
associated with intervention studies, 191, 203
for experiments involving human subjects, 28–29
and intervention studies, 206
Nuremberg Code, 12–14
and public health, 31, 154–55
redefining of by GIS, 218
of reporters and other mass media professionals, 51
and tuberculosis elimination, 88–90
"ethical foreign policy," era of, 100
ethnicity
and diabetes mellitus, 193
most important factor in shaping Afghanistan, 98
etiologic factors, 26, 49f
Evans, A. S., 168
expected numbers, 36
experimental population, 195
experimental studies. *See* intervention (experimental) studies
expert testimony, 178
exposed subjects, 67, 206, 207
exposure notification, as a "teaching moment," 32
exposure odds ratio (EOR), 232, 237–38
in a case/control study, point estimate for, 254
example of data that yield, 236t
numerical example of, 238t
true, 258
exposure of interest, 67
exposures
interactions among, 25
measuring, 25
routes and the dosages of, 10
exposure status
causes of death according to, 79–82
data, 209
quantifying variation in, 144
external validity, 195–96, 255, 256–57
extremely-low-birth-weight (ELBW) babies
ethical challenges associated with, 103
rights of, 104–5

F

false-negatives, 114, 118–20
false-positive results
  and cutoff point, 115
  mammograms, 122
  and predictive value positive, 116
  prostate cancer, 114
famine, in Afghanistan, 99
Farmworker Epidemiology Research Group, 268
Farr, William, 1, 21
fast-food industry
  advertising, 81
  "super-sizing," 80–81
fidelity, 31
filariasis, 84
Finn, S. B., 199
fireworks-related burn injuries, 36
fixed cohort, 207
flooding, in New Orleans, 40–41, 172
fluoride trial, 199–200
folic acid, 173
follow-up, 67, 208
fomites, 2
Food and Drug Administration (FDA), 9
  guidelines for establishing the therapeutic value
    of new drugs, 191
foodborne pathogen
  epidemic curve for *Escherichia coli* 0157 in
    Lanarkshire in 1996, 41f
  epidemics associated with, 43
  point exposure, 41
food consumption, 80
Ford Pinto, 174
forensic epidemiologist, 178–79
fourfold table, 237, 252
Fracastorius, Girolamo: *Des Res Conatagiosa,* 2
Frader, Joel E., 104
Framingham Heart Study, 173, 207, 209–10
Francois, I., 99
Frank, C., 153
frequency matching, 221, 261–62

G

Gamble, T. Jr., 11, 39
Gamblin, V. N., 49
Gandhi, Mohandas, 104
Gao, Y. T., 222
Garrett-Jones, C., 87, 240–41
gastric freezing, 155–56
gender-adjusted incidence rate, 75
gender-specific rates, 75

generalizability. *See* external validity
generalizability (in classical statistics), *vs.* external
  validity, 257
"genetic epidemiology," 177
Genetic Epidemiology of Lung Cancer and
  Smoking (GELCS) Study, 223–224f, 225f
genetic versus environmental causes of disease,
  176–77
"Geographic Identification of High Gonorrhea
  Transmission Areas in Baltimore,
  Maryland," 218
geographic information systems (GIS), 218–19
geographic variation, in mortality rates, 75–76
gestational diabetes, 194
giardia, 18
Global Eradication Initiative Polio Endgame
  plan, 91
Global Eradication of Malaria Program, 87
Goldberg, I. J., 10
Goodhand, J., 100
Goodson, L. P., 96, 99–100
Grady, D., 166, 266
Graunt, John, 1
  *Natural and Political Observations Made Upon
    the Bills of Mortality,* 20–21
Greenland, M., 265
green tea, and esophageal cancer, 222
Greenwood, M., 20, 21
grid of exposure versus health outcome, 159f
Grodin, M. A., 14

H

Hale, B. R., 97, 98
Halliday, S., 21
Harry, D., 182
health-care-management decision making,
  application of epidemiologic principles to, 55
health disparities, 50
health indicators, 47–48
health information, disclosure of, 29
Health Insurance Portability and Accountability
  Act (HIPAA), 29
health monitoring, 50, 53–54
health response, 152
health risks, communication of, 49
*Healthy People 2000: National Health Promotion
  and Disease Prevention Objectives,* 53
Healthy People 2010 (HP 2010), 53, 54
healthy worker effect, 214
"Heart and Estrogen-Progestin Replacement
  Study" ("HERS"), 266

heart disease. *See* cardiovascular disease; coronary heart disease
helicobacter pylori bacterium, 18
hemorrhagic fevers, viral, 45. *See also* dengue and dengue hemorrhagic fever
Henle, Friedrich Gustav Jacob, 2
Henle-Koch postulates, 2, 168
Hennekens, C. H., 165, 201
Hennessey, K. A., 36
hepatitis A, 8–9, 24
hepatitis C
    and liver cancer, 18
    and parenteral antischistosomal therapy (PAT) in Egypt, 152–53
Hernberg, S., 213
high-density lipoproteins (HDLs), 173
high-risk populations, 116
Hill, A. B., 25, 166, 222
Hippocrates: *On Airs, Waters, and Places,* 20
HIV/AIDS, 25
    divisive class culture of public concern for, 154
    in India, 172
    PS inappropriate as a prevention tool, 30–32
    in sub-Saharan Africa, 14, 50, 78
    transmission of, and syringe vending machines, 152
    tuberculosis associated with, 18
Hodgkin's lymphoma, 18
Holmen, T. L., 157
home health nursing, 61
homeland security, 25
homocysteine, 173
homogeneous health outcome, defining, 47
homophobia, 272
"Hong Kong influenza" pandemic of 1968, 49
hormone replacement therapy (HRT), and heart disease, 165–66, 265–66
host characteristics, 49
human experimentation, 13
human gene pools, purchasing, 181–83
human papillomavirus, 18
human populations, studying, 10–11
Human Subjects Committees, 27
hypergeometric distribution, 252
hyperglycemia, 193, 194
hypoglycemia, 193
hypotheses
    alternative, 251, 252, 253, 255
    components, 188
    epidemiologic, defined, 148–49
    formation of using descriptive studies, 148–53

generation versus evaluation, 229–31
null, 251, 252, 253, 255
hypothesis testing, 228, 252, 253

I

iatrogenic transmission, 153
Iceland, 182, 183
immunization, 60
incidence rate difference (IRD)
    defined, 232
    estimated from a series of strata, 238
    numerical example of estimating, 235t
    range of possible values of, 234
    from a simple analysis, 238
incidence rate (IR)
    absolute, 237
    age-adjusted, 73–75
    age-specific, 69, 73
    calculation of, 67–69
    category-adjusted, 75
    components of, 64
    crude, 69, 73, 74
    defined, 63
    estimating denominator with census data, 66–67
    formulae and interpretation, 141
    function of, 133
    gender-adjusted, 75
    measuring of disease and injury frequency, 91
    measuring of how fast (new) cases of disease or of injury are occurring, 65
    pictorial representation of, 92
    relation to prevalence and duration, 123–24, 217
    restriction of, 64
    and risk status of the people contributing person-time, 66
    two parts, 64
    for uterine cancer for women in the United States, 66
    variable that affects the size of, 236
    variation in magnitude of, 92
incidence rate ratio (IRR), 232, 239
    associated with tobacco smoking and lung cancer, 239
    estimated from cohort studies with person-time denominators, 234
    numerical example of estimating, 235t
incident cases, 24, 47, 216
incubation period, 2, 42, 241
index case, 91
indicators
    CSI as, 159
    health, 47–48

Leading Health Indicators, 54
  risk, 261
  sentinel health, 52
  of variation in disease frequency, 48
indirect standardization, 263
individual matching, 261, 262
Infante-Rivard, C., 267
infant mortality rate (IMR), 21
  among African Americans, 36
  often predicts subsequent changes in the entire
      population's health status, 48
  in South and Central American countries in the
      1990s, 35–36
  in the United States in 1990s, 36
infectious diseases. *See* acute onset infectious
    diseases
infective person, 41
influenza
  association with poverty, 45
  chicken influenza, 49
  "Hong Kong influenza" pandemic of 1968, 49
  marked seasonal variation in occurrence, 36
  pandemic of 1857, 49
  pandemic of 1918-1919, 24, 49
  potential for new pandemics, 44
information biases, 257, 267–73
information control, 60
informed consent, 28, 182, 185, 195
  culturally appropriate, 181
insecticide resistance, 86
Institutional Review Boards (IRBs), 27, 28
insulin, 192, 193
intentional epidemics. *See* bioterrorism
internal validity, 255, 257–73
International Classification of Diseases Codes
    (ICD codes), 65
International Health Regulations (IHR), 44–45
international immunization practices, 60
interval estimate, 228
intervention (experimental) studies, 165, 188–205
  adherence to protocol, 196–97
  and confounding bias, 261
  ethical concerns, 203
  importance of random assignment, 189–90
  limited extrapolability of the results of, 179
  versus observational studies, 189–91
  random allocation of exposure, 26, 169
  two main types of, 143, 191
interviewer bias, 271–73
intrapartum asphyxia, 78
inverse (negative) association, 161
involuntary detention, 88–89
ischemic heart disease, 38

Ivinson, A., 184, 186
Ivy, Andrew, 12

J

Jacques, L., 267
Jennings, M., 218
Jin, C., 243
Julius Caesar, 178
"jumping genes," 202
justice, 31

K

Kangilaski, J., 183
Kerala, in southwest India, 4
Khan, I. M., 98
kidney disease, end-stage, 193
Kitzmiller, C., 194
"knock out" pigs, 184
Koch, Robert, 2
Kohn, L. T., 83

L

Laaser, U., 98
Lambert, M. L., 99
land-mine-caused disabilities, in Afghanistan, 99
landrace crops, 99
Lassa, 45
latent period
  associated with acute onset diseases, 23–24
  associated with chronic diseases, 24
  bias, 157
  of bladder cancer, 167
  and cross-sectional studies, 157
  defined, 158
  determining, 159
latent TB infection (LTBI), 89–90
late sequelae, 24
Lawton, E. K., 246, 247
leaded gasoline, 132
Leader, N., 100
Leading Health Indicators, 54
lead time, 120f–121, 124, 251
leishmaniasis, in Afghanistan, 98
lesbian relationships, studies of violence
    in, 272
Lewis, R., 183
Liao, Y., 10
life events/icon calendar

method of collecting occupational histories, 268–71

number of jobs and working months reported by migrant farmworkers using a traditional occupational history approach versus, 270t

two-year sample of for collecting occupational histories from farmworkers, 269f

lifestyle choices, 49

linear association, 159, 160, 161

literacy, in Afghanistan, 100

lost-to-follow-up, 68, 197–98, 212

Lotka, A. J., 240

low-birth-weight babies, U.S. prevalence of, 103

low-density lipoproteins (LDLs), 173

lumpectomies, 157

lung cancer
  deaths worldwide, 79
  epidemic/pandemic, 38

Lurie, P., 14

M

Macdonald, George, 87, 240, 241

MacKay, A. M, 243

MacMahon, B., 33, 50

Macrae, J., 100

mad cow disease, 25, 45

miasma theory of disease causation, 39

malaria
  basic reproduction rate, 241–42
  drug-resistant, 44
  elucidation of life cycle of, 240
  eradication campaign, 85, 86–88
  mortality from in U.S. in early 1800s, 39
  reproduction rate (R_0) of, 240–41

mammography
  false-positive results, 122
  nonclinical settings for, 109
  use of for women 40 years of age and over according to selected characteristics: United States, Selected Years 1987–2000, 128

managerial science, 27

Mann, C. J., 246, 247, 248

Mannvernd, association of Icelanders for ethics in science and medicine, 183

Manson, J. E., 165, 201

Maori, 185

marker, 160

Markowitz, G., 132

mastectomies, 156, 157

matching
  frequency matching, 221, 261–62
  individual matching, 261, 262
  over-matching, 221

mathematical relation, between p-values and confidence intervals, 255

Mather, Cotton, 39

McCaffrey, I., 199

McDowell, N., 99

McLellan, K., 185

mean, 161

measles
  after-action report for the August 2003 investigation in Corvallis, Oregon, 57–62
  eradication program, Western Hemisphere, 90
  major problem in Afghanistan, 97
  in Romania, 36

measures
  difference, 232, 236
  of disease frequency, 24–25, 63, 123, 141
  effect, 228, 232–33, 254
  quantitative, 50
  ratio, 232, 233, 236

meat-packing industry, 23

median family incomes, 77

Medicaid, reduced eligibility standards for, 247–48

medical errors, as cause of deaths, 83

medical experimentation
  on human beings, 12
  permissible, 13

Medicare, discarding of previous policy that obesity is not a "disease," 81n2

Melo, H., 184

meningitis, 44

meningococcal meningitis, 45

mental health needs of children in Benton County, Oregon, assessing, 150–51

Merck Lipha, 181

Merrill, Gregory, 272

meta-analysis, 178

miasma theory, 1, 39

Michels, K. B., 191

microchimerism, 185

Middle Eastern people, perceived as "Other," 155

migrant populations, in studies separating genetic from environmental/lifestyle causes of disease, 177

minimally exposed cohort, 210

misclassification, 65, 115, 267–73

modern epidemiology, 25

Mokdad, A. H., 79

monozygotic twins, 176

moral and/or religious turpitude, 1

morbidity, 15, 77–79

mortality

from acute respiratory disease in Afghanistan, 97
from cancer, for women, 39f
causes of according to exposure status, 79–82
consumer products as causes of, 174–75
from coronary heart disease, 159–160f
from dengue/DHF, 72
from heart disease for persons with diabetes, 193
leading causes of, 83–84
leading causes of among adults worldwide,
    2002, by age group, 78t–79
leading causes of in the United States in 2000, 79
from lung cancer worldwide, 79
from malaria in U.S. in early 1800s, 39
maternal, in Afghanistan, 96
from medical errors, 83
from obesity in U.S., 79
perinatal, in Kiev, 35
from prescription-drug effects, 83
proportionate, 139–40
from stomach cancer, 76, 79
in sub-Saharan Africa, 78
ten leading causes of in the United States, 72
ten leading causes of in the United States,
    preliminary data for 2002, 73t
from tobacco use in U.S., 79
See also child mortality
mortality rates (MR)
age-adjusted, 73–75
basic to understanding the dynamics of health
    and disease in human populations, 92
crude, 73, 75
defined, 65
differences in by "race," 77
examples of geographic variation in state-
    specific rates within the United States,
    preliminary data for 2002, 76t
formulae and interpretation, 141
geographic variation in, 75–76
pictorial representation of, 92
used as estimate of IRs, 72
variation in magnitude of, 91–92
worldwide, 77–79
See also infant mortality rate (IMR)
mosquitoes, resistance to insecticides, 87, 88
motor vehicle emissions, inorganic lead, 132–33
Mujahideen, 96
Mukamal, K. J., 10
multimodal epidemic curves, 42
multivariate analysis, 262, 265
Muslims, perceived as "Other," 155
mycobacterium tuberculosis
as necessary component cause of
    tuberculosis, 169

transmission as mirror of socioeconomic
    conditions of a society, 97
myocardial infarction (MI), 173

N

National Cancer Institute, 268
National Center for Health Statistics (NCHS),
    50, 52
    Early Release program, 52–53
National Health, Lung, and Blood Institute
    (NHLBI), 195
National Health and Nutrition Examination Survey
    (NHANES), 80
national health goals, 53
The National Health Interview Survey (NHIS),
    50, 52
National Institutes of Health (NIH), 17, 195
National Welfare Reform Act of 1996, effects on
    children's health in the United States,
    246–49
natural history, of human diseases, 11, 15
Nazi Germany, "Euthanasia" Program, 12
necessary component cause, 169, 170f, 171f
negative (inverse) association, 161
neonatal tetanus, in Afghanistan, 98
neuropathy, 194
New Orleans, 40–41, 172
Newburgh-Kingston Dental Caries Trial, 199–200
news reporters, and epidemiology, 51
"New World" West Nile virus, 17
Nicholson, D., 182
nonadherence, to treatment regimens, 88–89
nonsystematic error. *See* random error
normally distributed variables, depiction
    of, 161
Northern Alliance, Afghanistan, 96
nosocomial infections, 18, 83
notifiable disease, 72
null hypotheses, 251, 252, 253
    "two-sided," 255
null values, 234
numerator, 64–65
Nuremberg Code, 11, 12–14, 28
    history of, 12
    permissible medical experiments, 13–14
Nurimen, M., 213
nurses' health study, 213
nutritional anthropometrics survey, Kono District,
    Sierra Leone, 145–48
nutritional epidemiology, 25
nutritional factors, 49

O

Obadia, Y., 152
obesity/overweight
   by body mass index, 82t, 83f
   deaths from in U.S., 79
   health problems from surpassed tobacco-related
      health problems in 2003, 81n1
   and incidence of Type 2 diabetes, 193
   and the super-sized industry, 80–81
   in the United States, 80, 82–83
observational studies, 26
   as analytic studies, 143, 189, 206
   case/control studies, 206, 214–17
   cohort studies, 206, 207–14
   confounding bias, 167, 190–91, 203, 206,
      250, 267
occupational diseases/injuries, 23, 132, 268
occupational epidemiology, 25
occupational histories, alternative method for
   collecting, 268–71
odds, 236
odds ratio. *See* exposure odds ratio (EOR)
Office of Homeland Security, 17
"Old World" West Nile virus, 17
oogonic cycle, 241
oral contraceptives (OCs), and embolisms, 259
oral-health screening program, Wisconsin,
   109–12
organ transplantation, 183–84
Orme-Zavalete, J., 8
outcome evaluation, 240
over-matching, 221

P

P. aeruginosa, 37
P. falciparum, 87
Pakistan, Islamic schools in, 100
Pan American Health Organization (PAHO), 90
Panama Canal, 41
pandemics
   "Hong Kong influenza" of 1968, 49
   influenza of 1918-1919, 24
   lung cancer, 38
Papanicolaou Smears (PAP smears), 109
Paradis, K., 184
parasite index, 88
Paredes, S., 99
Partner Counseling and Referral Service, 30
Partner Notification, 30
Partner Services (PS), 30–32
passive consent, 110

passive smoking, effects of on young infants'
   respiratory health, 243
Pasternak, D., 11
Pasteur, Louis, 2
pasteurization, 2
pathogens, 2
Pearce, N., 4
People's Republic of China (PRC), SARS
   epidemic, 43
perinatal conditions, and child mortality, 78
perinatal mortality rate, in Kiev, 35
period at risk, 46
peripheral neuropathy, 194
peripheral vascular disease, 194
permissive environmental conditions, 2
person, place, and time, 2
personal interviews, concerning exposure status, 209
Personal Responsibility and Work Opportunity
   Reconciliation Act (PRWORA), 246
   direct impact on children's health, 248
   effect on poverty, 246–47
   effects on women's health, 247–48
   restrictions placed on children, 247
person-time, 39, 46
person-year (P-Y), 6, 235
   denominators, 233
Peto, R., 165
phenylketonuria (PKU), 55, 113
physical agents, 49
Physician' Desk Reference, 266
Physicians' health study, 200–201
Piedagnei, J. M., 97
pigs, cloned, 184–85
placebo effects, 156
placenta previa, 78
plague, 45
point estimate, 228, 232, 233, 234, 254
point exposure, 24, 41, 131
polio
   campaign against, 87
   containment, 90–91
   major problem in Afghanistan, 98
   methods of studying, 24
   outbreak in Minnesota, 91
   polio syndrome diseases, 24
   sentiments about the safety of vaccine, 90
   vaccine trial of 1954, 199
"Polio Endgame," 91
polyp prevention trial study, 201
pooled measures of effect, 264
population-based epidemiology, 10–11, 14–15, 25
populations
   and attack rate, 24

high-risk, 116
reference, 195
at risk, 21, 46
vulnerable, protecting, 31
porcine endogenous retroviruses (PERV), 184, 185
positive linear relationship, 161
postcertification immunization policy, 91
post-traumatic stress disorder, 156
poverty
and children's health/mortality, 78, 248–49
diseases associated with, 45, 84–85
effect of welfare reform on, 247
and epidemics, 49
power, defined, 254t
precision, 250, 251
preclinical disease, 108, 119, 124
predetermined probabilities, of being in a certain
exposure group, 190
predictive value negative, 116
predictive value positive, 116–17
preexisting exposures, 26
pregnancy, and diabetic women, 194
premature birth, 78, 105
premature infants, care of, 104–5
premenstrual syndrome
and consumption of caffeine-containing
beverages, 157–58
and placebo effects, 156
Prentice, R. L., 266
prescription-drug effects, as cause of deaths, 83
prevalence/prevalence rate (P)
based on incidence rate of disease or injury and
average duration of disease or injury, 124
basic measure of disease frequency, 123
calculating, 107–8
comparison of estimates based on the full or
approximate formula, 108t
cross-sectional survey for measuring, 103f
defined, 102
expressed as a percentage, 102
formula based on the IR and D, 105–7
formulae and interpretation, 141
helps to determine which populations to
screen, 116
measuring, 103–8
referring to existing cases of preclinical
disease, 124
relation to incidence rate and duration, 217
used to refer to the proportion of a population
that has a certain risk factor, 102–3, 141
prevalent number of cases, 106
prevalent (previously diagnosed) cases of disease,
64, 65, 92, 216
preventive trials. *See* community (preventive) trials

Principles of Epidemiology (MacMahon and
Pugh), 3
privacy, 31
probability, reasonable, 179
probability distributions, 161, 252, 254
process evaluation, 239
program evaluation, 239–40
program planning, difficulty in relying on an
exposure-outcome relation for, 4
proportion
attack rates, 46
case fatality, 139
cumulative incidence (CI), 141
prevalence (P), 102–3, 141
proportionate mortality, 139–40
prospective cohort study, 207, 208
prospective studies, 33
prostate cancer screening, 122–23
prostate-specific antigen (PSA), 113–14
cutoff point, 115
high false-positive rate, 123
Pseudomonas, multi-drug resistance, 37
psychology, 26
*Psychosocial Effects of Screening for Disease
Prevention and Detection* (Robert T.
Croyle), 123
public health perspective, 15
public health system
ethics, 31, 154–55
evaluation of, 239–40
involving the public early in the discussion of
issues, 185
knowing when an epidemic is "real," 55
response to changes in sentinel predictors of
epidemics or to epidemics, 55
public schools, funding through fast-food
marketing, 81
Pugh, T. F., 50
pulmonary anthrax, 17
p-value, 251–53
one-sided and two-sided, 255

Q

quality-adjusted life years (QALYs), 103, 105
quantitative measures, need for development of, 50
quinine, 86

R

rabies
in Afghanistan, 98
vaccine for, 2

"race," differences in MRs by, 77
radiation experiments, 11
radioactive contamination, descriptive studies of
    from the Chernobyl plant, 145
random assignment, of exposure/treatment, 26,
    169, 189–90, 196, 203, 261
random error
    arises from statistical considerations, 196,
        232, 250
    associated with effect measures estimated from
        simple data analysis, 239
    and confidence intervals, 253, 255
    in intervention and observational studies, 190, 203
    and p-values, 251, 253, 255
random variables, 254
rates, true, 46–47
ratio measures, 232
    in case/control studies, 233
    versus difference measures, 236
    direction of, 236
reasonable probability, 179
recall bias, 267, 271
records review, 209
reemerging (resurging) diseases, 43
reference population, 195
Region of the Americas ministers of health, 90
relative frequency
    comparisons, 21t
    defined, 38
    of health outcomes in different populations, 21
relative magnitude
    of the incidence rates, 237
    vs. absolute of rates and differences, 236f
relative numbers, of health events, 21t
Report on an Inquiry into the Sanitary Condition
    of the Labouring Population of Great
    Britain, 40
reproduction rate (R_0), of malaria, 240–42
residual insecticidal activity, 86
residual noncomparability, 167
restriction, 256, 261
retrospective cohort study, 208, 258
review exercises, sample answers to, 277–84
Ridker, P. M., 173
Rift Valley, 202, 203
risk, 15, 130, 141
risk factors, 48, 112–14
risk indicators, 261
risk ratio. See cumulative incidence ratio (CIR)
risk reduction education, 32
Rivers, T. M., 168
Rocchini, A. P., 193
Rockett, I. R. H., 267
Rosner, D., 132

Ross, Ronald, 86, 240–42
Rossignol, A. M., 94, 157, 243
Rossignol, P. A., 8
Rothman, K. J., 169, 191, 243, 265
Roughan, P. D., 181
Ruffin, J. M., 156

S

Sabin vaccine, 91
Salk vaccine trials, 199
salmonella, 97
Salort, C., 99
sanitary movements, 1
SARS. See severe acute respiratory syndrome
    (SARS)
Schatzkin, A., 201
Scherzer, Teresa, 272
schistosomiasis, 152
Schnyder, G., 173
Screening in Chronic Disease (Allan S. Morrison),
    121, 123
screening programs, 108–12
    characteristics of a good disease or risk factor
        for which to screen, 112–14
    characteristics of a good program, 116–20
    evaluating, 121, 239–40
    importance of determining durations of
        preclinical forms of a disease, 124
    numerical example demonstrating the
        importance of specificity in determining
        the predictive value positive of, 117–18
    provisions for following up on people who
        screen positive, 121
    weighing the risks and the benefits of, 122–23
screening test
    characteristics of a good, 113, 114
    identifies prevalent cases of preclinical
        discern, 109
    should be designed to identify early, preclinical
        disease, 119
seasonal variation, in the frequency of disease,
    21, 106
secondary infection, 71
secular trends, 76
selection bias
    in case/control studies, 258t
    comparison biases, 257–60
    and individual matching, 262
    oral contraceptives and embolisms, 259f–260
self-extinguishing cigarettes, 175
Senituli, L., 181, 182
sensitivity
    definitions of, 114t

estimating from people with and without overt
        disease, 119t–120
numeric example estimating sensitivity of a
        screening test using a cohort approach,
        119–20t
of screening tests, 114, 116–17
sentinel health indicators, 52, 55
sentinel surveillance, 89
September 11, 2001, 17, 155
Sertoli cells, 185
serum cholesterol
    and cardiovascular disease, 173
    coronary heart disease mortality in relation to
        cholesterol-saturated-fat index, 159–160f
serum homocysteine, 76
severe acute respiratory syndrome (SARS), 18, 25
    bimodal epidemic curve, 41
    probable cases of by week of onset worldwide, 43f
    web of causation, 7f
sexually transmitted infections (STIs)
    and exposure notification, 28, 29–32
    prophylactic antibiotic treatment of, 30
Shapiro, S. B., 65
Sherburne, H. R., 94
shigella, 97
shingles, 24
Shuster, E., 11
Shyrock, R. H., 40
"sick building syndrome," 156
Sierra Leone, nutritional anthropometrics survey,
        Kono District, 145–48
signed digraph
    defined, 4
    of a Lyme disease vector-host community, 8f
silicosis, 169
simple analysis, 228–42
    case/control studies, 236–38
    cohort studies, 233–35
    data analysis, 232
    data layout for case/control data, 251, 252t
    data layout for cohort data with person-time
        denominators, 252t
    measures of effect, 232–33
    ratio measures versus difference measures, 236
Sinclair, Upton: The Jungle, 23
skewed to the left, 41
sleeping sickness, 202
smallpox
    bioterrorism and, 18
    epidemic, 39
    vaccination, 39
    worldwide eradication program, 85, 87
Smith, Theobald: Parasitism and Disease, 2
smoking. See tobacco smoking

Snow, John, 1, 21, 22–23, 204
social sciences, 26
Society of Professional Journalists Code of Ethics, 51
sodium intake, reduced, 76–77
software programs, 27
Soper, Fred, 86
South Asia, 172
specificity
    definitions of, 114t
    estimating from people with and without overt
        disease, 119t–120
    of screening test, 114, 116–17, 119–20t
spina bifida, 55
St. Louis encephalitis, 240
Stallones, R. A., 196
standard deviation, 253
standard error units, 253
standardization, 262–63t
standard normal deviate, 252
statistical power, 253
statistical significance, 251, 253
statistics, 25–26
steady state, 106f
stomach cancer
    large decrease in mortality from, 76
    mortality worldwide, 79
stomach ulcers, 18
strata, 238, 251, 263
stratification, 262, 263–64t
stratified analysis, 251
Struewing, J. P., 15
stroke mortality, decline in, 76–77
strong association, between an exposure and a
        health outcome, 165
study design
    analytic studies, 189
    data analysis, 212
    options in, 143f
study participants, 189, 195
subsets, 196, 198, 256
sufficient cause, 169–70f, 171f
suicide prevention programs, teenage, 154
"super-sizing," 80–81
Susser, E., 4
Susser, M., 4
synergy, 264
syringe vending machines, and reduced
        transmission of HIV, 152
systematic error. See biases (systematic errors)

T

Taliban, 96, 100
Tamil Nadu, India, 84

tamper-resistant drug containers, 174
Tay-Sachs disease, 55, 113
Tecumseh Heart Study, 173
teenage suicide prevention programs, 154
telephone language translation lines, 61
termination rate, 106
terrorist events, 17
See also 9/11 attacks; bioterrorism
tetanus, in Afghanistan, 98
tetraethyl lead, 132, 133
"theory of happenings," 240
Thomas, B. M., 267
Thompson, I. M., 114
Thun, M. J., 10
time-response, 149, 152, 157
tobacco advertisements, banning from television, 15
tobacco exports, 38
tobacco smoking
    and carcinoma of the lung, 76, 167, 222–23
    as a confounder in studying the association
        between coffee consumption and the
        incidence rate of myocardial infarction,
        260–61
    deaths from in U.S., 79
    difficulties in measurement, 209
    impact on the numbers of cases of coronary
        heart disease, 239
    in low- and middle-income countries, 79
    passive smoking, effects of on young infants'
        respiratory health, 243
    prevention of exposure to among asbestos-
        exposed people, 171
    prohibitions against, 1
tobacco studies, 25
Tolonen, M., 213
Tonga
    culturally sensitive issue of group decision
        making in the consent process, 183
    genetically homogeneous population, 181
    National Health Ethics and Research
        Committee, 182
    unique processes for group decision making, 182
Tonga Human Rights and Democracy Movement
    (THRDM), 182
torch sweaters, 174
toxic tort cases, 178
traffic-related trauma, 49
trials
    "Doctors Trial," 12
    drug, of HIV/AIDS treatment and transmission
        in sub-Saharan Africa, 14
    fluoride trial, 199–200
    intervention, 165
    polyp prevention trial study, 201

See also clinical (therapeutic) trials; community
    (preventive) trials
triglycerides, 173
tropical diseases, as cause of poverty, 84–85
true rates, 46–47
tsunami, in South Asia, 172
tuberculin skin test, 89
tuberculosis (TB)
    in Afghanistan, 98
    among people living in the U.S.-Mexico border
        region, 36
    drug-resistant, 44, 55
    elimination, and ethical considerations, 85,
        88–90
    and increases in the numbers of
        immunocompromised individuals, 55
    involuntary detention of cases, 88–89
    latent infection (LTBI), 89–90
    mycobacterium tuberculosis, 92, 98, 169
    and overcrowded living conditions, 49
    as reemerging disease, 17, 18, 25, 172
Tuskegee Syphilis Study, 11, 30
twins, monozygotic, 176
"two-sided" null hypotheses, 255
two x two tables, 237, 252
Type 1 diabetes, 193
Type 2 diabetes, 193
Type I error, 253, 254t
Type II error, 189, 253, 254t

U

unbiased measure of effect(s), 232
unexposed cohort, 67, 206, 207, 210–11
uniformity, 136
United Nations, 87
United States Bureau of the Census, 66
United States Holocaust Memorial Museum, 12
United States Preventive Services Task Force
    (USPSTF) on PSA testing, 113–14
unvaccinated, and poliovirus, 91
urban sprawl, 44
USA vs. Karl Brandt et al., 12
utilitarian theory, 15
Utz, G. C., 97, 98

V

vaccines
    polio, 90–91, 199
    rabies, 2
    smallpox, 39
    and social change, 202
Valdes, Rafael, 185

validity, 250
  and biases, 255
  external, 195–96, 255, 256–57
  internal, 255, 257–73
variables, 160–61
  confounding effects of, 162–63
  independent cause of the health outcome under
    study, 260
  normally distributed, 161
  random, 254
  that affect the size of cumulative incidence, 236
  that affect the size of incidence rate, 236
Vassilia, K., 36
vector-borne diseases, 38, 86, 240
vectorial capacity, 242
vectors, 86
veracity, 31
Victoria, Queen, 22
Vinten-Johansen, P., 22
viral hemorrhagic fevers, 45
vitamin B_6, 173
vitamin B_{12}, 173
Volterra, Vito, model of the predator-prey
    relationship, 240
voluntary consent, 13. *See also* informed consent
vulnerable people and populations, protecting, 31

W

Wallace, M. R., 97, 98
Wangensteen, O. H., 155
Wartenberg, D., 218
watch-dial painters, bone sarcoma, 131
Weber, W., 181
web of causation, 3–4
  causes of low birth weight in Yemen, 148, 149f
  diabetes Type II, 5f
  profile of the *Titanic* disaster, 6f
  severe acute respiratory syndrome (SARS), 7f
  and signed digraphs, 4
  theoretical, for ergonomic-related disability, 134f
Weeramanty, H., 184
weighting, 75
welfare reform, effects on children's health,
    246–49
West Nile virus, 17–18, 25, 55, 172, 240
Wharry, S., 186
wild-type polioviruses, 90–91
Wilson, B., 94

Wisconsin Division of Public Health (DPH),
    110–12
Wise, Amy J., 272
Wolfe, S. M., 14
women
  African American, breast cancer mortality
    rates, 65
  breast cancer incidence rate, 216f
  cancer mortality rates, 39f
  decisions about participating in a scientific study
    in some cultures, 28
  diabetic, and pregnancy, 194
  effect of Personal Responsibility and Work
    Opportunity Reconciliation Act on health
    of, 247–48
  and mammography, 128
  in Southwest India, literacy and family size, 4
  unprotected sexual activity, 48
  uterine cancer incidence rate, 66
Women's Health Initiative (WHI), 195, 266
workplace diseases/injuries, 23, 132, 268
World Health Assembly, 44
World Health Organization (WHO)
  coordinating center for worldwide health
    campaigns, 87
  malaria eradication campaign, 241
  recognizes obesity as one of the top ten global
    health problems, 80
World Trade Center attacks. *See* 9/11 attacks
World Vision International (WVI) Primary Health
    Care (PHC), 146
worldwide disease surveillance, 43, 44–45
Wright, J., 186

X

Xenotransplantation (XTP) studies, 184–86

Y

yellow fever, 38, 40, 44, 86
Yemen, causes of low birth weight in, 148, 149f

Z

Zahm, S. H., 268
zoological indices, 88